Pathology A to Z
- a Handbook for Massage Therapists

Second Edition

Pathology A to Z
– a Handbook for Massage Therapists

Second Edition

Dr. Kalyani Premkumar
MBBS MD MSc(Med Ed) CMT

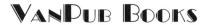

VanPub Books

Publishing division of
Meducational Skills, Tools & Technology Inc.
Calgary - Canada

Notice to Reader:

This publication is intended as a reference book only, not as a medical manual. The information imparted is to help you make informed decisions in the practice of massage therapy. It will be prudent to seek medical advice, when in doubt.

First Edition 1996 - 12,000 copies
Second Edition 2000

Published by
VanPub Books
(publishing division of Meducational Skills, Tools & Technology Inc.)
Calgary, Canada

Distributed by
Lippincott Williams & Wilkins
351 West Camden Street, Baltimore, MD 21201-2436
227 East Washington Square, Philadelphia, PA 19105
Toll free 1-800-638-3030
www.Lww.com

Canadian Cataloguing in Publication Data

Premkumar, Kalyani, 1959-
  Pathology A to Z

  Includes bibliographical references and index.
  ISBN 0-9680730-5-0

  1.Pathology--Handbooks, manuals, etc. 2. Massage therapy--
Handbooks,manuals, etc. 1. Title.
RB118.P73 2000   616.07   C99-911287-2

Produced in Canada

Preface

In the recent past, there has been a tremendous change in health care systems around the world, particularly in North America. There is a demand by the public for holistic care, with complementary medicine gaining acceptance and importance. A recent report to the National Institutes of Health on Alternative Medical Systems and Practices in the United States indicates that in 1990, 61 million Americans used alternative medicine. More total visits were made to alternative practitioners than conventional medical practitioners, with approximately $13.7 billion being spent on alternative medicine in that year. The time is therefore ripe for alternative health professionals to claim their place in the health care team.

Undoubtedly, to become fully accepted members of the health care team, it is vital for Holistic Health Practitioners to equip themselves with the knowledge about diseases and their causes that has been painstakingly accumulated over years of scientific research. It is also important to understand and be fluent with the language of medicine, in order to communicate effectively with other members of the team. This is the first step that has to be taken to bridge the gap that exists between medical and alternative health practitioners. Several measures are being taken to help this process especially in the field of Massage Therapy. For instance, the curriculum in Massage Therapy Colleges is being scrutinized in many provinces of Canada and USA and more stringent licensing procedures are being introduced.

While these changes are taking place, there is a growing realization that there is a deficiency of printed resources that cater specifically to the needs of Body Workers. At present, many students and practitioners wade through the voluminous literature of medicine to discover simple but important details relevant to their practice. What is the cause of a disease they encounter? Is it infectious? Can the client be harmed by therapy? Can the therapist be harmed by contact with the client? What are the precautions that should be taken? are just few of the questions that race through the mind of the therapist. Realizing this urgent need, the first edition of the book was published in 1996.

Encouraged by the overwhelming positive response from students and therapists, and feedback from the users, the 2nd edition has been published. Heeding the feedback – the number of color plates of skin disorders has been increased; the illustrations have been significantly improved and increased in number and information on more pathologies added. In addition, references have been included for every pathology addressed. The size of the book has been changed and the format altered, to improve clarity. The binding has been changed to enable the user to refer to the book even while they work on the client.

One of the grievances of users outside North America has been the lack of addresses of contacts in their country. Addresses from UK and Australia have been added. Many users have confirmed that they found the appendices describing Drugs/Therapies and the section on strategies for infection prevention particularly valuable. In this edition, examples and side effects of more Drugs, Therapies and Procedures are given. The section on strategies for infection prevention and safe practice has been markedly improved to provide more information. Changes have been made to the index and glossary to enhance usefulness.

This new edition aims to provide the body worker with all the relevant information they need on pathologies, to practice with confidence and serve their clients better.

Acknowledgements

This book could not have been written without the support of my husband and team mate, Prem, who knows and believes in my capabilities even better than myself. While he had to goad me to complete the first edition, I have revised and completed the second edition with excitement, encouraged by the overwhelming response of the users. I wish to thank my loving children Vivian and Kamini, for being participants in the project rather than onlookers, this time.

- Kalyani Premkumar

Foreword

The changes and additions made to the second edition of "Pathology A to Z – a Handbook for Massage Therapists" are a reflection of the growing need for more and more detailed resource material by massage therapists (and other holistic practitioners) all around the world. In response to feedback from its users, Dr. Kalyani Premkumar has expanded each section of the handbook to not only include additional information, but to update the existing material. The second edition, therefore, is a much more valuable tool to have in the clinic for quick reference than the first.

There are few people as qualified as Dr. Premkumar to produce this type of reference guide. She has the medical training to give her the expertise in explaining pathologies, as well as the massage therapy training which enables her to make the relevant connections for massage therapists to understand those pathologies and provide appropriate treatments.

It is exciting to see this book in such great demand, as it indicates the growing recognition on the part of massage therapists for being as knowledgeable as possible and targeting their skills towards specific therapeutic treatments. This bodes well for their clients, as maximum benefits will be derived from well-educated and experienced therapists.

Sylvia Muiznieks, B.Sc., R.M.T.
Secretary,
Canadian Council of Massage Therapy Schools
Program Administrator,
Centre for Complementary Health Education
Mount Royal College, Calgary, Alberta, Canada

About the Author

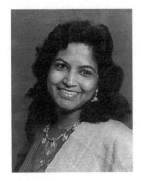

Dr. Premkumar is a Physician and a Medical Educator with over 15 years experience in teaching.

Currently she instructs at the Centre for Complementary Health Education, Mount Royal College, Calgary, Canada and is an Adjunct Assistant Professor at the University of Calgary in the Department of Cell Biology and Anatomy, Faculty of Medicine. She is presently working towards her doctorate in Educational Technology.

She is also the President of Meducational Skills, Tools & Technology Inc., Canada and Meducational Skills, Tools & Technology Pvt. Ltd., India.

She is a recording artist and has two Christian music albums to her credit.

Contents

Introduction to the book

The book has been organized alphabetically, according to diseases. As well, it has indices by word and body-system. The word index will help the reader in locating diseases with more than one name. Every disease has been dealt with using a uniform format for better readability and quick reference.

Each disease has a short description followed by the Cause, Signs and Symptoms, Risk factors, Caution and Recommendations to Therapists, Notes and Reference for further reading for every disease. The primary body system affected by the disease has also been indicated. Space has been allocated beside each disease for recording individual observations and notes. This space can also be utilized for noting other forms of treatment for that particular disorder - such as Aromatherapy, Acupressure etc., that the Holistic Practitioner is familiar with. Color plates have been included to illustrate some of the common skin ailments. Also, Figures have been inserted wherever appropriate beside the description of diseases.

The Glossary provided, for medical terms used in the book, will be helpful to understand unfamiliar terminology. The side effects of some of the common drugs and descriptions of therapies is an additional feature to alert Therapists while treating clients under medical and surgical management. Addresses of relevant organizations and support groups in Australia, Canada, UK and United States, have been added to enable Practitioners to access information on recent advances made and locate local support groups for clients. A separate section on Strategies for prevention of infection and safe practice gives details of infective agents and simple precautions that can be taken to combat infectious diseases.

The objective of this book is to help the reader understand more about diseases that have been **diagnosed by a Physician**, and to serve as a guideline, so that the client can be urged to a state of total well-being using non-invasive and alternative forms of therapy. It is envisaged that this book will help Holistic Practitioners broaden their attitude and outlook and make them feel comfortable as an accepted member of the health care team.

IT IS EMPHASIZED THAT THIS IS NOT A MEDICAL MANUAL TO HELP HOLISTIC PRACTITIONERS DIAGNOSE AND TREAT DISEASES, AND IT MAY NOT BE USED FOR SUCH PURPOSES.

- Author

Abortion (Miscarriage)

The spontaneous or induced expulsion of the products of conception from the uterus before 20 weeks of pregnancy.

Cause:

Abortion could occur spontaneously or may be induced. Spontaneous abortions may present in may ways. *Threatened abortion* is the condition when there is slight bleeding from the vagina. About 50% of such pregnancies are not aborted. *Inevitable abortion* is when the cervix dilates and abortion is definite. When parts of the products are retained in the uterus, it is termed as *incomplete abortion*. *Complete abortion* indicates complete expulsion of the products with minimal bleeding. *Missed abortion* is when the fetus is retained in the uterus for two months or more even after its death.

A person is said to have *habitual* or *recurrent abortion* when there is spontaneous loss of three or more pregnancies. When there is infection associated with abortion, it is termed *septic abortion*.

Spontaneous abortion could be due to many reasons. Abnormal development of the embryo due to genetic defects, faults in the implantation of the embryo, and abnormal positioning of the placenta are some of the causes. Maternal factors such as infection, severe malnutrition, abnormal reproductive organs such as incompetent cervix, injury, hormonal imbalances and blood group incompatibility may also produce spontaneous abortions.

Termination of pregnancy may be induced to safeguard the mother or on an elective basis. See also Ectopic pregnancy and Abruptio placenta

Signs and Symptoms:

Abortions may be preceded by a pink or brown discharge from the vagina before the onset of cramps, severe bleeding and expulsion of the contents of the uterus. If all the products are not expelled, the cramps and bleeding continue for days.

Infection and bleeding are some of the common complications. There is a risk of premature delivery in a mother who has had recurrent induced abortions.

Risk Factors:

See Cause. Spontaneous abortions are usually due to abnormalities in the chromosomes or development of the fetus. This type of abortion is more common if the parents are older, if the mother has had many children or has conceived within 3 months of giving birth. Abortions occurring in the second trimester are more likely to be due to disease in the mother such as infections, endocrine abnormalities or uterine factors. Smoking and alcohol consumption have been linked to increased rate of spontaneous abortions.

Caution and Recommendations to Therapists:

In general, do not massage the lower abdomen in the early stages of pregnancy.

Notes

Treatment varies according to the type of abortion. In threatened abortion, if pain and bleeding persists, and if there is evidence of fetal death, the uterus is evacuated. Curettage (a procedure where the inner lining of the uterus is scraped off) is done in cases of incomplete, inevitable, missed or septic abortions in order to remove any products of conception.

Abortion may be induced by suction curettage - a procedure where the products are aspirated via the cervix. If induced later in pregnancy it may be done through the cervix by suction or use of destructive forceps. Prostaglandins may be used as injections into the amniotic cavity, or by vaginal suppositories. Infusion of saline or urea solutions into the uterine cavity, are other methods used to induce abortions. For a more detailed description see Appendix C: Curettage; Suppositories.

If a client is prone to spontaneous abortions and is pregnant, always consult the Obstetrician before massaging. If the client has just had an abortion, consult the Obstetrician and avoid massage till bleeding has stopped completely.

During pregnancy, massage increases venous return and thereby helps the work of the heart. It stimulates the parasympathetic nervous system and has a calming effect. It reduces stress on the lower back and other weight-bearing joints temporarily. The Massage Therapist can be a source of emotional and physical support at this time. With themselves experiencing the benefits of touch, the massage session can motivate the client to learn and use infant massage after the baby is born.

Pregnancy massage with the client seated, lying on the side or any other comfortable position, can be done if cleared by the Obstetrician. In the first trimester, the positioning of the client could vary, as the abdomen is not large. However, deep work should be avoided in the abdomen. In the second and third trimester, the client may feel more comfortable lying on the side with a pillow supporting the leg and arm away from the table. Overstretching should be avoided as the connective tissue and ligaments are softened by the hormonal changes during pregnancy. The abdomen should be supported with pillows during the later part of the pregnancy. In the third trimester, due to the pressure of the uterus on the abdominal veins, there is a tendency for edema in the legs. If edema is excessive refer client to the doctor.

References

Fritz S. Mosby's fundamentals of therapeutic massage. New York: Mosby-Year book Inc; 1995. p. 145-146.

Waters B. Massage during pregnancy. Fuquay-Varina, NC: Research Triangle publishing; 1995.

Osporne-Sheets C. Pre- and Perinatal Massage Therapy. San Diego, CA: Body Therapy Associates; 1998.

Dodson MG. Bleeding in pregnancy. In: Aladjem S, editors. Obstetrical practice. London: CV Mosby Co; 1980. p. 451-458.

In general, the massage should be gentle and relaxing, and for a shorter duration. Fascial techniques to the low back should be avoided as also the use of potent essential oils. Lavender (for its calming effect), neroli (for its relaxing effects on smooth muscles of the gut), tangerine (for its uplifting effect) in a 1% dilution, have been recommended by some for use during pregnancy.

Other conditions in clients that have to be promptly referred to the doctor are: pain of any kind, vaginal bleeding, uterine contractions that persist; persistent dizziness, numbness, tingling; visual disturbance; faintness; shortness of breath; palpitations; leaking amniotic fluid; decreased fetal activity; generalized edema; headache; calf pain or swelling.

Reproductive system

Abruptio placenta (Placental abruption)

The premature separation of the placenta that has been normally implanted in the uterus.

Notes

The mother and fetus have to be carefully monitored if abruption is suspected. Delivery is the treatment of choice in most cases. Blood transfusion may be needed, depending on the severity. For more details see Appendix C: Blood transfusion.

Cause:

The cause is not known.

Signs and Symptoms:

It presents as abnormal uterine bleeding, excessive activity of the uterus and fetal distress, usually in the third trimester of pregnancy. Depending on the

Pathology A to Z -

severity, the mother may show signs of bleeding such as drop in blood pressure and increase in heart rate.

Risk Factors:

It is more common in older mothers, mothers who smoke or use cocaine, who have hypertension and are undernourished. External trauma can also cause this. The incidence is higher in those who have had abruptio placenta in previous pregnancies. See also Hypertension

Caution and Recommendations to Therapists:

Massage is definitely contraindicated in clients with this condition. Massage should be avoided in any pregnant client who complains of vaginal bleeding. See also Abortion.

References

Dodson MG. Bleeding in pregnancy. In: Aladjem S, editors. Obstetrical practice. London: CV Mosby Co; 1980. p. 462-467.

Abscess

A localised, pocket of infection composed of dead tissue, white blood cells and microorganisms.

Integumentary system

Cause:

The bacterial organism causing the infection varies according to the location the abscess is found. Usually, the organism is introduced into the dermis or subcutaneous tissue by injury or other mechanisms. Sometimes, they may reach an area through blood or lymphatics draining another infected site.

Signs and Symptoms:

It appears as a painful, tender and reddish soft tissue swelling that is filled with pus. There may be painful enlargement of lymph nodes that drain the site. Apart from the skin, abscesses may be formed in the brain, peritoneal cavity, pelvic cavity etc.

Risk Factors:

Wounds that are inadequately cleaned can lead to formation of abscess. It is more common in immunodeficient individuals.

Caution and Recommendations to Therapists:

Massage should be avoided locally. Massage around the abscess can help reduce the swelling, but it should be ensured that the region is covered. The lymph nodes draining the area may be enlarged. Encourage the client to take the full course, if on antibiotics. Since it is an infective condition, care should be taken to prevent spread. Refer to the section on 'Strategies for infection prevention and safe practice'.

Notes

In most people, incision and drainage of the abscess is adequate. If the infection has spread to the surrounding area, or if the person is immunodeficient, antibiotic therapy is necessary. For more details see Appendix C: Antimicrobial - antibacterial agents.

References

Larco M. Inflammation and immunity. In: Porth CM, editor. Pathophysiology - concepts of altered health state. 4th ed. Philadelphia: JB Lippincott Co; 1994. p.249.

Achalasia

A condition where the smooth muscle of the lower end of the esophagus does not relax properly while swallowing. The contraction of the esophagus is abnormal.

Cause:

It is due to a defect in the innervation of the lower esophageal sphincter. The cause of the defect is usually unknown. Sometimes, the defect may be produced by gastric cancer (see Cancer - stomach) infiltrating the lower end of the esophagus, damage by irradiation or certain toxins and drugs.

Signs and Symptoms:

There may be difficulty in swallowing, chest pain and regurgitation of food. The pain may be increased ar rest, while swallowing or by emotional stress. Since there is a large volume of saliva and ingested food retained above the defect, the contents may inadvertently enter the respiratory passage and result in lower respiratory tract infection.

Risk Factors:

Achalasia affects both sexes and people of all ages.

Caution and Recommendations to Therapists:

The client may be more comfortable if positioned with the head end raised. Avoid using deep pressure in the abdomen. In some clients it may be better to avoid abdominal massage altogether. See Appendix D for organizations and support groups.

Notes

Drugs that relax the sphincter may be used. However, they are of limited value. Sometimes mercury-filled dilators may be used to produce symptomatic relief. For more details see Appendix C: Cholinergic drugs; Sympatholytic drugs.

References

Orringer MB. Disorders of esophageal motility. In: Sabiston DC, editor. Textbook of Surgery - the biological basis of modern surgical practice. 14th ed. London: WB Saunders Co; 1991. p. 666-670.

Achondroplasia (Chondrodystrophia fetalis)

A type of hereditary disorder of skeletal growth that results in dwarfism with abnormal proportion of body.

Cause:

It is due to mutation of a gene that codes for proteins that form the matrix of cartilage. As a result there is failure of longitudinal growth in the cartilage of bones.

Signs and Symptoms:

The person is of short stature with abnormal body proportions. Usually the limb is disproportionately shorter than the trunk. The bones are thick and often deformed with abnormal angulation at the knee/elbow joint (valgus/varus deformities). Lumbar lordosis may be present. Mental functions are normal.

Notes

There is no specific treatment. Symptomatic treatment for arthritis and eye problems may be necessary. Counseling for the serious psychological problems of short stature may be needed along with referral to support groups. For more details see Appendix C: Genetic testing / counselling.

Risk Factors:

It is hereditary. Cleft palate, eye problems such as retinal detachment and cataract are often associated.

Caution and Recommendations to Therapists:

These clients may benefit greatly by the emotional support given by a caring Therapist. Due to their stature and deformity, they may be a point of ridicule and discrimination. The Therapist should ensure that steps are provided for the client to access the table. Suitable arrangements should be made for other areas of the clinic (eg. water fountain; sinks etc.) that may be accessed by the client.

Many clients have bony deformities that result in bad posture, excessive stress on weight-bearing joints and strain on ligaments and tendons. The Therapist should identify the muscles and joints that are stressed and focus more on these regions. Heat and hydrotherapy may be beneficial. For clients with arthritis see the section Caution and recommendations to Therapists under Arthritis – osteoarthritis.

References

Prockop DJ, Kuivaniemi H, Tromp G. Heritable disorders of connective tissue. In: Isselbacher KJ et al, editors. Harrison's principles of internal medicine. 13ᵗʰ ed. New York: McGraw-Hill Co; 1994. p. 2114-2115.

Acidosis

Renal, Respiratory, Gastrointestinal systems

A condition where the pH of the extracellular fluid is below normal (normal: 7.35-7.45).

Cause:

Acidosis is classified as *metabolic* or *respiratory* depending on where the problem lies. Normally, pH alterations are minimised by the lungs and kidneys. Metabolic acidosis is caused by a) increased production of acids eg. ketoacidosis following diabetes, alcohol intake, starvation, poisoning etc. b) decreased acid excretion by the kidney (kidney disease) or c) loss of alkali eg. diarrhea.

Respiratory acidosis may be caused by failure to ventilate properly. This may be due to depression of the respiratory center by cerebral disease or drugs, neuromuscular disorders and chronic pulmonary diseases. (

Notes

The primary cause of the acidosis has to be treated. The treatment depends both on the cause and severity. Oral alkali such as sodium bicarbonate or sodium citrate may be given.

Signs and Symptoms:

Diarrhea is common. There may be hyperventilation. Nonspecific symptoms like fatigue may be present. The person may go into a stupor and coma.

Risk Factors:

See Cause.

Caution and Recommendations to Therapists:

This condition is treated in a hospital setting. The client is usually too ill to seek a Massage Therapist.

References

Porth CM. Alterations in acid-base balance. In: Porth CM, editor. Pathophysiology –concepts of altered health states. 4ᵗʰ ed. Philadelphia: JB Lippincott Co; 1994. p. 629-644.

Acne

A chronic inflammatory skin disorder affecting the sebaceous glands and hair follicles.

Cause:

Notes

Acne is treated to prevent scarring or to reduce the psychological trauma suffered by the person. In most cases, acne clears as the person grows older. Keeping the skin dry and clean, use of moisturizing soap and dietary changes are some of the treatment options. In more severe cases, application of specific lotions - antibiotic or otherwise is resorted to. For more details see Appendix C: Antimicrobial - antibacterial agents.

Irritation produced by components of sebum from the sebaceous glands escaping into the dermis is responsible for the inflammation. The cause of acne is unknown and many factors influence its course (see Risk factors).

Signs and Symptoms:

Acne is of many types. *Acne vulgaris* is the common condition seen in young adults, where lesions are seen in the face and neck and sometimes in the back, shoulders and chest. *Acne conglobata* is more common in middle age, with a higher incidence in men. The lesions may be seen in any area of the face, trunk and thighs. *Acne rosacea*, also occurring in middle-aged and elderly adults, results in lesions over the nose, cheeks and forehead. In chronic cases, it may result in irregular thickening of the skin over the nose (rhinophyma).

Acne is characterized by a combination of blackheads, pustules, abscesses, nodules and cysts in the affected area. The secretions from the lesions may be foul-smelling, watery or pustular. Scars may be seen from previous lesions. Acne tends to flare up in cycles. In girls, it is usually worse before the menstrual period. There may be seasonal variations, with most cases becoming better in summer.

Scarring of tissue and infection are common complications. See Appendix A: pages 349 & 353 (Keloid).

Risk Factors:

High fat diet, food products such as chocolate, makeup, infection by *Propionibacterium acnes* organism, stress, increased activity and proliferation of sebum-producing cells are all predisposing factors. There is a tendency for acne to develop in families especially if one or both parents have oily skin.

Caution and Recommendations to Therapists:

Acne is not contagious; neither can it be spread from one region of the body to another by touch. Wash hands thoroughly before massaging the face of such clients as super infection can be introduced by unclean, oily hands. Avoid massaging the affected area if there is extensive inflammation. Some clients may like light massage of the face without oil, so judgment should be made on an individual basis. Do not use ointments and lotions that may clog the opening of the sebaceous glands. Friction and deep tissue pressure should be avoided. For the rest of the body, water-based lotion may be used as an alternative to oil in clients who are concerned. Avoid hot or cold packs in clients with Acne Rosacea as it may worsen the condition.

Many clients with acne are self-conscious, with low self-esteem because of its appearance. Therapists need to treat such clients with special care. Clients may be on oral steroid therapy for the condition and the overall immunity may be lowered as a result. The Therapists should not treat such clients if harboring any kind of infection, as it may spread to the client.

References

Plewig G, Kligman AM. Acne: Morphogenesis and treatment. New York: Springer-Verlag; 1975. Cullen SI, editor. Focus on Acne Vulgaris. London: Royal Society of Medicine Services Ltd; 1985. p. 1-176.

Acquired Immunodeficiency Syndrome
(AIDS; Human Immunodeficiency Virus infection)

A viral infection that progressively destroys the immunity of the individual.

Lymphatic, Cardiovascular, Respiratory, Nervous systems

Cause:

It is caused by the RNA virus - Human Immunodeficiency Virus Type I/ Type II (HIV). The virus primarily affects the T lymphocytes that are responsible for cell-mediated immunity (the type of immunity that comes into play in skin graft rejection etc.). However, it does affect other forms of immunity too. AIDS victims become vulnerable to infections that do not affect normal individuals. Also, infections that produce only mild symptoms otherwise may result in severe symptoms in them. They are also prone to unusual cancers.

AIDS is transmitted by contact with infected blood or body fluids. Intercourse (anal/vaginal), transfusion of contaminated blood or blood products, sharing of contaminated needles, transmission to the fetus from infected mothers through the placenta are some of the routes through which the virus is transmitted. There is growing evidence that it is not transmitted by casual social or household contact. There is no report of the virus being transmitted by insect bites.

On an average, the time between exposure to the virus and diagnosis is 8-10 years. But the incubation period may be shorter or longer. Initially, the presence of the virus is detected only by laboratory tests. Later, symptoms due to the deficient immune state is seen. There is a wide variation in the way the disease presents itself and the time between acute infection and onset of symptoms.

Signs and Symptoms:

The signs and symptoms are variable. Initially, the person may exhibit only flu-like symptoms and remain asymptomatic for many years. Later, the infection process may present as opportunistic infections (infections that do not affect normal individuals) and unusual cancers (See Appendix A: page 352). Some of the common infections and cancers that are seen in AIDS infection are fungal infections, Tuberculosis, Herpes virus infection, pneumonia, sarcomas and lymphomas. In some, it presents as autoimmunity where the body's immune cells attack self eg. as arthritis, or as neurological problems - encephalitis, dementia or peripheral neuritis. There may be generalized enlargement of lymph nodes, weight loss, fatigue, night sweats and fever.

Notes

The quality of life of an AIDS patient is improved by using specific antiviral therapy and drugs to prevent/treat opportunistic infections. Counselling and education are important components of the management plan. The patient should be made aware of the potential to infect others and sexual practices and intravenous needle use need to be discussed frankly.

One of the tests performed to indicate exposure to AIDS is the Enzyme-Linked ImmunoSorbent Assay test (ELISA). This identifies the presence of antibodies to the AIDS virus. If this is positive more sophisticated tests are performed. However, testing for antibodies alone is not reliable as it may take from a few weeks to many months for antibody production to reach detectable levels. For more details see Appendix C: Antimicrobial - antiviral agents.

Risk Factors:

Homosexual and bisexual individuals, intravenous drug users, those requiring recurrent transfusions of blood or blood products and heterosexual partners of the above groups are all at risk. There is a high incidence of AIDS in infants born to infected mothers.

There is a risk of infection in healthcare workers who handle infected specimens especially if their skin is punctured and the wound comes in contact with the infected specimen.

Though there is no evidence that transmission of the virus occurs via contact with other body secretions such as tears, saliva, sweat and urine, care should be taken in handling all secretions of infected individuals.

Caution and Recommendations to Therapists:

The HIV epidemic has challenged the thinking about fundamental ethical and legal issues such as confidentiality, right to privacy, informed consent etc. It has challenged the codes that require health professionals such as nurses and doctors to provide service to all people without regard for socioeconomic status or nature of health problems.

Although it is unlikely for Massage Therapists to come in contact with blood or body fluids of clients, in general, special precautions have to be taken. It is advisable for Therapists to wear gloves, or refrain from treating any client if the Therapist has an open wound. Open wounds and lesions in the client should be avoided even with gloved hands. Ensure that those lesions are covered at all times. Since the disease affects the immunity of the individual, it should be ensured that the client is not exposed to any form of infection in the clinic. AIDS clients may have diseases like tuberculosis, herpes, and hepatitis B, among others. Special precautions have to be taken to prevent spread of such diseases to the Therapist.

If there has been an exposure to blood or body fluids inadvertently, immediately scrub the site vigorously with a disinfectant solution such as 10% povidone iodine and wash under running water for 10 minutes (this may help remove the HIV cells from site). Report immediately to a Medical Service. Refer to the section on 'Strategies for infection prevention and safe practice' for more information (Appendix B).

The treatment regime has to be individualized as AIDS presents in very many ways. Also, the client may have exacerbations and remissions from time to time. Further, the client may be on medications, which have their own side effects. It is important to take a proper history before each session. A full body relaxation massage of short duration is recommended.

It is possible for the Therapist to transmit negative feelings to the client through touch. If the Therapist is uncomfortable massaging an individual diagnosed to have AIDS, it may be better to refer the client to another Therapist who is comfortable, rather than force oneself to give an ineffective massage. Massage by a caring Therapist can be a tremendous source of emotional support to these clients with a social stigma.

References

Fineberg, HV. The social dimensions of AIDS. Sci Am. 1988: 259 (4): 128-134.

Fauci AS, Lane HC. Human immunodeficiency virus (HIV) disease: AIDS and related disorders. In: Isselbacher KJ et al, editors. Harrison's principles of internal medicine. 13th ed. New York: McGraw-Hill Co; 1994. p. 1566-1618.

Pathology A to Z -

Many support groups are available for those affected by AIDS. Refer client to a local support group (see Appendix D).

Adhesive capsulitis (Frozen shoulder; Scapulocostal syndrome; Calcific tendinitis of the rotator cuff; Subacromial fibrosis; Pericapsulitis; Acromioclavicular arthritis)

Musculoskeletal system

A disorder of the shoulder joint caused by tightening of the joint capsule.

Cause:

The cause is not known in most situations. It may be caused by misalignment of the scapula with the humerus as in individuals with kyphosis. It may also be due to the spread of inflammation from lesions of the rotator cuff coupled with fibrosis of the capsule. Rarely, degenerative shoulder joint disease, rheumatoid arthritis, and prolonged immobilization can cause this condition.

Signs and Symptoms:

There is a slow restriction of movement of the arm to the point of affecting daily activities such as combing hair. The patient finds it difficult to abduct and

Notes

Most individuals improve spontaneously within 12 to 18 months after onset of disease. The onset of the disease can be prevented if an injured shoulder is mobilised early. Manipulation under anesthesia may also help.

In severe cases it may be treated surgically. Injection of steroids or anti-inflammatory drugs into the joint capsule may help relieve symptoms.

For more details see Appendix C: Antiinflammatories - steroidal drugs; Antiinflammatories - non steroidal drugs.

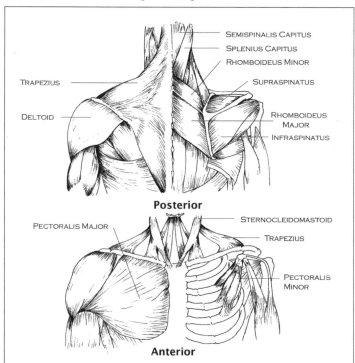

Some muscles of the neck and shoulder

flex the arm and has difficulty moving the arm to the back. There is limitation of external rotation, abduction, flexion and internal rotation of shoulder. It may be associated with gradual onset of a dull ache. Pain is referred to the C5, C6 area. In acute frozen shoulder, the pain may radiate to below the elbow. Nocturnal pain is common. In chronic conditions, nocturnal pain is absent and pain is felt only on stretching the capsule.

Risk Factors:

This condition is more common in women over the age of 50.

Caution and Recommendations to Therapists:

In acute frozen shoulder, ice or superficial heat reduces pain and muscle guarding. The aim is to maintain and slowly increase the range of movement. Use capsular stretching procedures with the client's arm hanging over the side of the table. In the chronic stage, the aim is to stretch the capsule - especially the antero-inferior area. Moist hot packs can be used around the shoulder joint to increase tissue elasticity by raising the temperature. It is best to use it before stretching. Muscle spasms of the back should also be addressed. Specifically, the muscles around the shoulder girdle, pectoralis major and minor, and rotator cuff muscles should be focussed upon. The biceps, triceps, subscapularis and deltoid should be thoroughly massaged. Improvement occurs very slowly and awareness of this reduces frustration in the part of the Massage Therapist and the client.

Work in close conjunction with a physiotherapist. Encourage client to do stretching and strengthening exercises to improve the range of motion and strength of muscles. Some of the effective exercises include standing beside a wall and walking the fingers up the wall as high as possible. This helps with abduction of the shoulder. Another effective exercise is the pendulum swing where the client leans forward waist down while holding onto a support about a foot away from the body, while the affected arm hangs loose. The arm is then slowly moved in circles of different diameters. Schedules lasting for half an hour, three times a week for three weeks followed by twice a week for two weeks, and modified thereafter according to improvement is the recommended regimen.

References

Hall CM, Brody LT. Therapeutic exercise moving toward function. Philadelphia: Lippincott Williams & Wilkins; 1999. p. 614-617.

Donatelli RA. Physical therapy of the shoulder. 3rd ed. New York: Churchill Livingstone; 1997.

Wine ZK. Russian Medical massage: shoulder dysfunctions. Massage 1995; 53 (Jan/Feb): 36-39.

Endocrine, Reproductive systems	# Adrenogenital syndrome
	It includes a spectrum of disorders resulting from abnormality in the synthesis of adrenocortical hormones.

Cause:

Notes

The cause is identified and treated accordingly. The deficient hormones have to be replaced by daily administration. Counselling is an important component of the management plan. For more details see Appendix C: Genetic testing / counselling.

It is usually caused by a lack of specific enzymes required for the synthesis of the steroidal hormones produced by the adrenal cortex. The condition is transmitted to a child from a parent with the defective gene (*congenital adrenal hyperplasia*). Since many enzymes are required for synthesis and the synthesis is in the form of a cascade, lack of even a single enzyme results in accumulation of the precursors. Thus there is an excess of androgens (hormones that are responsible for development of the reproductive organs). Aldosterone (hormone regulating sodium and water levels in the body), and corticosteroids (hormones regulating metabolism of fat, carbohydrate and protein) levels are low.

Signs and Symptoms:

The symptoms vary according to the sex, age and the enzyme that is deficient. In newborn females, the external genitalia appear abnormal. The clitoris is enlarged and resembles a penis, and the labia majora may be fused to each other. At puberty, females do not start menstrual periods. There is deepening of voice and growth of facial hair. The skin is oily and acne is common. The loss of fluid and sodium produces signs of dehydration.

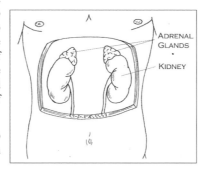

In newborn males, there is no obvious abnormality. The condition is difficult to diagnose in males.

Risk Factors:

It is more common in females.

Caution and Recommendations to Therapists:

Encourage client to take the prescribed replacement hormonal therapy regularly.

References

Ganong WF. Review of medical physiology. 15th ed. California: Appleton & Lange; 1991. p. 339-343.

Adult Respiratory Distress Syndrome

(ARDS; Shock lung)   **Respiratory system**

Difficulty in breathing brought on by stiffening of the lung by fluid accumulation.

Cause:

The lung capillaries become more leaky allowing fluids to get into the spaces between the cells with resultant stiffening of the lung. This leads to difficulty in inflating the lung and reduced exchange of oxygen. ARDS may be the result of any condition that results in such lung pathology.

Signs and Symptoms:

It presents as difficulty in breathing (dyspnea), noisy, rapid and labored respiration. It progresses to restlessness, mental disorientation and if left uncorrected, to heart failure and death.

Notes

The condition has to be treated in hospital under close monitoring of respiratory rate and other vital signs. Oxygen may have to given along with mechanical ventilatory support.

Risk Factors:

Entry of stomach contents into the respiratory tract, trauma, pneumonia, smoke or chemical inhalation that produce inflammation and drowning are risk factors. Rarely, it may be a complication of tuberculosis.

Caution and Recommendations to Therapists:

The client will invariably be hospitalised. Massage can help maintain joint mobility and range of motion of various joints while the individual is confined to bed. A half-lying or position with support below the knees, the arms (slightly abducted at the shoulder and flexed at the elbow), and head may be comfortable as there is less weight on the back and pressure on the diaphragm by the abdominal organs is minimised. A gentle relaxation massage can help reduce stress in these highly stressed individuals. More time should be spent on massaging the accessory muscles of respiration including the sternocleidomastoid, pectoralis, latissimus dorsi and neck muscles. See Appendix D for organizations and support groups.

References

Ingram R. Adult respiratory distress syndrome. In: Isselbacher KJ et al, editors. Harrison's principles of internal medicine. 13th ed. New York: McGraw-Hill Co; 1994. p. 1240-1243.

Albinism

Integumentary system

A congenital disorder resulting in reduced melanin pigment in the hair, eyes and skin.

Notes

There is no specific treatment. The person should be educated regarding use of sunscreens and protection from ultraviolet irradiation. Genetic counselling is also necessary. For more details see Appendix C: Sunscreen; Genetic counselling / testing.

Cause:

It is inherited from the parents. It is usually due to a defect in the melanin synthetic pathway.

Signs and Symptoms:

The iris of the eye is translucent. The person has photophobia, nystagmus (abnormal movement of the eyeball), reduced visual acuity and may have strabismus (cross-eye). The color of skin and hair varies according to the type of albinism, race and ethnicity of the person. In the more severe type, the person is very sensitive to the sun as they do not tan. In less severe types, the pigmentation of the hair and skin may improve with age. In a type of albinism which is temperature sensitive, the person may have white skin and hair and blue eyes at birth but pigmentation may be seen at puberty. Darker hair may be seen in cooler areas of the body (extremities) but remain light-colored in warmer areas like the scalp and axillae.

Albinism may predispose to skin cancer.

Risk Factors:

See Cause.

References

Fitzpatrick TB et al, editors. Dermatology in general medicine. 3rd ed. New York: McGraw-Hill; 1987.

Caution and Recommendations to Therapists:

Massage by a caring Therapist can be a tremendous source of emotional support to these clients who may feel ostracized because of the skin discoloration. Enquire about the sensitivity of the skin to varying temperatures if heat treatment is being considered.

Alcoholism (Alcohol dependence)

A condition where a person has a strong compulsion to use alcohol, exhibits increased tolerance or has physical signs on withdrawal from alcohol.

Nervous, Gastrointestinal, Reproductive, Cardiovascular systems

Cause:

The cause is multifactorial with interaction of genetic, biologic and environmental factors. The effects of alcohol is related to the genetic vulnerability, use of other drugs at the same time and other underlying disease that may interfere with the metabolism of alcohol and past experience with alcohol.

Ethanol is a central nervous system depressant that decreases the activity of neurons. It is easily absorbed through the cell membrane with most being absorbed in the small intestines. While it is excreted through the lungs, urine and sweat, maximum metabolism occurs in the liver. With constant use, the body compensates by increasing the rate of metabolism and chemical changes at the cellular level leading to addiction and dependence.

Signs and Symptoms:

Some of the effects of alcoholism are due to nutritional deficiencies and almost all systems are affected. Alcohol alters the sleep stages. Many experience "alcohol blackout" where recent memory is lost for a short period. Permanent impairment of the central nervous system can occur too. Alcoholism is termed as "the great mimicker" as any psychiatric syndrome can be seen during heavy drinking. Peripheral neuropathy is common. The effect of alcohol on nervous system is responsible for a large number of accidents in roads and industries.

Alcoholism can cause gastritis, esophagitis, cirrhosis and esophageal varices. Pancreatitis, hepatitis, liver failure and cancer of head and neck, esophagus, stomach, liver, pancreas and breast can all be caused by prolonged alcohol use. Anemia and vitamin deficiencies are common. Arrhythmias, thrombus formation are some of the effects on the cardiovascular system. Prolonged use reduces immunity and increases susceptibility to infection. Pneumonia is common.

It can affect the reproductive system producing menstrual abnormalities in women and reduced sex drive and impotence in men. The fetus of an alcoholic mother is also affected (*fetal alcohol syndrome*) with reduction in growth, nervous system dysfunction and signs of dependence on alcohol, among others. Physical symptoms apart, alcoholism impacts the life of the family and society as a whole.

Risk Factors:

Family members are more at risk implying a genetic predisposition.

Notes
Many support groups exist for people with this problem.

Caution and Recommendations to Therapists:

Do not massage an individual who is under the influence of alcohol. Never massage a client when you are under the influence of alcohol. Ensure that at least twelve hours have elapsed since the last drink before you start work.

Massage with its calming effect can be of benefit to those withdrawing from addictions. Refer client to support groups (See Appendix D for organizations and support groups).

References

Fritz S. Mosby's fundamentals of therapeutic massage. Mosby Year Book Inc. 1995. p. 343-344.

Integumentary system	# Alopecia
	A condition where there is reduced hair in the scalp (baldness).

Cause:

There are many causes of alopecia. *Common baldness* or *androgenetic alopecia* affects genetically predisposed men and women in their late adolescence and early twenties and is dependent on androgen levels. *Alopecia areata* is due to problems with immunity, where antibodies to hair follicle antigens are increased. Alopecia may be induced by intake of certain drugs. Drugs given to treat cancer (chemotherapy) produce hair loss as they suppress mitosis (cell duplication). Vigorous scalp massage and brushing, hair weaving, excessive use of hair care products, use of brush rollers or hot combs can result in hair loss (*traction alopecia*). Other conditions like systemic lupus erythematosus, syphilis and thyroid disorders can cause alopecia.

Signs and Symptoms:

There is increased hair shedding during washing or combing in the predisposed individual. In women, loss of hair occurs more in the crown while men tend to loose along the hair-line. In alopecia areata, there is a patch of baldness on the scalp. This may progress to total scalp hair loss, or loss of all hair in the body. It may be associated with changes in the nails.

Risk Factors:

Androgenetic alopecia is inherited.

Caution and Recommendations to Therapists:

Since many different conditions cause alopecia, a proper history has to be taken. The Therapist should also enquire about medications that are being taken eg. steroids and take into consideration the side effects of these drugs.

Notes

Topical application of 2% minoxidil has been shown to improve hair growth. Drugs that inhibit androgen are tried by some, but they are not approved treatment options. Hair transplant is one of the recent forms of treatment. Anti-inflammatory therapy, steroid application and education about autoimmune diseases are additional modes of treatment for alopecia areata.

For more details see Appendix C: Antiinflammatories - steroidal drugs; Antiinflammatories - non steroidal drugs.

References

Fitzpatrick TB et al, editors. Dermatology in general medicine. 3rd ed. New York: McGraw-Hill; 1987.

Alzheimer's disease (Primary degenerative dementia)

A progressive form of mental disorder that results in deterioration of the intellect (dementia), severe enough to affect the performance of the person socially and in their occupation.

Nervous system

Cause:

The cause is unknown, but various factors have been implicated. It could be due to deficiencies of certain neurotransmitters such as acetylcholine, norepinephrine and somatostatin. Viral factors, hereditary, immunological and environmental factors have also been implicated. There is slow loss and atrophy of brain tissue particularly in the temporal and frontal lobe. There is accumulation of a protein (beta amyloid precursor protein) in and around neurons and blood vessels of the brain that interfere with the transmission of nerve impulses.

Signs and Symptoms:

It starts very slowly with forgetfulness, learning difficulties, difficulty in concentrating and lack of personal hygiene. It then progresses to language, communication difficulties and lack of motor coordination. It is accompanied by personality changes. Finally, the individual has urinary and fecal incontinence and is unable to recognize family and friends. Seizures may occur. The person also becomes more susceptible to infection.

Risk Factors:

There may be a family history of the disease. It occurs in middle and late life. It is more common in people with Down's syndrome. Increased intake of aluminium - as in cooking in aluminium utensils, excessive use of aluminium containing antacids have also been implicated as risk factors.

Caution and Recommendations to Therapists:

Alzheimer's disease is not infectious. A full body relaxation massage helps to soothe the individuals. Vary the duration of massage according to individual tolerance. As the disease progresses the motor function deteriorates. The aim should be to prevent joint stiffening and contractures and to maintain mobility. Passively move all joints. Moist hot packs can be used to increase tissue extensibility. Use transverse friction around joints to reduce adhesion formation. Do not overstimulate hypertonic muscles. Massage to antagonist muscles can help relax affected muscles. Since these individuals are bedridden in late stages, watch for bedsores.

Avoid massaging over a wide area around bedsores. Research has shown that massaging over and around bed sores worsen the condition and causes more damage to tissues. Since these individuals are more susceptible to infection, do not massage when you have even a mild infection. Encourage client to exercise. If the client is mentally incapacitated, an informed consent from the guardian of the client has to be taken. In such cases, the Therapist may have to take cues

Notes

There is no known cure yet. Drugs are given to increase the levels of neurotransmitters and increase blood flow and thereby oxygen to the brain. As the dementia progresses, it may be necessary for the individual to be cared for in a nursing home. Since the individual with Alzheimer's disease may live in this state for a long time, it is important to give attention to the needs of the caregiver.

References

Beal MF, Richardson EP, Martin JB. Alzheimer's disease and other dementias. In: Isselbacher KJ et al, editors. Harrison's principles of internal medicine. 13th ed. New York: McGraw-Hill Co; 1994. p. 2269-2275.

Davies DC. Alzheimer's disease: Towards an understanding of the aetiology and pathogenesis. In: Current problems in Neurology II. London: Libbey; 1989.

from verbal and non-verbal forms of communication. Keep addresses of local support groups handy (Refer to Appendix D).

Amnesia

Loss of memory.

Cause:

Amnesia usually results from involvement of the temporal lobes of the brain. Significant loss of memory occurs if both the temporal lobes are affected. If the lesion is unilateral and involves the speech-dominant temporal lobe, problems with verbal memory occur. If the lesion is in the nondominant lobe, then deficits in visual and nonverbal recall is seen.

Causes include chronic alcoholism, head injury, after temporal lobectomy, herpes simplex encephalitis, strokes or brain tumors, Alzheimer's disease, seizures, classical migraine, certain drugs, electroconvulsive therapy etc. Transient global amnesia, where the individual suddenly becomes confused and amnesic may follow immersion in cold or hot water, physical exertion etc. The attack may last from 2-12 hours. The cause of this is not known.

Signs and Symptoms:

A classic example of amnesia is that seen as a complication of chronic alcoholism. Here the person is unable to recall new information. Memory of situations that occurred before the onset of illness is remembered, but memory of new events is severely impaired.

Risk Factors:

See Cause.

Caution and Recommendations to Therapists:

If a client has amnesia, ensure that you have proper written records of treatment plan and treatment given.

Notes

The cause of amnesia should be investigated and treated. If the investigation is negative, reassurance is the only measure. A course of thiamine may help some individuals.

References

Brown MM, Hachinski VC. Acute confusional states, amnesia, and dementia. In: Isselbacher KJ et al., editors. Harrison's principles of internal medicine. 13th ed. New York: McGraw-Hill Co; 1994. p. 141-142.

Amputation

Removal of part of a limb when its survival compromises the health or life of the individual.

Cause:

Amputations are often done when the blood supply to parts of the body is severely compromised leading to gangrene formation or infection.

Signs and Symptoms:

After amputation, patients often have *Phantom Limb* pain. Phantom limb has been described as having a tingling feeling or a feeling of a definite shape of the

Notes

Phantom limb has been treated with anaesthetic blockage of trigger sites, or by excessive stimulation. Vigorous vibration of the stump has also been used successfully. Other modes of treatment include placement of electrodes in the dorsal column of the spinal cord. For

Pathology A to Z -

amputated limb. The shape may take the form of the real limb initially, but later change in shape. Cramping, shooting, crushing or burning pain may be felt in this area, starting immediately, or days or months later. Later, other zones may become sensitized and act as triggers for phantom pain. Emotions, stress, urination or defecation may aggravate the pain.

more details see Appendix C: Anaesthetics.

The cause of Phantom Limb pain in amputees cannot be fully explained by a single mechanism. It has been attributed to changes in the peripheral, autonomic and central nervous system after amputation.

Risk Factors:

Amputation may be done on patients with a) arteriosclerosis where the diminished blood supply has resulted in gangrene; b) malignant tumors and c) complications of diabetes leading to gangrene and d) after severe trauma to the limb.

Caution and Recommendations to Therapists:

Since the pain mechanism changes with time, the therapeutic approach also has to be modified according to individual needs. Some clients may be self conscious about the absence of limbs and the Therapist should make an extra effort to put them at ease. History of the reason for amputation should be obtained. If due to gangrene complicating diabetes mellitus, other complications of diabetes may be present. The client may also be on medications for the condition. (See Caution and Recommendations to Therapists under Diabetes mellitus). Ask the client if they would like the prosthesis on or off during the massage and obtain permission before massaging the stump.

Obtain a detailed history of triggers that produce Phantom limb pain. Even gentle touch, warmth and other painless stimuli in an area away from the amputation site can be triggers. Application of ice or quick light percussion strokes of the amputated limb and stump may help relieve phantom pain. Massage is given after the stumps have healed completely. Avoid inflamed or ulcerated areas. Use passive movements to loosen the stiffened joints in the area. Effleurage is used to reduce edema and increase the circulation. Massage muscles of the shoulders, back, arms and trunk to reduce fatigue and pain in muscles that are used for working with crutches or prosthesis.

References

Clippinger FW. Amputations and limb substitutions. In: Sabiston DC. editor. Textbook of Surgery – the biological basis of modern surgical practice. 14 ed. Philadelphia: WB Saunders Co; 1991. p. 1345-1350.

Jenson TS, Krebs B, Nielsen J et al. Phantom limb, phantom pain, and stump pain in amputees during the first 6 months following limb amputation. Pain. 1983; 17: 243.

Amyloidosis

A condition where there is extracellular deposition of a fibrous protein - amyloid in one or more sites.

Renal, Gastrointestinal, Cardiovascular, Nervous, Respiratory, Musculoskeletal systems

Cause:

In many cases the cause is unknown. In some it may be associated with multiple myeloma, chronic infectious diseases like osteomyelitis, tuberculosis, leprosy, chronic inflammatory diseases like rheumatoid arthritis and aging. It may be seen after long-term hemodialysis.

Notes

There is no specific therapy for amyloidosis. Various drugs are being tried out to decrease the formation of amyloid and promote lysis of existing amyloid deposits.

Signs and Symptoms:

The signs and symptoms depend on the organ affected and the extent to which it is affected. If the kidney is affected, it can present as proteinuria or kidney failure in late stages. Functional abnormalities are seen in late stages, if the liver is affected. Lesions in the heart present as cardiac failure or cardiomegaly. Gastrointestinal lesions may present as obstruction, ulceration, bleeding, diarrhoea etc. Joints, nervous system and respiratory system may be affected and no area is spared.

Risk Factors:

See Cause.

Caution and Recommendations to Therapists:

References

Damjanov I, Linder J. editors. Anderson's pathology. 10th ed. Philadelphia: Mosby Year book Inc; 1996. p. 448-459.

Since the condition can affect different organs and symptoms vary accordingly, the Therapist should obtain a detailed history to individualize the treatment plan. It may be necessary to consult the treating physician.

Amyotrophic Lateral Sclerosis

Nervous system

(ALS; Lou Gehrig's disease)

A progressive disease of the motor neurons that produces atrophy of muscles.

Cause:

Notes

There is no treatment as yet that can stop the progress of the disease. Only supportive treatment such as physiotherapy and splinting are available. More recently, motor neuron trophic factors that have been identified are being used in clinical trials. The average survival time is 2-5 years.

Since many other treatable conditions may present with symptoms and signs similar to ALS, care should be taken by the Physician to rule them out.

The cause is unknown. It has been found to be hereditary in a few cases where the onset of the disease has been in childhood or early adulthood. The disease produces death of the lower motor neuron (neurons from the brain and spinal cord that go directly to the muscle) as well as upper motor neurons (neurons from the brain that modify the actions of lower motor neurons). The sensory neurons, the autonomic regulation, control of movement and the intellect are intact.

Signs and Symptoms:

Due to the death of the upper motor neurons, the person has increased tone of muscles, exaggerated reflexes, weakness, and lack of fine control over movements. The lesion in the lower motor neuron results in flaccidity (lack of tone), atrophy and weakness of muscles. Typically this disease begins with weakness and atrophy of the small muscles of the hand. It progresses to affect other limbs, neck and face. In severe cases the muscles of the pharynx, palate, tongue and other regions are affected producing difficulty in speech and swallowing. If the respiratory muscles are affected, it can result in labored breathing and death.

Risk Factors:

It usually begins between the ages of 40-70 years. It affects men more than women. In the early-onset disease, which is hereditary, both men and women are affected equally.

Caution and Recommendations to Therapists:

Take time to assess the client thoroughly. Since both upper and lower motor neurons can be affected, the tone may be increased in some groups of muscles while others are flaccid with marked atrophy. Contractures may also be present. Remember that the intellect as well as the sensory system is intact. This is one disease that will pose a tremendous challenge to the Massage Therapist, as the treatment options have to be varied since the presentation changes from day to day.

The aim is to reduce tone in regions with increased tone - so a relaxation massage is required here with increased use of strokes like effleurage and gentle friction. In regions with decreased tone a stimulatory massage is required with more use of pétrissage. Use friction strokes to prevent adhesions. Perform passive range of motion movements of all joints to prevent joint stiffness. Massage has been shown to increase circulation in these muscles. This may help alleviate the muscle cramps that these clients often get. Encourage clients to join support groups in the local area. Refer to Appendix D for resources.

References

Smith RA. editor. Handbook of Amyotrophic Lateral Sclerosis. New York: Marcel Dekker; 1992.

Wine ZK. Russian medical massage: Lou Gehrig's disease. Massage. 1993; 44(July/August): 18,20.

Anaphylaxis

A systemic response to specific antigens when a sensitized individual is exposed to the antigen.

Cardiovascular, Lymphatic, Respiratory, Integumentary systems

Cause:

It is the result of acute and severe antigen-antibody reactions in a previously sensitized individual.

Signs and Symptoms:

The signs and symptoms are seen within minutes of exposure to the antigen. There is difficulty in breathing and the person goes into shock (see Shock).

Notes

The best form of treatment is to prevent exposure of the person to the antigen s/he is sensitized to. Skin testing before use of new agents can help prevent a fatal reaction. It is very important to diagnose anaphylaxis early since death can occur within minutes to hours after the onset of symptoms. Prompt administration of adrenaline can reduce the symptoms dramatically. Administration of oxygen, intubation and tracheostomy may be necessary in some cases. Individuals prone to anaphylaxis should wear an informational bracelet and have immediate access to an epinephrine kit. A different form of therapy is the administration of blocking antibody to the specific antigen (immunotherapy).

For more details see Appendix C: Adrenergic drugs; Intubation; Tracheostomy; Immunotherapy.

Itching, redness and swelling of the skin may accompany it. This is due to the release of histamine from mast cells. Gastrointestinal manifestations such as nausea, vomiting, abdominal cramps and diarrhea may be seen. Edema of the larynx can present as hoarseness, and noisy breathing. Bronchial spasm may present as tightness in the chest. The condition is life-threatening as edema in the larynx can lead to obstruction of the air passages.

Risk Factors:

Hormones such as insulin, vasopressin etc, enzymes, pollen extracts (grass, trees), food (eggs, seafood, nuts, grains, chocolate), venom (bee, wasp, hornets etc), antiserum (certain vaccines), local anesthetics, antibiotics (eg. penicillin) and diagnostic agents can all cause anaphylaxis in previously sensitized individuals.

Caution and Recommendations to Therapists:

It is important to get a history of allergy from every client treated and flag the records of clients with allergy. Anaphylaxis is an emergency and can be fatal if not treated promptly. Prevention is best. It is important to ensure that there are no antigens in the clinic that can precipitate an attack. A diluted drop of lubricant that is to be used can be first tested in a very small area of skin to see if an inflammatory reaction occurs locally. Remnants of detergents in sheets can cause allergic reactions in some individuals. A well ventilated, dust free room should be used for massaging any client with a history of allergy. See Appendix D for organizations and support groups.

References

Austen F. Diseases of immediate type hypersensitivity. In: Isselbacher KJ et al, editor. Harrison's principles of internal medicine. 13th ed. New York: McGraw-Hill Co; 1994. p. 1632-1634.

Cardiovascular system

Anemia

A condition where the hemoglobin level in the blood is below normal.

Cause:

Notes

It is important to identify the cause of anemia before treating it. Nutritional deficiency anemias can be prevented by the intake of a well balanced diet that includes red meats, green vegetables, eggs, whole wheat, milk etc. Iron supplements are required when the needs are increased as during pregnancy and in nursing mothers.

Anemia may be due to various causes. The causes include those conditions that a) affect production of hemoglobin/red blood cells b) result in blood loss and c) lead to rapid destruction of red blood cells.

Conditions that destroy the bone marrow such as tumors and exposure to radiation result in *aplastic anemia*. Here the production of platelets and white blood cells are affected in addition to red blood cells. Production of red cells may also be affected by inadequate secretion of erythropoietin (hormone that stimulates red cell production) by the kidneys. Anemia may also result if the components for manufacture of hemoglobin are inadequate. Protein, iron, vitamin B12 or folic acid deficiency can lead to this type of anemia. Protein deficiency can be seen in malabsorption syndrome or malnutrition. Iron deficiency can occur due to reduced intake or increased need as during pregnancy. Deficiency of vitamin B12 or folic acid can follow reduced intake or lack of intrinsic factor in the stomach. The intrinsic factor secreted in the stomach is required for proper absorption of vitamin B12 in the ileum. This type of anemia is called *pernicious anemia.*

Conditions that lead to excessive blood loss can also cause anemia. The blood loss could be acute as after injuries, vomiting of blood (esophageal varices rupture), coughing of blood (can occur in Tuberculosis; lung cancer), blood loss in the feces (hemorrhoids, colon tumors, peptic ulcers, ulcerative colitis, worm infestation, etc.), or profuse menstruation in women (endometriosis, fibroids, etc.). As well, bleeding disorders like hemophilia where there is a lack of clotting factors can result in excessive blood loss and anemia.

Increased destruction of red cells can also lead to anemia. This occurs when the spleen is overactive, or if the red cells are abnormal. In certain genetic disorders like *thalassemia* and *sickle cell anemia*, the structure of the hemoglobin is abnormal and the red cells are destroyed prematurely (*hemolytic anemia*).

Most often, anemia may be seen in individuals with chronic disease such as chronic inflammation; cancer; liver disease; rheumatoid arthritis etc.

Signs and Symptoms:

Initially, there are no specific symptoms. The person fatigues easily, is listless, irritable and is unable to concentrate. There is also a greater susceptibility to infections. Pallor may be seen. The nails tend to become brittle and spoon-shaped. Cracking of the corners of the mouth and smoothness of tongue are other symptoms. In severe cases, there may be numbness and tingling of the fingers. Other associated symptoms and signs are seen depending on the type of anemia.

Risk Factors:

See Cause.

Caution and Recommendations to Therapists:

Advice clients who appear abnormally pale to see a physician and get their hemoglobin levels checked. If the anemia is due to bleeding disorders, care should be taken not to use excessive pressure as they tend to bruise easily and bleeding can occur under the skin. It should also be remembered that anemic individuals are susceptible to infections especially those who have bone marrow failure. In the case of those with aplastic anemia the physician should be consulted. It should be ensured that clients with anemia are not exposed to any infection in the clinic. Refer to Appendix D for resources.

References

Gaspard KJ. The red blood cell and alterations in oxygen transport. In: Porth CM, editor. Pathophysiology concepts of altered health states. 4th ed. Philadelphia: JB Lippincott Co; 1994. p. 323-339.

Aneurysm

An abnormal localized dilatation of an artery.

Cardiovascular system

Cause:

Any condition that causes weakening of the arterial wall can lead to an aneurysm. Dissecting aneurysms - the type which results in hemorrhage into the vessel wall are common in patients with hypertension and those with connective tissue disorders (eg. Marfan's syndrome).

Notes

Surgical obliteration is one of the treatment options used.

a Handbook for Massage Therapists

Signs and Symptoms:

Often, aneurysms are asymptomatic and may only be diagnosed on rupturing. With aneurysms of the thoracic aorta, the patient may have pain in the back, neck, or behind the sternum. Difficulty in breathing, dry cough, noisy breathing and hoarseness of voice may be present due to the pressure of the dilated vessel on the surrounding tissue.

Pressure on the superior vena cava may result in edema of the face and neck and engorgement of neck veins. Sometimes, the patient may present with a pulsating mass.

Aneurysm can occur in any artery. Rupture of an aneurysm in an artery in the brain can be a cause of sudden death. Unruptured

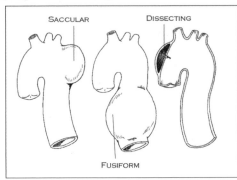

Aorta showing types of Aneurysms

aneurysms in the brain may present as palsy of certain cranial nerves (dilatation of pupil, pain behind the eye; loss of sight, etc.) or as sudden unexplained headache.

Risk Factors:

Congenital defects, trauma, infections, arteriosclerosis, hypertension and connective tissue disorders predispose to this condition.

Caution and Recommendations to Therapists:

Consult physician before embarking on deep abdominal massage, on clients with history of hypertension or atherosclerosis. Heavy abdominal massage in clients with abdominal aortic aneurysm can result in rupture, extensive bleeding and death. Avoid massage over any mass that is pulsating. See Appendix D for organizations and support groups.

References

Sabiston DC. Aneurysms. In: Sabiston DC. editor. Textbook of Surgery – the biological basis of modern surgical practice. 14 ed. Philadelphia: WB Saunders Co; 1991. p. 1539-1577.

Angina pectoris (Ischemic heart disease)

Cardiovascular system

It is a form of heart disease produced by inadequate blood supply to the walls of the heart.

Cause:

Notes

Treatment varies from individual to individual. Treatment should be aimed to reduce the risk factors and treat conditions that may precipitate an attack. The person is also advised to make life

The classical type of angina (Latin - to choke) is associated with narrowing of the coronary arteries by atherosclerosis. The symptoms are usually precipitated by exercise. The variant type of angina is brought on by spasm of the coronaries and can occur at rest or at night. Angina may also be present in individuals

Pathology A to Z -

where there is an abnormal oxygen demand as in aortic stenosis (narrowing of the aorta near the aortic valve) or hypertrophy of the heart. Rarely, severe reduction in the oxygen carrying capacity as in severe anemia may precipitate the condition.

Signs and Symptoms:

The disease presents as recurring pain lasting for a short duration. The pain or pressure sensation may be felt over the chest or posterior to the sternum and may radiate to the shoulder, arm, jaw, or other areas of the chest. The pain is usually described as constricting, squeezing or suffocating. In the classical types, exertion or emotion precipitates the symptoms. In the variant type, the pain can occur at rest or at night. In the unstable type the pain becomes progressively severe, lasting longer. This type can lead to myocardial infarction.

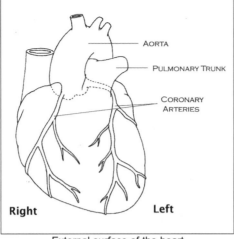

AORTA

PULMONARY TRUNK

CORONARY ARTERIES

Right   **Left**

External surface of the heart

Risk Factors:

Family history of angina, hypertension, obesity, smoking, diabetes mellitus, stress, sedentary life-style and high cholesterol levels in the blood are all risk factors. There is a lower incidence of angina in premenopausal women.

Caution and Recommendations to Therapists:

Massage can help clients with a history of angina by reducing stress levels. Stress predisposes to an anginal attack. Massage also reduces the activity of the sympathetic nervous system, which is partly responsible for coronary vasoconstriction. Sudden exposure to extreme cold or heat can bring on an attack. So keep the client warm, and avoid extreme fluctuations in temperature when using hot or cold packs.

If a client has an attack on the table, bring him/her up to a sitting or standing position as this reduces the load on the heart and call for help. If the client has the prescription drug it should be taken promptly. Always make sure that a client diagnosed to have angina has the prescription drugs handy while coming for massage. Keep the telephone number of the client's physician in your records. A contact address should be obtained as well. See Appendix D for organizations and support groups.

style changes such as weight reduction, changes in diet, exercise etc. to minimize attacks.

Drugs given for angina dilate systemic veins and coronary vessels thereby reducing the load on the heart and increasing oxygen supply respectively. Since the drugs such as nitrates are absorbed quickly via mucous membranes they are often placed under the tongue. They may also be given as patches under the skin, as ointments or swallowed. Other drugs that reduce heart rate and contractility of the heart are also available. Aspirin is often given as it prevents the activity of platelets.

Surgery may be done in selected individuals. *Angioplasty* is a method where a flexible guidewire is passed into the coronary artery and another balloon catheter is passed over the guidewire. The balloon is inflated at the point where there is narrowing until the stenosis is reduced or relieved. A newer procedure - *stent implantation* may be done to relieve angina. In this case, a small, latticed, stainless steel tube is introduced on the balloon catheter. The steel tube is left in place at the site of the narrowing, to keep the blood vessel open.

In the case of *coronary artery bypass grafting*, a section of a vein is used to connect the aorta with the coronary artery beyond the narrowing. Sometimes the internal mammary arteries (the artery deep to the sternum) may be anastomosed to the coronary artery beyond the obstruction.

For more details see Appendix C: Antiinflammatories - non steroidal drugs; Angioplasty; Bypass grafting; Catheterization; Anticoagulants.

References

Goldman L, Braunwald E. Chest discomfort and palpitation. In: Isselbacher KJ et al, editors. Harrison's principles of internal medicine. 13th ed. New York: McGraw-Hill Co; 1994. p. 55-60.

Angioedema

A cutaneous vascular reaction involving the deeper dermal and subcutaneous tissue, often occurring in association with urticaria (hives).

Cause:

There is dilation of cutaneous blood vessels with leakage of fluid into the surrounding tissue (edema). The lymph vessels are also dilated. White blood cells are seen in the extracellular fluid in the region. The release of chemical mediators from basophils and mast cells are responsible for the reaction.

It is believed that both immunological and non-immunological factors can result in the release of chemical mediators. In rare cases, the condition may be inherited and may affect the respiratory and gastrointestinal systems. Oral and parenteral drugs are common causes of this condition. In some, it may be a reaction to certain food proteins or to various substances added for coloration or preservation. Nuts, fish, shellfish, eggs, milk, chocolate, tomatoes and berries are some of the food products commonly implicated. Pollen, animal dander may cause this condition. Sometimes, certain infections can produce angioedema. Insect bites and various substances in contact with the skin are other causes. It may be associated with other systemic diseases like systemic lupus erythematosus, rheumatoid arthritis, viral hepatitis, infectious mononucleosis etc.

Some forms of urticaria and angioedema are precipitated by physical factors like cold, heat, exposure to the sun, pressure etc. In some, emotional stress or exercise may produce urticaria and angioedema. *Dermographism* is a response seen along the region of the skin that has been briskly stroked.

Signs and Symptoms:

The skin reaction is transient and appears as red, edematous patterns on the skin. They may vary in size from a few millimeters to many centimeters. The lesions last from 4 to 24 hours. Urticaria can be distributed in any part of the body while angioedema tends to occur in regions where there is loose connective tissue like the eyelids or lips.

Risk Factors:

See Cause.

Caution and Recommendations to Therapists:

Since angioedema is one form of allergy, a thorough history with details of allergens has to be recorded and the record flagged for future sessions. Heat, cold or pressure may precipitate the condition in some clients. The skin may turn red and edematous along the lines of the stroke and can be a cause for alarm. Since angioedema can predispose to anaphylaxis this condition has to be taken seriously.(see Caution and Recommendation to Therapists under Anaphylaxis). See also Appendix D for organizations and support groups.

Notes

The ideal management is to identify the cause and remove it. Factors that produce the condition should be avoided. Usually antihistamines are given orally. Drugs that block the release of chemical mediators by mast cells are of benefit. Epinephrine and corticosteroids are active forms of treatment required if the condition deteriorates and anaphylaxis is imminent. For more details see Appendix C: Antihistamines; Adrenergic drugs; Antiinflammatories - steroidal drugs.

References

Austen F. Diseases of immediate type hypersensitivity. In: Isselbacher KJ et al, editors. Harrison's principles of internal medicine. 13th ed. New York: McGraw-Hill Co; 1994. p. 1634-1636.

Ankylosing spondylitis (Spondylitis; Ankylopoietica;
Marie-Strumpell disease; Bechterew's disease)

Musculoskeletal system

An inflammatory disease of the axial skeleton.

Cause:

The cause is unknown. The presence of large macrophages in the acute stages suggests an immune response.

Signs and Symptoms:

It affects the sacroiliac joints, intervertebral disk spaces and costo-vertebral joints commonly. Rarely, it affects the large synovial joints like hips, knees and shoulders. Fibrosis, calcification, ossification and stiffening of the joints are seen. The spine becomes rigid and appears bamboo-like in the X-ray. The disease has exacerbations and remissions.

Notes

There is no definitive treatment option. The individual is encouraged to follow an exercise regime geared to improving mobility and maintaining range of motion. Antiinflammatory drugs may be given to reduce pain and stiffness. In severe cases of arthritis in large synovial joints like the hip, replacement therapy may be resorted to. For more details see Appendix C: Antiinflammatories - non steroidal drugs.

Typically, the patient complains of persistent or intermittent low back pain. The pain becomes worse at rest and is reduced by mild activity. The pain may also radiate to the thigh. There is reduced mobility of the vertebral column and the curvature of the lumbar region is slowly lost. In late stages the spine gets

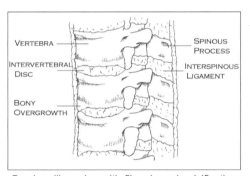

VERTEBRA

INTERVERTEBRAL DISC

BONY OVERGROWTH

SPINOUS PROCESS

INTERSPINOUS LIGAMENT

Bamboo-like spine with fibrosis and calcification

fixed. If the costovertebral joints are fixed it can affect the lung volume. Kyphosis is present when the thoracic or cervical regions are affected and the weight of the head compresses the vertebral bodies and bends the spine forward. The head is therefore hyperextended to help maintain the field of vision.

Ankylosing spondylitis may be accompanied by weight loss, fever and fatigue. Osteoporosis may also be present. Complications include fractures, subluxation of the spine and spinal cord compression.

Risk Factors:

It is more common in North America. The disease is more severe in men. It occurs at any age but the incidence is higher in the 20-30 age group. There is a high genetic predisposition to the disease.

Caution and Recommendations to Therapists:

The client should be positioned according to individual comfort with ample support using pillows. In clients with kyphosis extra cushioning in the neck region may be needed. Pillows placed under the knee can relieve the tension on

References

Adams JC. Hamblen DL. Outline of orthopaedics. 11th ed. London: Churchill Livingstone; 1990. p. 179-181.

the hamstrings and iliofemoral ligament and cause the pelvis to tilt backwards and straighten the lumbar spine.

The aim is to retain the mobility of the joints, to strengthen weak muscles and to stretch tight ones. Do not try to forcibly mobilize ankylosed joints. Spinal manipulations should be avoided altogether. Since osteoporosis is common, deep pressure should not be used. Gentle massage should be given to the back and limbs. Hot packs are very helpful to ease the pain. Advice clients to sleep in a supine position if possible. Encourage client to do breathing exercises regularly to mobilize the thorax.

The client may be on painkillers and give inadequate feedback. Avoid massage if the area is inflamed. The Physician should be consulted in clients with severe deformities.

Anterior compartment syndrome

Musculoskeletal system

A collection of signs and symptoms produced by increased pressure and consequent reduced blood flow to a closed muscle compartment in the leg.

Cause:

In the anterior aspect of the leg a compact compartment is formed between the tibia and fibula and an unyielding fascia around the muscles. The muscles tibialis anterior, extensor hallucis longus, extensor digitorum longus, peroneus

Notes

The condition is diagnosed by measuring the pressure in the compartment. If the symptoms are chronic or severe, surgery may be done to reduce the pressure.

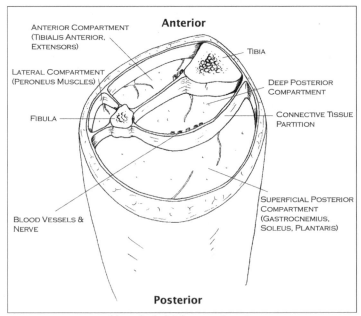

Anterior

ANTERIOR COMPARTMENT (TIBIALIS ANTERIOR, EXTENSORS)

TIBIA

LATERAL COMPARTMENT (PERONEUS MUSCLES)

DEEP POSTERIOR COMPARTMENT

FIBULA

CONNECTIVE TISSUE PARTITION

SUPERFICIAL POSTERIOR COMPARTMENT (GASTROCNEMIUS, SOLEUS, PLANTARIS)

BLOOD VESSELS & NERVE

Posterior

Musculoskeletal compartments

Pathology A to Z -

tertius, the peroneal nerve and blood vessels lie in this compartment. Any condition that increases the pressure in the compartment compromises the blood supply to the soft tissue resulting in the characteristic symptoms.

Signs and Symptoms:

There is a tight feeling in the calf region with pain, tenderness, numbness and tingling. The symptoms develop slowly but progress steadily and are pronounced on using the leg. Like angina pectoris, the pain begins on using the limb to the same extent every time. The pain may be produced even on stretching the muscle.

Risk Factors:

Overuse and repetitive stress to the muscles in this compartment usually cause it. The stress results in inflammation and swelling of the tissue in this confined space.

Caution and Recommendations to Therapists:

The limb should be positioned in level with the heart. Elevation may reduce the blood flow to the already compromised tissue. Placing the limb in a dependent position may increase the venous congestion due to the effect of gravity. In the acute stage, measures to reduce the inflammation and swelling are helpful. Rest and ice application have been found to be beneficial. The thighs should be massaged well, using broad strokes like effleurage and pétrissage to increase venous and lymphatic drainage. In the subacute stage, heat can be applied to soften the connective tissue. Suitable strokes such as cross fibre friction are used to stretch the tight fascia followed by ice application. However, such techniques should be avoided if it is too painful. In those with lowered sensation, care should be taken not to use excessive pressure, as the feedback from the client is likely to be inadequate.

References

Mercier LR, editor. Practical orthopedics. 4th ed. New York: Mosby-Year book Inc; 1995. p 305-306.

Anthrax

An acute bacterial infection that is introduced into the body of humans by contact with infected animals.

Integumentary, Respiratory, Cardiovascular, Gastrointestinal systems

Cause:

It is caused by the *Bacillus anthracis*. The bacillus is present most frequently in herbivorous animals. Humans get infected if they come in contact with, inhale or ingest the spores present in infected animals, animal products or through insect bites. The spores can survive for years in dry earth, but are destroyed by boiling for 10 minutes or by the use of hydrogen peroxide and formaldehyde, among others.

Signs and Symptoms:

In the cutaneous form (common) the person has a localized skin lesion with nonpitting edema around it. The lesion is characteristically described as a

Notes

Penicillin G injections is the best form of treatment. Other antibiotics may be given to those sensitive to penicillin. Improvement of working conditions for handlers of animal products has reduced the incidence drastically. Agricultural workers, veterinary personnel and those at risk may be given vaccines against anthrax. There is a need for improved anthrax vaccines as the current vaccines are impure, provide incomplete protection and have side effects. In addition, anthrax bacillus may be used in biological warfare. For more details see Appendix C: Antimicrobial - antibacterial agents; Immunization.

'malignant pustule'. It appears as a red macule which, with time progresses to a papule, vesicle and pustule and finally ulcerates. It is usually painless. Small vesicles may surround the initial lesion and the lymph nodes draining the area may be enlarged. If the spores are inhaled (*woolsorter's disease*), it presents as inflammation of the mediastinum which quickly spreads to other systems. The person has fever, difficulty in breathing and hypotension. It is associated with a very high mortality. If the spores have been ingested, the person may present with fever, nausea and vomiting, abdominal pain and bloody diarrhea.

Risk Factors:

Occupations that involve contact with animals and animal products put a person at risk. Skinning, butchering, dissecting, exposure to hides, wool or bones are some examples of occupations at risk.

Caution and Recommendations to Therapists:

This is an infective conditon. If you have come in contact with an animal or human diagnosed to have anthrax, report to a medical center immediately for treatment. See Appendix D for organizations and support groups. Also see Appendix B for Strategies for infection prevention and safe practice.

References

Holmes. RK. Diphtheria, other corynebacterial infections, and anthrax. In: Isselbacher KJ et al, editors. Harrison's principles of internal medicine. 13th ed. New York: McGraw-Hill Co; 1994. p. 628-630.

Turnbull PCB. Anthrax vaccines: Past, present and future. Vaccine. 1991; 9: 533.

Aphasia

Nervous system

A condition where there is disturbance in comprehension/production of speech and language.

Cause:

Aphasias may be caused by cell death in specific areas of the brain due to insufficient blood flow, hemorrhage, encephalitis, trauma or tumor. Lesions in the dominant (the left side in right-handed individuals) frontal, parietal and superior temporal lobes produce aphasia. Lesions in the posterior part of the brain can result in some defects.

Aphasias are classified in many ways - according to the anatomical location affected, physiologic or psychological basis. Prognosis and type of therapy adopted is related to the classification. *Dysarthria* is a defect in articulation and occurs due to problems with muscles in the oropharynx and respiratory apparatus. *Dysphonia* is a defect in production of voice and is due to disease of the larynx or innervation of the laryngeal muscles. *Dysgraphia* is faulty writing skills and is due to problems with the muscles used in writing.

Signs and Symptoms:

Global aphasia is characterised by minimal speech, nonfluent aphasia (slow, incorrectly articulated words and sentences), poor comprehension of written and spoken language. *Broca's aphasia* manifests as nonfluent aphasia, agrammatic sentences and poor articulation. The person may be mute. In *Wernicke's aphasia* (*sensory aphasia*), there is fluent speech but total

Notes

Treatment varies according to the type of aphasia and it is important to identify the type by various reading, comprehension and written tests. Various techniques are used by trained specialists to improve function. The prognosis depends on the extent of lesion and the underlying problem.

Pathology A to Z -

incomprehension of spoken speech. The person is unable to read or to repeat sounds or words.

In minor types of aphasias such as *conduction aphasia*, the person has difficulty in repetition of speech and in reading aloud, but has adequate comprehension of written and spoken words. Some people have pure *word deafness* and are unable to repeat a sentence or write a dictation. Others have mainly visual problems where visual language is more compromised than hearing. They cannot read or write. Yet others have pure *word blindness* where they have normal spoken and written language but are unable to read. In some people with certain types of lesions in the temporal lobe, there is difficulty in recalling names of objects or parts of objects and with recent memory.

Aphasias may be associated with hemiplegia, eye or ear defects.

Risk Factors:

See Cause.

Caution and Recommendations to Therapists:

It is important for the Therapist to understand the type of aphasia in the client and to establish suitable ways of communication with regards to feedback during the session. Associated problems such as hemiplegia have to be addressed as well. Refer to resources for information on Disability etiquette. Additional training may be required for those wishing to work with people with mental disabilities in order to fully understand the pathophysiology of the disorders and the challenges the client faces. See Appendix D for organizations and support groups.

References

Mohr. JP. Disorders of speech and language. In: Isselbacher KJ et al, editors. Harrison's principles of internal medicine. 13th ed. New York: McGraw-Hill Co; 1994. p. 158-161
Albert ML et al. Clinical Aspects of dysphasia. New York: Springer-Verlag; 1981.

Appendicitis

Gastrointestinal system

The inflammation of the vermiform appendix.

Cause:

Appendix is a worm-like structure of 3-6 inches in length that is attached to the cecum. The inflammation is a result of obstruction to the lumen of the appendix by faeces, or due to twisting. The appendix becomes swollen and red. If the obstruction persists, death of tissue occurs with perforation of the appendix and spilling of the contents into the abdominal cavity producing toxic reactions.

Notes

The pain produced by appendicitis can resemble that of many other conditions like gastritis, renal stones, pancreatitis, ovarian cyst, diseases of the uterus and inflammation of other areas of the bowel. The best treatment is early operation - appendicectomy. Immediate surgery is required if complications of abscess formation, peritonitis or spread of infection to other areas are to be combated. For more details see Appendix C: Appendicectomy.

Signs and Symptoms:

The person experiences a vague pain below the sternum and around the umbilicus. The location of the pain is different from the actual position of the appendix as the pain is referred to this area. The pain intensifies over a few hours and becomes colicky (spasmodic) in nature. When the inflammation spreads to the peritoneal covering, the pain is localized to the right lower quadrant of the abdomen. The abdominal muscles over the area go into spasm and become

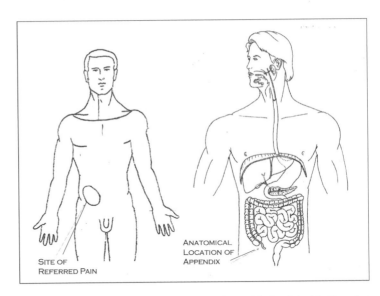

ANATOMICAL LOCATION OF APPENDIX

SITE OF REFERRED PAIN

board-like. The person walks bent over, or lies with the right hip flexed, to reduce the pain. Fever, nausea and vomiting accompany the pain.

Risk Factors:

It can occur at any age but is frequent between 5-30 years of age.

Caution and Recommendations to Therapists:

Do not massage the abdomen if a person complains of pain resembling that of appendicitis as massage can rupture the inflamed appendix. Refer to a Physician immediately.

Avoid abdominal massage in clients who have recently had appendicectomy until clearance has been obtained from a physician.

References

Condon RE, Telford GL. Appendicitis. In: Sabiston DC, editor. Textbook of surgery – the biological basis of modern surgical practice. Philadelphia:WB Saunders Co; 1991. p. 884 – 898.

Arrhythmias

Cardiovascular system

Conditions where the heart beat - rate and/or rhythm is abnormal.

Notes

Sinus node dysfunction is treated with placement of permanent pacemakers. Premature complexes are left untreated. If the arrhythmias produce symptoms, they may be treated with antiarrhythmic drugs. The primary cause of arrhythmias has to be treated. In most clients with Wolff-Parkinson-White syndrome, bypass tracts can be surgically destroyed. Some cases of arrhythmias require the use of cardioverters/

Cause:

In a person with a healthy heart, the rate and rhythm of the heartbeat is initiated in the sinoatrial node (part of the conducting system of the heart). At rest, the normal sinus rate is between 60-100 beats per minute. If the beat is less than 60, *sinus bradycardia* is said to exist. This may be considered as normal in trained athletes. When it is more than 100 it is termed *sinus tachycardia*. Sinus node dysfunction may be seen in the elderly, in those with hypothyroidism, advanced liver disease, hypothermia, acute hypertension, and typhoid fever, among others. In many cases, the cause is not known.

Pathology A to Z -

The action potential initiated in the sinoatrial node is conducted via the atrium to the atrioventricular node (AV node). From here, the impulse travels through the bundle of His, right and left branches and the Purkinje fibers to stimulate the rest of the heart. Problems can arise as a result of defects in the conduction of the impulse. Such disturbances are called *conduction defects*. Depending on the location and extent of the block, it is termed as *first-degree AV block*, *second-degree heart block* or *third-degree heart block*. Sometimes, another area of the heart takes the function of the sinoatrial node and initiates impulses (*ectopic impulse*).

The cause of tachycardias may be due to increased level of adrenaline/ noradrenaline, electrolyte imbalances (eg. increased potassium levels - hyperkalemia), reduced oxygen availability, drugs and mechanical stretch. Tachyarrhythmias are usually associated with palpitations. Abnormal action potentials originating from the atrium or the ventricle are called *atrial* and *ventricular premature complexes* respectively. In sinus tachycardias the beats do not increase more than 200 per minute and may be a physiologic response to fever, anxiety, exercise, thyrotoxicosis etc.

Atrial flutter - a condition where the atrium beats 250-350 beats per minute and *atrial fibrillation* - a condition where the atrium beats 350-600 beats per minute may be seen following surgery, emotional stress or acute alcoholic intoxication and in people with heart disease and those suffering from thyrotoxicosis.

Wolff-Parkinson-White syndrome is due to a congenital abnormality where impulses from the atrium bypass the AV node through abnormal tracts. Flutter and fibrillation may be seen in the ventricles too.

Signs and Symptoms:

The person with sinus bradycardia may feel fatigued due to the reduced cardiac output. They may complain of dizziness and fainting spells. *Ventricular flutters* and *fibrillations* are dangerous and may result in sudden death. Often, arrhythmias are identified in EKG tracings.

Risk Factors:

See Cause.

Caution and Recommendations to Therapists:

If a client with a history of arrhythmias complains of dizziness, palpitation or has a fainting spell call for help immediately. Ensure that you have a record of the address and telephone number of the treating Physician.

If a client has a permanent pacemaker implanted, avoid the area of the pacemaker pocket. It is usually below the clavicle on the nondominant side. It is also important to find out what environmental factors can affect the functioning of the pacemaker. Most pacemakers use radiofrequency signals. See Appendix D for organizations and support groups.

defibrillators. Defibrillators depolarize all or most of the myocardium, so that normal rhythm may resume. Some of the devices can be implanted and they recognise and terminate life-threatening arrhythmias. For more details see Appendix C: Antiarrhythmic drugs; Defibrillators.

References

Lowe JE. Cardiac pacemakers. In: Sabiston DC, editor. Textbook of surgery – the biological basis of modern surgical practice. Philadelphia: WB Saunders Co; 1991. p. 2074-2095. Josephson ME, Marchlinski FE, Buxton AE. The bradyarrhythmias: disorders of sinus node function and AV conduction disturbances. In: Isselbacher KJ et al, editors. Harrison's principles of internal medicine. 13th ed. New York: Philadelphia: McGraw-Hill Co; 1994. p. 1011-1036.

Musculoskeletal system

Arthritis - gouty (Gout)

A joint disorder due to deposition of crystals.

Cause:

Gout is caused by deposition of monosodium urate or uric acid crystals in the joint cavity. The crystals attract leukocytes, which release lysosomal enzymes that trigger inflammation. The deposition of crystals in joints is due to the higher levels of urate in the serum either due to increased production, decreased elimination or both. Urate production is influenced by dietary intake of purines, breakdown and salvage of nucleic acid (found in the nucleus of cells). The urate formed is normally excreted via the kidney and intestines.

Signs and Symptoms:

There is an acute onset of pain, redness and swelling of the joint. It affects the peripheral joints - commonly the metatarsophalangeal joint of the big toe.

Risk Factors:

Primary gout is more common in men between the ages of 40 and 60. In women, those who are postmenopausal are affected. It has been associated with genetic defects in the metabolism of purine. Certain drugs, food or alcohol may precipitate the attack of gout. Drugs such as aspirin affect the elimination of the uric acid by the kidneys and increase the chances of gout. Other drugs that increase the acidity of urine and kidney disease reduce elimination of urates and predispose to gout. Foods such as liver, kidney and anchovy that have a high purine content tend to increase uric acid levels in the blood. Excessive alcohol increases breakdown of ATP and increased lactic acid production, thus affecting both production and excretion of urates. As well, alcoholic beverages such as beer have a higher content of purines.

In cases where there is a rapid breakdown of cells as in leukemia, chemotherapy for cancer, hemolysis etc, blood urate levels increase with a predisposition to gout. Strenuous physical activity with excessive breakdown of ATP (adenosine triphosphate) and myocardial infarction are other predisposing factors.

Caution and Recommendations to Therapists:

Advice the client to reduce intake of purine rich diets such as liver, kidney, sardines, anchovies and sweet breads and encourage him/her to follow the physician's orders. Do not massage during the acute stage. In any case, the client is under severe pain and is unlikely to seek a Massage Therapist. Passive range of motion is also contraindicated as repetitive movements may increase inflammation. The joint should be rested in this stage. Cold packs may be beneficial.

In the subacute stage, light massage may be done in surrounding areas. Range of motion and local massage should not be done.

In the chronic stages, the aim should be to increase circulation by light to medium brisk massage. However, the duration should be short. See Appendix D for organizations and support groups.

Notes

It is important to determine the cause of the hyperuricemia ie. increased production or decreased elimination in a client with gout. In acute cases, anti-inflammatory drugs or injection of steroids into the joint is resorted to.

Treating obesity, diabetes mellitus and hypertension - all conditions that may predispose to an attack, may control hyperuricemia. Reduction in alcohol intake should be encouraged. Drugs that specifically lower uric acid levels in the blood, or those that alkalinise the urine and thereby increase solubility of uric acid may also be used. For more details see Appendix C: Antiinflammatories - steroidal drugs; Antiinflammatories - non steroidal drugs.

References

Hall CM, Brody LT. Therapeutic exercise moving toward function. Philadelphia: Lippincott William & Wilkins; 1999. p 185-198.

Wine ZK. Russian medical massage: Arthritis. Massage 1995; 57 (September/October): 90-92.

Kelly WN, Wortmann RL. Hyperuricemia. In: Kelley WN et al, editors. Textbook of Rheumatology. 4th ed. Philadelphia: WB Saunders Co; 1993.

Arthritis - infective (Septic arthritis)

It is an inflammation of joint structures due to infection.

Cause:

It can be caused by a variety of bacterial diseases including gonorrhea, scarlet fever, enteric fever, or spread of infection directly from the surrounding area or blood-borne from another infected part of body.

Signs and Symptoms:

There is a sudden swelling and inflammation of the joint with the joint cavity filled with pus or fibrinous fluid. The infection may spread to the bone, ligaments and cartilage in that area. The patient may complain of severe pain. Muscles around the joint may go into spasm. This may be accompanied by fever. In the chronic type of arthritis, healing occurs by fibrosis that in turn leads to stiffening of the joint.

Risk Factors:

Bacterial infection of any kind in other regions, or chronic illness like diabetes, rheumatoid arthritis, increases the susceptibility. Alcoholics and elderly people are more prone. Any disease that depresses the immune system or use of immunosuppressive drugs puts an individual at high risk.

Caution and Recommendations to Therapists:

Do not massage till the inflammation has subsided and the infection has been controlled. Very gentle massage may be given far away from the inflamed joint when fever has subsided. After recovery heat application with vigorous and deep massage should be given along with passive stretching to prevent fibrosis and maintain range of motion. The client should be encouraged to exercise to strengthen the muscles and surrounding structures that atrophy due to disuse during the acute period. See Appendix D for organizations and support groups.

Notes

Potent antibiotics are given to fight the infection. To reduce adhesions, intra-articular drainage is done and the pus removed from the joint cavity. This condition is considered as a medical emergency as the infection can destroy the articular cartilage and bone. For more details see Appendix C: Antimicrobial - antibacterial agents.

References

Adams JC. Hamblen DL. Outline of orthopaedics. 11th ed. London: Churchill Livingstone; 1990. p 105-107.

Arthritis - osteoarthritis (Osteoarthrosis;

degenerative joint disease)

A chronic degenerative joint disease.

Cause:

It is the most common joint disease in man. The cause is unknown in the *primary type*. The *secondary type* may occur after injury to the joint, ligament or cartilage. Excess mechanical stress placed on the joint due to developmental defects or overweight can also produce osteoarthritis.

Signs and Symptoms:

Osteoarthritis typically affects single large synovial joints. It affects joints asymmetrically. There is a progressive loss of articular cartilage and inflammation

Notes

There is no cure for osteoarthritis. However, treatment is given to reduce pain, maintain range of motion and to minimize disability. Drugs may be given to reduce pain and inflammation. Correction of posture and factors that overload specific joints have to be addressed. Obese individuals are encouraged to loose weight. Physical therapy plays an important role. Application of ice, heat, transcutaneous electrical nerve stimulation (TENS) and exercise (isometric) to strengthen adjacent muscles has been found to be helpful. Joint replacement surgery or arthroscopic removal of debris from joints may be done for those clients with severe osteoarthritis, in whom medical and other interventions have failed.

For more details see Appendix C: Antiinflammatories - non steroidal drugs; Pain killers; TENS; Arthroscopy.

of the synovial membrane. There is joint pain, stiffness, limitation of motion, joint instability and deformity. Typically, pain is produced on using the joint and is relieved at rest. As the disease progresses, pain may persist and occur at rest and several hours after use. Though the articular cartilage does not have nerve fibres, pain is produced due to inflammation of the synovial membrane, damage to adjacent bone, stretch of ligaments/ joint capsule or muscle spasm.

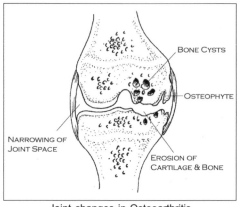

BONE CYSTS

OSTEOPHYTE

NARROWING OF JOINT SPACE

EROSION OF CARTILAGE & BONE

Joint changes in Osteoarthritis

There may be stiffness of the joint after a prolonged period of inactivity. Cracking sounds are produced in the affected joint on movement. It commonly affects the hips, knees, lumbar and cervical vertebrae, ie. primarily the weight bearing joints.

If the cervical spine is affected the patient complains of localized stiffness. In lumbar spine involvement, there is low back pain and stiffness, muscle spasm and loss of mobility. There may be pain due to the compression of nerve roots.

Osteoarthritis of the hip causes pain in the groin region or the inner aspect of the thigh. The pain may be referred to the gluteal region or knee. Movement of the hip is restricted. The patient may hold the hip flexed, externally rotated and adducted. The gait may be affected. There may be difficulty getting up after sitting. The muscles around the hip may be atrophied.

In the case of knee, the joint may be swollen with fluid and movement may be limited.

Risk Factors:

The incidence increases with age. There is a genetic predisposition in some individuals. Immunologic factors have also been implicated in accelerating the changes in the primary type. Trauma to and repetitive use of a joint can predispose to osteoarthritis.

Caution and Recommendations to Therapists:

Deep moist heat application improves the circulation around the joints. Passive movement and friction of the joint are indicated when pain is minimal. Trigger point therapy, lymphatic drainage techniques are other forms of treatment that have been used.

The Therapist should work in close conjunction with a Physiotherapist. Therapeutic exercise is an important component that is used to increase

References

Bennet K. Therapeutic exercise for arthritis. In Hall CM, Brody LT. Therapeutic exercise moving toward function. Philadelphia: Lippincott Williams & Wilkins; 1998. p 185-199.
Adams JC. Hamblen DL. Outline of Orthopaedics. 11th ed. London: Churchill Livingstone; 1990. p 116-119.

flexibility, strength and endurance and to reduce pain. It is also used to improve the overall well being of the person. Isotonic and isometric exercises may be used. Isometric contractions where intraarticular pressure and shear is minimal may be used in the acute stage followed by isotonic and isometric exercises during the subacute and chronic stages. See Appendix D for organizations and support groups.

Arthritis - others

An inflammation of the synovial joints.

Cause:

Arthritis is a term given to describe rheumatic disorders where there are inflammatory and degenerative changes in the joints. More than 100 types of arthritis exist, some of them primary while others are secondary to systemic diseases. Arthritis may be associated with: diffuse connective tissue disease (eg. Systemic lupus erythematosus); spondylitis (eg. Ankylosing spondylitis); degenerative joint disease (eg. osteoarthritis); infection (eg. bacterial, viral, fungal or parasitic); metabolic and endocrine diseases (eg. Gout, Amyloidosis etc); neoplasms; neuropathic disorders (eg. carpal tunnel syndrome); bone and cartilage disorders (eg. osteoporosis); myofascial pain syndromes (eg. fibromyalgia) and with many other conditions such as psoriasis.

Signs and Symptoms:

One or more joints may be affected with inflammation, pain and limitation of movement.

Risk Factors:

See Cause.

Caution and Recommendations to Therapists:

It is important for the Therapist to know the cause of the arthritis before working with a client. Avoid local massage if the joint is inflamed. Ice, compression, rest and elevation is most helpful at this point. Isometric exercises of muscles overlying the joint may reduce the effects of disuse during this stage. During the healing process, passive movement of the joint, range of movement exercises and hot packs are beneficial. Passive stretch may be done to muscles that have shortened as a result of spasm, guarding or bad posture. Work in conjunction with a Physiotherapist.

The aim of treating any type of arthritis is to limit the progression of damage to the affected joint, to increase flexibility, to strengthen the muscles around the joint and to address the adaptive changes that may have occurred in neighbouring joints. See Appendix D for organizations and support groups.

Notes

The cause has to be identified and treated accordingly. Painkillers and antiinflammatory drugs are used to reduce the symptoms. For more details see Appendix C: Painkillers; Antiinflammatories - steroidal drugs; Antiinflammatories - non steroidal drugs.

References

Hall CM, Brody LT. Therapeutic exercise moving toward function. London: Lippincott William & Wilkins; 1999. p. 185-198.

Wine ZK. Russian medical massage: Arthritis. Massage 1995; 57 (September/October): 90-92.

Kelly WN, Wortmann RL. Hyperuricemia. In: Kelley WN et al, editors. Textbook of Rheumatology. 4th ed. Philadelphia: WB Saunders Co; 1993.

Arthritis - rheumatoid

One of the autoimmune diseases that affects multiple systems, producing degenerative changes in connective tissue and inflammatory vascular lesions.

Notes

The goals of treatment are to reduce the inflammation and pain, prevent contractures/deformities, maintain the range of motion and facilitate healing. Since the actual cause is known, the treatment is directed towards reducing inflammation and immune response. Anti-inflammatory drugs such as aspirin and glucocorticoids are used. Sometimes, glucocorticoids are injected into the joint.
Immunosuppressive drugs are given to minimize immune reactions. In those whose joints are severely damaged, surgery may be done to reconstruct or replace joints.

For more details see Appendix C: Antiinflammatories - steroidal drugs; Antiinflammatories - non steroidal drugs; Immunosuppressants; Joint replacement.

Cause:

The actual cause of the disease is not known. It has been postulated that it may be due to the response of the body to an infectious agent in a person who is genetically susceptible. The process by which the infective agent causes inflammation in the joint is a controversy. It is believed that the microorganism or the response of the body to it, induces an immune response to components of the joint as the components have similar antigenic properties as the microorganism. Some consider it as an autoimmune disease where antibodies called *rheumatoid factors* are produced against the body's own antibodies.

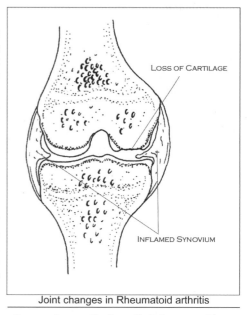

Joint changes in Rheumatoid arthritis

The antigen-antibody reaction that takes place in the synovial tissue of joints attracts lymphocytes and macrophages to the area along with the stimulation of thecomplement system.

Signs and Symptoms:

In long standing arthritis of the joints of the finger, the finger appears spindle-shaped.

In most patients, it begins with fatigue, loss of appetite, weight loss and generalized weakness. The characteristic joint pain follows this. Diagnosis is made based on specific criteria. Typically, the patient complains of morning stiffness for at least one hour over 6 weeks, swelling of more than three joints for over 6 weeks, with symmetrical joint swelling. There is loss of motion in the affected joints. In arthritis of the hand, the metacarpophalangeal joints are flexed, the first interphalangeal joints hyperextended, and the second interphalangeal joint flexed. Rheumatoid arthritis can affect any joint, but the small joints of the limbs are more commonly affected.

Apart from the joints, nodules - *rheumatoid nodules*, may be found around the joint, in the extensor surfaces or other areas exposed to external pressure. Many other organs such as the eye, lungs etc. may be affected by this disease.

Risk Factors:

It is more common in women in the older age group. There is also a genetic predisposition. Often, there is a family history of the disease. Exposure to cold and dampness are other predisposing factors.

Caution and Recommendations to Therapists:

Arthritis cannot be cured, but its relentless progress can be prevented. Stress reduction helps muscles to relax and reduce discomfort. In the early stages the aim should be to prevent contractures, deformity and to maintain joint range of movement. Hot packs help alleviate pain. Massage should not be given in the acute stages, but passive movements of the joints are encouraged.

In the chronic stages, general massage helps reduce stress. Brisk but gentle effleurage and kneading can be used in the limbs. Friction strokes can be used around the joints to reduce the thickening in the periarticular tissues. But make sure that there is no pain. In general, massage should be for a shorter duration.

For clients with this condition, maximum benefit is obtained if the Massage Therapist works in conjunction with the Physician and Physiotherapist. Individualized therapeutic exercises are used to reduce pain, increase mobility and improve muscle performance. The exercises used should have minimal or no joint stress and shock. Water exercises are beneficial as, for example, waist level water reduces the body weight to 50% of that in land. The clients may be on painkillers and/or anti-inflammatory drugs that suppress pain and symptoms. The suppressed pain sometimes may result in inadequate feedback from the clients. Care should be taken while massaging such clients as harm may be done to the joints inadvertently. Refer clients to local support groups (see Appendix D).

References

Bennet K. Therapeutic exercise for arthritis. In Hall CM, Brody LT. Therapeutic exercise moving toward function. Philadelphia: Lippincott Williams & Wilkins; 1998. p 185-199.

Adams JC. Hamblen DL. Outline of orthopaedics. 11th ed. London: Churchill Livingstone; 1990. p 107-112.

Arthropathy (Neurogenic Charcot's arthropathy)

Musculoskeletal system

A degenerative disease of the joint.

Cause:

The degeneration is due to the loss of sensory innervation of the joint. As a result, symptoms are masked when joint damage is caused by excessive stress put on it.

Notes

Treatment is purely supportive.

Signs and Symptoms:

There is swelling, warmth, hypermobility and instability of the joint. It may affect one or many joints. Although a deformity may be present, pain is minimal.

Risk Factors:

It is more common in men over the age of 40. Alcoholism has been shown to predispose to this condition. Loss of sensory innervation of the joint can occur in those with diabetes mellitus, syphilis, spinal cord injury, peripheral nerve injury and leprosy. Recurrent injection of corticosteroids into the joint for other reasons can result in this condition too.

Caution and Recommendations to Therapists:

Warm compresses may be used to relieve pain and spasm if present. Use caution while testing range of motion as the loss of sensation in the affected joint masks the stress that you may put on the joint. A whole body relaxation massage is recommended.

References

Adams JC, Hamblen DL. Outline of orthopaedics. 11th ed. London: Churchill Livingstone; 1990. p 121-122.

Asthma - bronchial

Respiratory system

A reversible, hyper-reactivity of the bronchi to a variety of stimuli, with narrowing and inflammation of the air passages and difficulty in breathing.

Cause:

Notes

Asthma is considered as one of the Chronic Obstructive Pulmonary Diseases along with Chronic Bronchitis and Emphysema. The best form of treatment is avoidance of precipitating factors. Attacks are treated with bronchodilators, corticosteroids and other drugs that prevent the release of bronchoconstriction-producing chemical mediators. For more details see Appendix C: Antiasthmatics; Antiinflammatories - steroidal.

The bronchospasm is caused by the release of mediators from cells in the lung such as mast cells, macrophages, basophils etc. The mediators produce hyperreactivity of the smooth muscles of the air passages, along with increased capillary permeability and local edema. In addition, white blood cells are attracted to the site, the secretions of which add to the local reaction.

The stimuli can be allergens such as pollens of various plants, grass, flowers, feathers of poultry, cat or dog hair, and dust mites, various proteins in food such as shellfish, eggs and milk. Exercise, anxiety and stress, coughing or laughing may be stimuli in some people. In some, asthma may follow an upper respiratory illness, with no history of allergy. In yet other individuals, drugs such as aspirin, indomethacin, drugs that block sympathetic nervous system action, food preservatives (eg. sodium/potassium metabisulfite) etc. may induce an attack. Climatic conditions that tend to concentrate air pollutants such as ozone, nitrogen dioxide, sulfur dioxide may cause asthma in susceptible individuals.

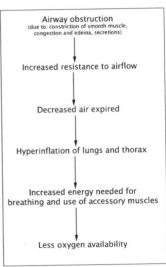

Airway obstruction
(due to: constriction of smooth muscle, congestion and edema, secretions)

↓

Increased resistance to airflow

↓

Decreased air expired

↓

Hyperinflation of lungs and thorax

↓

Increased energy needed for breathing and use of accessory muscles

↓

Less oxygen availability

Pathophysiology of asthma

Occupational asthma is a health problem in many people. Asthma may result from exposure to meat salts, wood and vegetable dusts, industrial chemicals and plastics, animal and insect dusts/secretions among others.

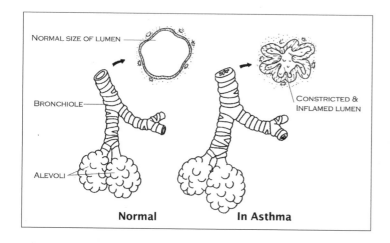

NORMAL SIZE OF LUMEN

CONSTRICTED & INFLAMED LUMEN

BRONCHIOLE

ALEVOLI

Normal   **In Asthma**

The spasm of bronchi, inflammation, edema and clogging by thick mucus produce the symptoms.

Signs and Symptoms:

The signs and symptoms are due to the sequence of events that follow the airway obstruction.

Typically, the patient develops airway obstruction within minutes after exposure to the allergen (if allergic asthma). This attack may resolve quickly. Later, bronchoconstriction may develop 6-10 hours after exposure. This has been labelled as the late reaction.

There is a history of recurrent difficulty in breathing and wheezing. Cough with thick sputum is also present. The individual uses the accessory muscles for respiration during an attack. In chronic asthmatics, the chest is barrel-shaped, with high shoulders and raised ribs as the individual tries to overcome the difficulty in expiration.

Risk Factors:

It occurs at all ages, but is more common in childhood. Usually there is a family history of asthma. Males are more often affected with this condition. Stress and anxiety can precipitate an attack. See Cause.

Caution and Recommendations to Therapists:

Obtain a detailed history - specifically the triggers that bring on an attack. If there is a history of allergy, ensure that the client is not allergic to the oil or other potential allergens in the clinic. It may be advisable for the client to have the required medications close at hand during the massage. A whole body relaxation massage helps to reduce bronchospasm. The client should be positioned as comfortably as possible. Most often this is a half-lying position

References

McFadden ER Jr. Asthma. In: Isselbacher KJ et al, editors. Harrison's principles of internal medicine. 13th ed. London: McGraw-Hill Co; 1994. p. 1167-1176.

Klimowitch P. Massage for sufferers of respiratory diseases. Massage therapy Journal. 1993; 32(2): 42-43.

Ewer TC, Stewart DE. Improvement of bronchial hyperresponsiveness in patients with moderate asthma after treatment with a hypnotic technique: a randomized control trial. British Journal of Medicine. 1986; 293: 1129-1132.

with pillows supporting the knees, head and arms. Work at relaxing the neck and muscles of the shoulder girdle. Concentrate on relaxing and massaging the abdominal, intercostal, pectorals, latissimus dorsi, sternocleidomastoid and scalene muscles. Massage the muscles of posture - these clients tend to develop kyphosis. Vibration can also be employed over the chest to loosen the thick mucus plugs. A disposable sputum mug with disinfectant may have to be provided. Ensure that the mug is disposed off in a leak proof bag. Deep breathing exercises are very beneficial to open up the alveoli. Ask client to take short inspirations and expire slowly through the mouth four or five times. The expiration should be complete but not be forced.

Consider keeping brochures from your local Asthma Research Council on remedial relaxation and mobility exercises for these clients (refer to Appendix D for available resources). The frequency of massage can be varied according to the clients' needs. A relaxation massage scheduled once a week has been found to be beneficial.

Ataxia (Asynergia)

Nervous system

Disturbance in movement.

Cause:

Notes

The primary cause has to be treated. Physical and occupational therapy are of benefit.

Normally, posture and gait are due to integrated activity of the basal ganglia, thalamus, cerebellum and spinal cord. Any condition that disrupts this integration can result in ataxia.

Signs and Symptoms:

Ataxias are characteristic depending on the site of the lesion. In people with hemiparesis where there is weakness of limbs on one side, the affected arm is kept adducted at the shoulder, with flexion at the elbow and wrist. The affected leg is extended at the hip, knee and ankle. Since there is difficulty in flexing the limb, the hip is swung outwards to prevent scraping of the foot on the floor. In people with paraparesis -where the function of both legs are affected, walking is laboured and consists of slow, stiff movements at the hips and knees. In some, the legs may cross with each step, producing the motion of scissors. The characteristic gait in Parkinsonism is described under Parkinson's disease. In cerebellar disease, the person stands with the legs apart and takes steps of different lengths, with the trunk lurching from side to side. It is typically described as a drunken gait.

Ataxias may be present in people who have lost sensations in the lower limbs due to disease of sensory nerves or sensory pathways. Since these individuals are unaware of the position of the lower limbs, they have difficulty in walking and standing. These individuals have a wide base and walk carefully, looking at the ground. The feet make characteristic slapping sounds as the feet are lifted higher than necessary and flung forward and outward. The gait worsens if the person tries to walk in the dark.

Ataxia may be seen in people with cerebral palsy, muscular dystrophy, frontal lobe disease, chorea and hydrocephalus, among others.

Risk Factors:

See Cause and Signs and Symptoms.

Caution and Recommendations to Therapists:

A detailed history and physical assessment should be done to identify muscle groups that are increased/decreased in tone and areas with loss of sensation. Massage Therapists should work in close conjunction with Physiotherapists.

References

Gilman S. Ataxia and disorders of balance and gait. In: Isselbacher KJ et al, editors. Harrison's principles of internal medicine. 13th ed. London: McGraw-Hill Co; 1994. p. 125-130.

Atelectasis (Collapsed lung)

Respiratory system

A lack of expansion of small or larger parts of the lung segments.

Cause:

Blockage of the bronchi/bronchioles by thick mucus secretions or foreign bodies causes lack of airflow into the area beyond the blockage. This leads to slow absorption of the little air remaining in the area, into the blood, and collapse of this segment of lung. The area may eventually expand after healing/removal of the blockage. If there is an inflammatory reaction, it may heal by fibrosis with permanent collapse and damage to the lung.

Notes

Treatment is directed towards alleviating the primary cause.

Signs and Symptoms:

There is difficulty and abnormal awareness of breathing (dyspnea). If only a small area is affected there may be no symptoms. If a very large area is affected while breathing, the ribs and intercostal regions are drawn inwards abnormally. The tips of fingers, toes and tongue may appear blue (cyanosis), along with a rapid heart rate.

Risk Factors:

Any chronic obstructive disease, cystic fibrosis and pulmonary edema can predispose to atelectasis. It is more common in heavy smokers. Any condition that makes deep breathing painful such as fractured ribs, upper abdominal surgery, obesity and prolonged immobility/bed rest can cause atelectasis.

Caution and Recommendations to Therapists:

Increase humidity and warmth of room before massaging these clients as it helps to loosen thick and plugged mucus. There should be proper air circulation and filtration in the clinic. The aim is to reduce the symptoms and help with the drainage of the excess mucus by dislodging them from the walls of the bronchi and to increase the mobility of the thorax. If the client has breathing

References

Porth CM. Alterations in respiratory function. In: Porth CM, editor. Pathophysiology – concepts of altered health states. 4th ed Philadelphia: JB Lippincott Co; 1994. p. 538-539.

difficulties, s/he will feel most comfortable in a half lying position with support beneath the knees, arms and head.

For those with no breathing difficulties, other positions may be used. Since the basal regions of the lungs are most affected, position the client with the head end lower than the rest of the body either by using pillows under the abdomen to raise it or tilting the table with the foot end higher than the head end.

Let the client relax for about ten minutes in this position before massage. Encourage clients to breathe deeply with slow and full expiration throughout the massage. Steam inhalation at this point helps loosen the thick sputum, if present. Do a whole body relaxation massage and use vigorous chest clapping, hacking and vibrations for 10 to 20 minutes. You may have to provide a sputum mug with disinfectant for the client. Use proper precautions while handling and disposing the mug and contents. Massage the tired respiratory muscles and the accessory muscles that are used for respiration. This should include the pectorals, the latissimus dorsi, trapezius, sternocleidomastoid and scalene muscles.

These clients are very prone to respiratory infection. Do not massage if you have any form of respiratory infection. Schedule these clients for a time when they are unlikely to come in contact with others with infection. Encourage client to loose weight if obese, and stop smoking, if a smoker.

Atherosclerosis

Cardiovascular system

Deposition of fibro-fatty substances in the inner lining of medium and large-sized arteries.

Cause:

Notes

Prevention of atherosclerosis, rather than treatment, should be the goal. Atherosclerosis can be prevented and even reversed by reducing the risk factors. Hypertension should be controlled and the public should be educated about weight reduction, exercise, proper diet and smoking.

The most important treatment option is diet control. The individual should be encouraged to reduce the intake of calories, cholesterol and saturated fat and lead a more active lifestyle. In those with a persistent increase in cholesterol levels, drugs are given. The drugs reduce cholesterol levels by decreasing synthesis and increasing excretion. Estrogen therapy in postmenopausal women is also beneficial. For more details see Appendix C: Antihypertensives; Hormone therapy / replacement.

There is hardening and narrowing of large and medium-sized arteries due to accumulation of lipids intracellularly and extracellularly (Greek: *atheros*-paste; *sclerosis*-hardness). There is proliferation of smooth muscle cells and formation of scar tissue in the vessels thus producing narrowing and facilitation of thrombus formation.

Signs and Symptoms:

The patient may have no symptoms and signs, as this disease is slow in onset. There may be a history of thrombosis, angina, myocardial infarction (heart attack), or stroke. Superficial arteries may be hard and thickened. Edema and discoloration of the skin may be seen in regions where blood flow is affected.

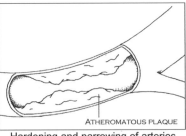

ATHEROMATOUS PLAQUE

Hardening and narrowing of arteries

Pathology A to Z -

Risk Factors:

It is more common in males over 35 and in postmenopausal women. The incidence is higher in African-Americans. Cigarette smoking, oral contraceptives, high srum cholesterol levels (>200mg/100ml) with high levels of low-density lipoproteins (type of proteins which help transport cholesterol in the blood) increase the risk. Patients with hypertension, diabetes, obese individuals, those leading a sedentary lifestyle, those of type A personality, and highly stressed individuals are all predisposed. There is a greater predisposition to atherosclerosis in family members of the patient.

Reduction of blood pressure has been shown to reduce the risk. Similarly, reduction or elimination of smoking decreases the risk. Pipe and cigar smokers are at risk too, though less, as less smoke is inhaled.

Caution and Recommendations to Therapists:

The Therapist should ensure that a detailed history including present medications has been taken. Obtain clearance from the treating Physician if the client has any complications of atherosclerosis.

Since these clients are prone for thrombus formation, deep strokes are likely to dislodge thrombus, if present, from their point of attachment. The thrombus can float as emboli and clog smaller arteries in the lungs, heart or brain leading to pulmonary edema and difficulty in breathing, infarction or stroke. If the client gives a history of previous strokes, chronic hypertension or thrombus, massage should be given only after consulting the Physician. Use gentle strokes in all clients with this condition.

Consider keeping brochures from your local Hypertension Society or Association in your waiting room (see Appendix D). Encourage high-risk clients to get their blood pressure and cholesterol levels checked regularly.

References

Porth CM. Alterations in blood flow. In: Porth CM, editor. Pathophysiology – concepts of altered health states. 4th ed Philadelphia: JB Lippincott Co; 1994. p. 357-362.

Autism

Nervous system

A condition characterized by failure to develop language skills or other forms of social communication.

Cause:

It is due to a primary defect in the brain. The actual cause is not known.

Notes

There is no specific treatment for this condition.

Signs and Symptoms:

The individual is unable to appreciate what is going on in the minds of other people. They are often preoccupied with specific objects. There may be associated mental retardation.

Risk Factors:

It is more common in males.

Caution and Recommendations to Therapists:

It is important to see the client as a person first. Their disability should take second place. Refer to resources for information on Disability etiquette. Additional training may be required for those wishing to work with people with mental disabilities, in order to fully understand the pathophysiology of the disorders and the challenges the client faces. See Appendix D for organizations and support groups.

References

Caviness VS. Neurocutaneous syndromes and other developmental disorders of the central nervous system. In: Isselbacher KJ et al, editors. Harrison's principles of internal medicine. 13th ed. London: McGraw-Hill Co; 1994. p. 2341-2342.

Nervous, Musculoskeletal systems	# Back pain (Low back pain)
	A chronic pain usually in the lower back.

Cause:

There are numerous causes of back pain. Four types of pain have been differentiated - *local, referred, radicular* and that *arising from muscular spasm. Local pain* is caused by anything that presses on or irritates the sensory nerve endings in the area. Fractures or tears of the periosteum, synovial membranes, muscles and ligaments in the region produce this type of pain.

Referred pain may be due to projection of pain from the abdominal and pelvic viscera or from the spine into the regions lying within the area of the lumbar and upper sacral dermatomes. Disease of the posterior aspect of the stomach or duodenum is often referred to the lower thoracic and upper lumbar regions. Disease of the pancreas often produces pain in the back. The pain is located to the right of the spine if the head of the pancreas is affected and to the left if the body or tail is affected. Pain in the lower sacral region below the sacroiliac joint may be due to pull on the uterosacral ligament that supports the uterus. In men, infection and carcinoma of the prostate may produce sacral pain. Problems in the colon often produce pain that is felt in the lower part of the abdomen between the umbilicus and the pubis or in the mid-lumbar region. If very severe, pain may be distributed around the body (belt-like).

Radicular pain is due to pressure on specific nerve roots. *Muscle spasm pain* is usually in relation to local pain and is due to muscles going into a protective spasm.

Some of the common conditions that cause low back pain are congenital defects (eg. spina bifida), fracture, dislocation, sprain of sacrospinalis muscles, disc prolapse, pressure on roots due to conditions producing narrowing of the spinal/intervertebral canal etc., arthritis - osteoarthritis, rheumatoid or ankylosing spondylitis and metastatic cancer, among others.

Unfortunately, in many cases, the cause of the low back pain cannot be identified and the patients are often classified as having 'postural' back pain or with psychiatric illness. Those with the former may find relief by bed rest. Exercise following the period of bed rest is beneficial.

Signs and Symptoms:

Local pain type - Local swelling may be present, but may be absent if the

Notes

A careful history and examination is very important for diagnosing the cause of pain.

When and what conditions cause the pain has to be determined. Prevention is best. Regular exercise to strengthen abdominal and paraspinal muscles are beneficial. Proper conditioning and warm-up before strenuous activity prevents strain on ligaments and spinal joints. Use of bed board or stiff mattress has been found to be useful. Sleeping with the spine hyperextended or sitting in badly designed chairs for long periods should be avoided. Correct posture while sitting and while lifting weight is important.

Most ligamentous and muscular strains are treated by bed rest for a few days to a few weeks. Lumbosacral support following the rest period may be beneficial. Muscle relaxants and painkillers are given. Heat, cold, diathermy or massage have to be complimented with exercises to strengthen the back muscles.

In the case of disk problems, complete bed rest is important and painkillers may be necessary. Traction may be beneficial. Following bedrest, active exercise, muscle relaxants and anti-inflammatory agents have been found to be useful. Surgical management is considered only if all else fail. Here, part of the lamina of the vertebra and the disk involved may be removed.

For more details see Appendix C: Muscle relaxants; Painkillers; Antiinflammatories - non steroidal drugs.

deeper structures are affected. The pain may be constant or intermittent and may be aggravated by specific positions or activity. The pain is sharp or dull and is felt near or in the affected part of the spine. The area is tender to touch and muscles in the region may go into protective spasm producing alterations in posture or deformity.

Referred pain type - Pain due to disease in the upper lumbar region are projected to the anterior aspects of the thigh and legs. Pain due to disease in the lower lumbar or upper sacral region is projected to the gluteal region, posterior aspect of the thighs, calves and occasionally the feet. The pain is usually described as diffuse, deep and aching. But it cannot be precisely localised as that of local type. Pain due to the viscera is felt deep in the abdomen and tends to radiate to the back. Visceral pain is not affected by movement of the spine and does not improve on lying down and is altered by activity of the viscera in question. However, if the pain is due to an aortic aneurysm that has eroded the spine, movement of the spine alters the intensity of pain.

Radicular or *root pain type* - the pain may be described as sharp and shooting, radiating distally. The pain is localised to the areas supplied by the spinal nerve root in question (see table). The pain is aggravated by stretching the spine and while involved in activities that irritate or distort the root. Coughing, sneezing, and straining increase the cerebrospinal fluid pressure and irritate the nerve root. Raising the leg with the knee extended, stretches the spine and aggravates the pain.

Location of pain when specific nerve roots are affected	
Root	*Region*
L1, L5	Inguinal
L2	Lateral aspect of thigh
L2,3	Knee (L3), Anterior thigh
L4	Anterior aspect of leg
L5, S1	Lateral and posterior aspects of calf
	Dorsum of foot (L5), Heel, lateral aspect of foot (S1)

Irritation of the fourth, fifth lumbar and first sacral nerve produces pain that radiates down the back of the thigh and posterior and lateral aspect of the legs and is termed *sciatica*. This pain typically stops at the ankle and may be associated with tingling and numbness in the region. Pain described as feeling of burning/cold, jabbing are usually due to nerve problems.

Muscle spasm type - the muscles are tense. Posture may be abnormal as a result of the spasm. The pain may be described as cramping or as a dull ache.

Risk Factors:

See Cause.

Caution and Recommendations to Therapists:

The Therapist should determine the cause of back pain in the client. If the pain is due to muscle spasm or bad posture or weak abdominal muscles, massage

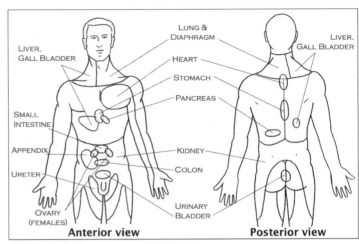

Anterior view   **Posterior view**

Locations of referred pain

may be beneficial. If it is due to nerve impingement with associated symptoms of tingling, numbness, muscle weakness or shooting, radiating pain, then the client has to be referred to a Physician, or the Physician should be consulted. Some of the 'red flags' that suggest serious spinal pathology in people with acute backache are: age of onset <20 or >55 years; pain not mechanical in nature; thoracic spine pain; past history of carcinoma; steroids; HIV infection; generally unwell with weight loss, night sweats; progressive neurological deficits; structural deformity; constant and/or progressive pain; inflammation; severe night pain and recent severe trauma. In these cases, it may be wiser to refer the client to a Physician and /or discuss with a Physician.

Exercise has been found to be beneficial in the management of any chronic pain. It has been shown to improve flexibility, mobility and decrease pain by inhibiting the transmission of pain impulses to the central nervous system. It enhances the sense of well being, controls weight and improves sleep. Many other physiological benefits have been identified. It is important for the Therapist to not only encourage clients with chronic pain to exercise, but also keep themselves fit by regular exercise. See Appendix D for organizations and support groups.

References

Brooker CK, Cooper RG. Management of the chronic pain client in primary and tertiary care. Reports on Rheumatic Diseases. Chesterfield: The Arthritis Research Campaign; 1998 September. Series 3, Practical Problems, No. 16.

Wright SM. The use of Therapeutic Touch in the management of pain. Nursing Clinics of North America 1987; 13(5): 635-648.

Taws S. Alleviating low back pain through soft tissue release. Massage 1994; 52 (Nov/Dec): 30-36.

Musculoskeletal system	# Baker's cyst (Popliteal cyst)
	A fluid-filled swelling behind the knee.

Cause:

Notes

No treatment is necessary. If the cyst interferes with the movement of the knee, the cyst may be excised.

The Baker's cyst or popliteal cyst is a swelling that develops in relation to the semimembranous bursa. It is filled with synovial fluid and often communicates with the knee joint through a hollow stalk.

Signs and Symptoms:

It seldom causes any symptoms. In children it may regress spontaneously. In adults who develop the cyst when there is excessive fluid in the knee joint, as in rheumatoid arthritis or other joint disease, the cyst may extend up to the calf.

Risk Factors:

It is more common in children and in people who have chronic knee joint disease.

Caution and Recommendations to Therapists:

Avoid massage over the cyst. If the cyst is too large it may press on the surrounding tissue including the small saphenous vein and result in edema and stagnation of blood distal to the cyst. If the part of the limb distal to the cyst is cold (as compared to the other limb) with indications of reduced circulation, avoid massaging the limb. Advice client to see a doctor to rule out complications of poor venous drainage such as venous thrombosis.

Many nerves and blood vessels lie superficially in the popliteal fossa – the location of the cyst. The branches of the sciatic nerve – the common peroneal and tibial, the popliteal vein and artery are some of the important structures traversing the fossa. Hence, deep pressure should be avoided in this location at all times – even in clients without Baker's cyst.

References

Werner R, Benjamin BE. A Massage Therapist's guide to pathology. Philadelphia: Williams & Wilkins; 1998. p. 92–95.

Benjamin B. Understanding Baker's cyst. Massage Therapy Journal. 1997; 32(3): 20.

Bell's Palsy (Facial palsy)

Nervous system

Disease of the VIIth cranial nerve - facial nerve that results in paralysis of one side of the face.

Cause:

The cause of Bell's palsy is unknown. It is commonly caused by inflammation around the nerve as it travels from the brain to the exterior. The facial nerve carries taste fibers from the anterior two-third of the tongue and motor nerves that control the facial muscles. A branch of the facial nerve supplies the stapedius muscle of the middle ear.

A picture similar to Bell's palsy (facial palsy) can be caused by pressure on the nerve by tumors, injury to the nerve, infection of the meninges or the inner ear or dental surgery. Diabetes, pregnancy and hypertension are other conditions where facial palsy may occur.

Signs and Symptoms:

The disorder comes on suddenly. The flaccid paralysis of the facial muscles result in drooping of the mouth on the affected side and difficulty in puckering the lips (due to paralysis of the orbicularis oris). The person has difficulty closing the eyes tightly (orbicularis oculi affected) and creasing the forehead (paralysis of occipitofrontalis). Paralysis of the buccinator prevents the patient

Notes

Eighty to ninety percent of individuals recover spontaneously and completely in 1-8 weeks. Corticosteroids are used to reduce the inflammation of the nerve. Electrotherapy may be used to reduce the speed of atrophy of the facial muscles.

Supportive measures include protection of the eye during sleep, massage of weakened muscles and splint to prevent drooping of the lower part of the face. For more details see Appendix C: antiinflammatories - steroidal drugs; Electrotherapy.

from puffing the cheeks and is the cause of food getting caught between the teeth and cheeks. Saliva may dribble from the corner of the mouth. There is also excessive tearing from the affected eye. Due to the incomplete closure of the eye these individuals are prone to conjunctivitis. Pain may be present near the angle of the jaw and behind the ear.

If the nerve has been affected proximal to the branch carrying taste sensations (eg. in the middle ear) from the anterior two third of the tongue, taste is diminished or lost. If the branch to the stapedius muscle is affected, the person is painfully hypersensitive to loud sounds (hyperacusis).

Risk Factors:

Exposure to cold and chills have been found to trigger Bell's palsy.

Caution and Recommendations to Therapists:

Massage should be done on the shoulders, neck, as well as the unaffected side. In the acute stage, the goal should be to relax the muscles of the normal side thereby relaxing the muscle on the opposite, affected side. Stabilise the client's head. Use light strokes from the middle of face to the sides. Some suggest that in the forehead, strokes should be directed from the middle of the forehead to the temporal area; from the upper edge of the eyebrows to the hairline; in the middle of the face strokes should be directed downwards from the nose and cheeks to the angle of the mandible; upwards from the side of the nose and mouth towards the earlobe and spiral strokes in the region of the temple.

In the subacute stage, in addition to the strokes described above, deeper, shorter strokes may be used in the direction of the muscle fibres of the facial muscles. It may be beneficial to seat the client in front of a mirror and work on both sides of the face while standing behind the client. To increase the tone on the affected side use kneading strokes with the fingertip. Light tapotement and vibration help stimulate the paralyzed muscles. Passive movement is very

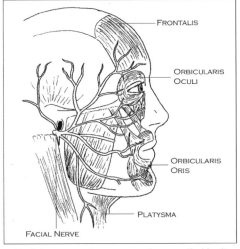

Facial nerve and some muscles supplied by it

beneficial. Since the facial muscles of both sides act in synergy, the movement on the normal side of the face can be mirrored passively using the fingers. This may speed up recovery.

References

Turchaninov R, Cox CA. Medical Massage. Scottsdale: Stress Less publishing Inc; 1998. p. 214-226.

In chronic stages, active exercises may also be used. To exercise the orbicularis oculi ask client to alternately close and open eyes with and without mild resistance to the eyelids. For the buccinator the cheeks should be puffed out and in. Ask client to try and whistle. For the orbicularis oris the mouth should be puckered. Ask client to smile as widely as possible. Saying words that use the letters P, B, M, N also exercise the labials. To exercise the frontalis ask client to raise and lower eyebrows. The strength of the muscles can be increased if some resistance is applied to the movement of each of the facial muscles. Knowledge of the action and direction of fibres of the facial muscles is required to effectively do so. The client can be taught to massage, passively/ actively move the muscles and apply resistance.

Application of moist heat to the affected side may help reduce the pain, if present. Spend about 15 minutes massaging the face. Teach client to massage the face regularly. To maintain the tone, massage can be done two to three times a day. See Appendix D for organizations and support groups.

Bends (Decompression sickness; Caisson disease)

A condition that results from sudden, rapid ascent to the surface of the water after very deep dives or rapid ascent in an unpressurized cabin of an airplane.

Musculoskeletal, Respiratory systems

Cause:

Divers have to breathe air or other gases at increased pressure to equalize the pressure on the body during dives. Since 100% oxygen causes symptoms of oxygen toxicity (lung damage, convulsions etc), the concentration of oxygen is kept to below 20% by mixing nitrogen or other gases. If a diver breathing 80% nitrogen ascends, the pressure of nitrogen in the alveoli drops. The nitrogen dissolved in the tissues diffuses to the lungs. No symptoms are seen if the ascent is gradual. If the ascent it rapid, the nitrogen forms bubbles in the tissue fluid and blood causing the symptoms.

Signs and Symptoms:

The bubbles in the tissue cause severe pain around joints. Bubbles in the nervous system can result in loss of sensation and weakness. Sometimes the bubbles in the blood can obstruct the arteries to the brain or other organs resulting in paralysis, respiratory failure or myocardial infarction. Bubbles in the pulmonary arteries cause difficulty in breathing -'*the chokes*'.

Risk Factors:

See Cause.

Caution and Recommendations to Therapists:

Education of divers and prompt treatment has played a significant role in reducing the incidence of bends. A Therapist may meet (very unlikely) a client who has residual neurological deficits due to bends. As in any neurological disorder, the sensory and motor function has to be assessed carefully and treatment individualized.

Notes

It can be prevented by ascending slowly from deep dives or by using compression chambers to slowly reduce pressure. The person should be promptly recompressed in a pressure chamber. This should be followed by slow decompression. If the nervous system is irreversibly damaged, some neurological deficits may be present.

References

Ganong WF. Review of medical physiology. 15th ed. California: Appleton & Lange; 1991. p 644-645.

Botulism

An infection that produces paralysis of nerves.

Cause:

The disease is caused by the toxins liberated by the microorganism *Clostridium botulinum*. The organism is found in soil all over the world. The toxin may enter the body through ingestion of food previously contaminated with the organism. In some, it is due to the contamination of wounds by the organism. In infants, it may be due to the ingestion of spores followed by liberation of toxin in the intestines of the infant.

The toxin enters the blood and is transported to peripheral nerves that liberate acetylcholine as the neurotransmitter. Here, it irreversibly blocks the release of acetylcholine. The incubation period for food-borne botulism is 18 to 36 hours. If it follows wound infection, the incubation period is longer.

The toxin can be inactivated by heat at 100°C for 10 minutes. The spores require a higher temperature - 120°C for inactivation.

Signs and Symptoms:

Following ingestion of contaminated food, the person presents with paralysis, usually beginning with one of the cranial nerves and descending to other nerves. It may result in respiratory muscle paralysis and death.

When the cranial nerves are involved the person may have difficulty talking and swallowing and have double vision. Soon it is followed by weakness of muscles of the neck, arms, thorax and legs. It may be associated with nausea, vomiting and abdominal pain, due to the involvement of the parasympathetic nerves. Dryness of mouth, dizziness and blurred vision are other common symptoms. There is no fever. The person is generally alert and oriented.

Risk Factors:

Eating food contaminated by spores or eating contaminated food that is not heated to a temperature that destroys toxins puts a person at risk. Improper canning or handling of food predisposes to the disease.

Caution and Recommendations to Therapists:

References

Morello JA, Mizer HE, Wilson ME, Granato PA. Microbiology in patient care. 6th ed. New York: McGraw-Hill; 1998. p. 346-348.

The general hygiene has to be maintained in the clinic. Prompt cleaning of wounds, proper storage and handling of food and eating cooked and uncontaminated food can prevent botulism. See Appendix D for organizations and support groups. Also see Appendix B: Strategies for infection prevention and safe practice.

Bronchiectasis

An abnormal dilation and destruction of the walls of the bronchi.

Cause:

It is caused by any condition that repeatedly damages the bronchial walls and supporting tissues and reduces the action of the cilia that help clear the mucus. There is a collection of mucus in the dilated bronchi. An inflammatory reaction results with further weakening of the walls. The ciliated epithelium is replaced by squamous epithelium hindering the clearance of mucus further. The dilatation may be confined to one or more lobes of the lungs.

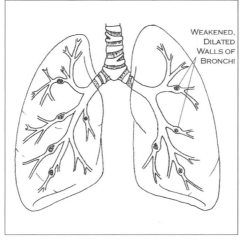

WEAKENED, DILATED WALLS OF BRONCHI

Notes

The treatment of bronchiectasis should target four areas - treatment of underlying problem, if any; improving the clearance of secretions; control of infection and reversal of airflow obstruction.

Chest physiotherapy plays an important role in clearing secretions. Vibration, percussion and postural drainage are of great help. Increasing humidity and warmth of air breathed may facilitate dislodgment of the thick secretions. Bronchiectasis is treated with antibiotics if an infection is suspected. Use of bronchodilators is another element of treatment. Sometimes surgery may be required to remove a severely affected lobe.

For more details see Appendix C: antimicrobial - antibacterial agents; Bronchodilators; Antiasthmatics.

Signs and Symptoms:

It is usually asymptomatic at the start. Frequent episodes of pneumonia or blood-tinged sputum follow. Classically, there is a persistent cough with large amounts of foul-smelling, yellow-colored sputum. Noisy breathing, difficulty in breathing, loss of weight, anemia, recurrent fever with chills are other symptoms.

Risk Factors:

It is more common in chronic smokers. Men are more often affected. Lung tumors, foreign body obstruction, recurrent respiratory infections, tuberculosis, fungal infections of lungs, cystic fibrosis, congenital malformation of bronchi and inhalation of corrosive gases are other predisposing factors.

Caution and Recommendations to Therapists:

The aim is to reduce the symptoms and help with the drainage of the excess mucus by dislodging them from the walls of the bronchi and to increase the mobility of the thorax. The client has to be positioned according to the lobe that is affected, for maximum benefit. The bronchi of the lobe affected should be facing downwards and towards the main bronchi so that gravity could also be used to drain secretions.

For lower lobe drainage (most common), position client with head end lower than foot end (see Bronchitis) with the help of pillows. For draining the middle lobe the client should lie flat on the back with pillows arranged to turn the body

References

Klimowitch P. Massage for sufferers of respiratory disease. Massage Therapy Journal. 1993; 32 (2): 42-43.

Davis AL, Salzman SH. Bronchiectasis. In: Cherniack NS, editor. Chronic Obstructive Pulmonary Disease. Philadelphia: WB Saunders; 1991. p. 316-338.

to left or right at an angle of 45 degrees away from the affected side. For upper lobe drainage, a seated position should be used.

Steam inhalation before treatment is beneficial. Alternately, increase the humidity and warmth of the room while treating such clients. Use hacking, clapping and vibration movements over chest for 20-30 minutes. Do a whole body relaxation massage. Massage the tired respiratory muscles and the accessory muscles that are used for respiration. This should include the pectorals, the latissimus dorsi, trapezius, sternocleidomastoid and scalene muscles. Encourage clients to breathe deeply with slow and full expiration. You may have to provide a sputum mug with disinfectant for the client. Use proper precautions while handling and disposing the mug and contents. See Appendix D for organizations and support groups.

Bronchitis

Respiratory system

An acute or chronic inflammation of the bronchi and trachea. It is one of the Chronic Obstructive Pulmonary Diseases (COPD).

Cause:

Notes

Chronic Bronchitis is considered as one of the Chronic Obstructive Pulmonary Diseases (COPD) along with Emphysema. Prevention of risk factors is the best form of treatment of COPD.

Treatment of chronic bronchitis varies according to the severity of the problem. Progress of the disease can be retarded by cessation of smoking. Antibiotics should be given promptly if infection is suspected. Exercise has been shown to increase work capacity and sense of well being. Exercise using muscles other than that of arms (many of which are accessory muscles for breathing) have been shown to be beneficial.

Bronchodilator drugs may be given to clients who respond to them. In those with severe and persistent problems continuous oxygen is supplemented. Lung transplantation may be considered in those who do not benefit from all other measures. Resection of carotid bodies (the structures that sense carbon dioxide and oxygen levels in the blood), negative pressure ventilation are some controversial measures advocated.

Many of the situations cited under risk factors result in impairment of ciliary action of the respiratory epithelium and reduced macrophage function in the airways. As a result the immunity is lowered locally. Also, the mucus is not cleared from the airways causing narrowing and plugging of the bronchioles. The mucus also serves as a nidus for bacteria to multiply making the individual more prone for infection. All of the above cause excess mucus production, inflammation and destruction of the alveolar septa. Healing around the bronchi occurs by fibrosis producing narrowing. This sequence of events is responsible for the chronic symptoms in those with bronchitis.

A person is diagnosed as having chronic bronchitis if there is excessive mucus production sufficient to cause cough with sputum for at least 3 months of the year for more than two consecutive years.

Signs and Symptoms:

Typically there is a history of smoking. The person has cough with sputum and has a reduced capacity to exercise or do strenuous work. Soon the symptoms progress to difficulty in breathing even on minimal exertion. Sounds may be heard over the chest as the air flows through the narrowed bronchi. There is recurrent respiratory infection and if left untreated, the disease progresses to respiratory failure and death.

Individuals with chronic bronchitis are referred to as "blue bloaters" as they are often cyanotic (due to reduced oxygen in blood) and overweight.

Risk Factors:

It is more common in individuals over 40. Men are more frequently affected with this condition. Bronchitis tends to recur in winter. Smoking, respiratory allergies and recurrent respiratory infections are commonly associated with bronchitis. This disorder can occur as a complication of tonsillitis, sinusitis or pharyngitis. Cold, moist environment, constant exposure to dust, smoke or fumes also predisposes to the condition. Chronic bronchitis is more common in children of parents who smoke. Increased incidence has been documented where air pollution is seen due to natural gas being used for cooking indoors.

Caution and Recommendations to Therapists:

The aim is to reduce the symptoms and help with the drainage of the excess mucus by dislodging them from the walls of the bronchi and to help with the mobility of the thorax. Proper air circulation and filtration in the clinic helps these clients. Higher humidity and warmth also helps with the drainage of mucus. Since the basal regions of the lungs are most affected, position the client with the head end lower than the rest of the body either by using pillows under the abdomen to raise it or tilting the table with the foot end higher than the head end. Let the client relax for about ten minutes in this position before massage. Steam inhalation at this point helps loosen the thick sputum.

Do a whole body relaxation massage and use vigorous chest clapping, hacking and vibrations for 10 to 20 minutes. You may have to provide a sputum mug with disinfectant for the client. (Use proper precautions while handling and disposing the mug and contents). Massage the tired respiratory muscles and the accessory muscles that are used for respiration. This should include the pectorals, the latissimus dorsi, trapezius, sternocleidomastoid and scalene muscles. Encourage clients to breathe deeply with slow and full expiration throughout the massage treatment.

These clients are very prone to respiratory infection so massage should be avoided if the Therapist has even a mild form of respiratory infection. Schedule these clients for a time when they are unlikely to come in contact with others with infection. Encourage client to stop smoking if smokers. See Appendix D for organizations and support groups.

References

Klimowitch P. Massage for sufferers of respiratory disease. Massage Therapy Journal. 1993; 32 (2): 42-43.

Josephson. GD et al. Airway obstruction. New modalities in treatment. Med Clin North Am 1993; 77: 539.

Reid LM. Chronic obstructive pulmonary diseases. In: Fishman AP, editor. Pulmonary diseases and disorders. 2nd ed. New York: McGraw-Hill Book Co; 1988. p. 1247-1272.

Brucellosis

A bacterial infection that produces nonspecific symptoms.

Musculoskeletal, Respiratory, Cardiovascular systems

Cause:

It is a bacterial infection caused by the genus *brucella* that is transmitted to humans from an infected animal or from ingestion of infected milk, milk products or tissues. Sometimes, the infection is spread by contact with the organism by injured skin, through the conjunctiva or by inhalation. Animals get the infection sexually or by ingesting contaminated milk or infected tissue.

After entering the body, the organism is ingested by white blood cells. The organism multiplies within the cells and destroys them. The infection spreads

Notes

It is treated with antibiotics for 3-6 weeks.

Brucellosis can be prevented by eradicating the disease in animals. Vaccines are available for animals (not humans). Use of pasteurized milk and milk products can be a form of prevention. Those who are at risk should take precautions to prevent entry via injured skin, inhalation or through the conjunctiva by covering injured skin, wearing

protective clothing, gloves and goggles.
For more details see Appendix C:
Antimicrobial - antibacterial agents;
Immunization.

to the lymph nodes via the lymphatic vessels and may enter the bloodstream. Organs such as the liver, spleen and bone marrow get infected. The incubation period is from 7-21days.

Signs and Symptoms:

Low-grade fever, weakness, fatigue, headache, backache, muscle pain, loss of appetite and weight are some of the symptoms. Very few physical findings are seen. If the infection is localised, there may be enlargement of the spleen, liver and lymph nodes. The lungs, bone and heart are other organs that may be affected.

Brucellosis is difficult to diagnose as the signs and symptoms mimic many other diseases.

Risk Factors:

It is more common in those working with animals such as butchers, farmers and veterinarians.

Caution and Recommendations to Therapists:

Infectious diseases can be prevented in many ways and Massage Therapists can play an important role in preventing spread of diseases in the clinic by using simple strategies. (Refer to Appendix B: Strategies for infection prevention and safe practice). Also see Appendix D for organizations and support groups.

References

Morello JA, Mizer HE, Wilson ME, Granato PA. Microbiology in patient care. 6th ed. New York: McGraw-Hill; 1998. p. 353-359.

Buerger's disease (Thromboangiitis obliterans)

Cardiovascular system

An inflammatory disorder of the small and medium-sized arteries of the arms and legs that can result in thrombus formation.

Cause:

The cause is not known. The linkage of this disease to smoking indicates that it may be due to hypersensitivity to nicotine.

Notes

It is diagnosed using Doppler techniques to measure blood flow in the limbs. There is no specific treatment except for stopping to smoke. As part of the treatment, the sympathetic system may be blocked in order to increase blood flow. Surgery may be done to destroy the sympathetics in the lumbar region (lumbar sympathectomy). In severe cases with gangrene, amputation may be required. Rarely, arterial bypass of the larger vessels may be done. For more details see Appendix C: Doppler techniques; Surgical sympathectomy; Amputation; Arterial bypass.

Signs and Symptoms:

The patient may present with pain and weakness of the calf muscles and/or the foot on using it. The pain is relieved by rest. However in those with prolonged disease, pain may be present even at rest. The skin may be pale or blue in color. It may be thin and shiny, with loss of hair due to poor nutrition. The nails may be thick and malformed. In severe cases, ulcers or gangrenous areas may develop. The arterial pulsation may be reduced or not felt in the limbs.

Risk Factors:

It affects men between the ages of 25 and 40 who are heavy cigarette smokers. Attacks may be precipitated on exposure to extreme temperatures, emotional stress and trauma.

Caution and Recommendations to Therapists:

Massage is beneficial as it helps reduce stress, improve peripheral circulation and reduces sympathetic stimulation. Since the condition predisposes to thrombus formation, the Therapist should ensure that there is no scope of them dislodging already formed thrombi. It may be wise to get clearance from a Physician. If cleared, keep leg slightly elevated during the treatment. Use gentle effleurage and kneading. The effleurage may be painful due to the dragging of the skin. If it is painful, use only kneading strokes making sure that you keep the hand stationary on the skin and lifting it off the client when moving from one area to the next. More than normal pressure may injure the poorly nourished, thin skin. Avoid areas of ulcer and gangrene.

Do not apply heat or cold to the limbs as the local vasodilatation - without increase in blood flow to the whole limb, can damage the tissues. Heat to the lumbar or abdominal region may help improve the overall blood supply to the limbs by the inhibitory effect of the warm blood from the lumbar region on the vasomotor center in the brainstem.

Encourage client to stop smoking. Keep brochures giving details on the health hazards of smoking in the waiting room. Keep telephone numbers of local 'quit smoking' associations handy. See Appendix D for organizations and support groups.

References

Wheeler BH. Thromboangiitis obliterans (Buerger's disease). In: Sabiston DC, editor. Textbook of Surgery - the biological basis of modern surgical practice. 14ᵗʰ ed. Philadelphia: WB Saunders Co; 1991. p. 1637-1640.

Bunion

Musculoskeletal system

Formation and inflammation of an adventitious bursa over the first metatarsal bone due to excessive friction and pressure.

Cause:

It is caused by chronic, repetitive pressure over the medial part of the head of the first metatarsal bone.

Signs and Symptoms:

Due to repeated friction, the bursa that is formed becomes inflamed. The walls thicken and more fluid fills the bursa. The inflamed bursa may become infected. When inflamed the site is painful, red and edematous.

Risk Factors:

It is common in ballet dancers (from demi pointe and rolling in). It is also common in people who wear improper shoe size and in dancers and catchers who wear shoes with improper flexibility. People with deformity of the first toe (hallux valgus) - where the toe is angulated laterally, are more prone.

Caution and Recommendations to Therapists:

Encourage the client to identify the irritant that produced/aggravates the problem and remove it. Do not massage the local area if the bunion is inflamed. Massage

Notes

The inflammation subsides if the friction over the site is avoided. If the bursa is very large, surgery may be required to excise the bursa. Antiinflammatory drugs and local injection of steroids are other forms of treatment. For more details see Appendix C: Antiinflammatories - steroidal drugs; Antiinflammatories - non steroidal drugs.

References

Mercier LR, editor. Practical orthopedics. 4ᵗʰ ed. New York: Mosby-Year book Inc; 1995. p. 251.

the surrounding muscles that may go into spasm because of the pain. Elevation and support of the affected leg during the massage may be beneficial.

Integumentary system	# Burns
	Injury to the skin by heat.

Notes

Depending on the severity, the wound is closed with autografts and skin substitutes within the first week of a burn. It is important to remove dead tissue to facilitate drainage of secretions and prevent superinfection. Topical and systemic antibiotics are necessary.

The nutrition and electrolyte balance of the individual have to be monitored. For more details see Appendix C: Antimicrobial - antibacterial agents.

Cause:

Dry heat, hot liquids or steam, electricity and contact with acids or chemicals can cause Burns.

Signs and Symptoms:

The signs and symptoms depend on whether the burn has affected partial or full skin thickness. Burns are classified into three types according to the severity: *first degree* when only reddening of the skin is seen; *second degree* - where there is blistering of the skin and destruction of the top of the epidermis; *third degree* - where both dermis and epidermis of the skin is destroyed. In the latter, regeneration of the skin is not possible and skin graft may be required. If the burn is extensive and severe it results in loss of plasma fluids and shock. The first and second-degree burns are more painful as the pain receptors are intact.

Risk Factors:

Occupations that expose individuals to any form of heat.

Caution and Recommendations to Therapists:

Massage should be given only when the tissue is fully healed and can withstand pressure. Unhealed skin looks pink, thin and delicate. Avoid massaging over these areas as it may blister on applying even the least pressure. In burns of the hand, support should be given to the hand while massaging and the joints of the fingers and wrist should be moved very gently. No movements should be forced. Uncontaminated cream or oil should be used for massage. Use frictions or finger kneading over the healed and scarred tissue. Give light and stimulating massage to the rest of the limb above the site of injury without dragging the injured area.

References

Wittlinger H, Wittlinger G. Introduction to Dr. Vodder's manual lymphatic drainage. Vols I & II. Heidelberg: Karl F Haug Verlag GMH & Co; 1982.

Pruit BA, Goodwin CW, Pruitt SK. Burns including cold, chemical, and electric injuries. In: Sabiston DC, editor. Textbook of Surgery - the biological basis of modern surgical practice. 14th ed. London: WB Saunders Co; 1991. p. 178-209.

Boswick JA. The art and science of burn care. Rockville: Aspen publishers; 1987.

In clients with old healed burns, massage can be deep, with transverse friction over healed scars. Do not use violent stretching techniques over joints. Ensure that the sensations are intact as nerve damage may have occurred. If there is loss of sensation, it is important to remember that client feedback will be inadequate and you may do damage to the tissue inadvertently. Olive oil has been found to be effective in treating clients with burns. In treating clients with healed skin graft, the principle should be to soften and loosen the graft and improve the circulation. Massage over the graft only after complete healing has occurred.

Manual lymph drainage, a technique that requires training may be beneficial in facilitating lymph flow. See Appendix D for organizations and support groups.

Bursitis

An inflammation of a bursa.

Cause:

A bursa is a fluid-filled sac that is lined with synovial membrane. It is present in the connective tissue surrounding a joint. It functions to reduce the friction that is seen between bone and muscle, muscle and muscle, tendon and bone and bone and skin. Trauma, gout or infection from adjacent structures may cause bursitis.

Signs and Symptoms:

Bursitis can be acute, subacute or chronic. The patient complains of pain and stiffness of the joint adjacent to the bursa. In superficial bursitis, redness and swelling of the bursa is present. Fluid can be felt in the bursa. In inflammation of bursa located in deeper areas, no redness or swelling may be seen. The muscles crossing the bursa may go into spasm due to the pain.

The pain is increased if a particular movement exerts more pressure on the bursa. However, there is no pain in the joint.

Risk Factors:

Repeated stress and trauma over the bursa are risk factors. Bursitis can be produced secondary to a fracture, dislocation or tendinitis. Rarely, it may be seen in gout, rheumatoid or infective arthritis. It can occur in occupations that involve repetitive movements as in assembly line workers.

Caution and Recommendations to Therapists:

Treatment should be aimed at identifying and eliminating the primary cause. The aim should be to reduce the pain, inflammation and decrease the muscle spasm. Cold packs applied lightly over the area help reduce the pain. Direct compression of the bursa and on-site massage should be avoided in acute stages. However, the rest of the body can be massaged. When the inflammation has subsided, massage may be given to the surrounding muscles with friction directly over the joint. Ice packs should be used after friction techniques. Passive movement of joint close to the bursa can be done within the pain-free range. In the acute stage treatments lasting for half an hour, two times a week is recommended. The frequency may then be reduced to once a week until the inflammation has fully subsided and the full range of motion has been obtained.

Notes

Bursitis can be a recurring problem if the primary cause is not addressed. It is treated by rest to the involved part, use of nonsteroidal anti-inflammatory drugs and sometimes injection of steroids into the local area. For more details see Appendix C: Antiinflammatories - steroidal drugs; Antiinflammatories - non sterodial drugs.

References

Adams JC. Hamblen DL. Outline of orthopaedics. 11th ed. London: Churchill Livingstone; 1990. p. 98.

Bursitis - Achilles

An inflammation of the bursa located above the insertion of the common tendon of the gastrocnemius and soleus muscles to the calcaneus.

Notes

See Bursitis.

Cause:

Injury or irritation to the bursa by overuse of the Achilles tendon. Wearing tight shoes may also cause inflammation of this bursa.

Signs and Symptoms:

The pain is localized to the posterior aspect of the ankle and is worsened on plantar or dorsiflexion. Both movements put pressure on the bursa.

Risk Factors:

Occupations involving repeated, plantar flexion predispose to this condition.

References

Adams JC. Hamblen DL. Outline of orthopaedics. 11th ed. London: Churchill Livingstone; 1990. p. 98.

Caution and Recommendations to Therapists:

See Bursitis.

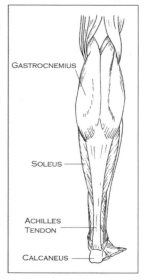

Bursitis - anserine

An inflammation of the sartorius bursa located over the medial side of the tibia just below the knee.

Notes

See Bursitis.

Cause:

Injury or irritation to the bursa by repetitive use of the sartorius muscle.

Signs and Symptoms:

The pain is experienced on climbing stairs. There is tenderness over the insertion of the conjoint tendon of the sartorius, gracilis and semitendinosus muscles.

Risk Factors:

Occupations involving repeated extension and flexion of the hip predispose to this condition.

References

Adams JC. Hamblen DL. Outline of orthopaedics. 11th ed. London: Churchill Livingstone; 1990. p. 98.

Caution and Recommendations to Therapists:

See Bursitis.

58

Bursitis - iliopectineal

An inflammation of the iliopectineal bursa.

Cause:

Injury or irritation to the bursa by repetitive flexion and extension of the hip.

Signs and Symptoms:

The pain is localized to the groin region and is worsened on passively or actively moving the hip. Movements put pressure on the bursa. The pain may radiate to the L2, L3 segments ie. to the front of thigh and knee joint and lower lumbar region.

Risk Factors:

Occupations involving repeated movement of the hip predispose to this condition.

Caution and Recommendations to Therapists:

Use heat/cold packs to reduce pain. Later use friction massage in the inguinal area. Massage deeply, the thigh muscles and the gluteal region to reduce muscle spasm. Gentle massage over the lower back, thigh and knee ie. L2, L3 segment relieves pain, by reducing transmission of pain impulses to the brain. (Also see Bursitis).

Notes

See Bursitis.

References

Adams JC. Hamblen DL. Outline of orthopaedics. 11th ed. London: Churchill Livingstone; 1990. p. 98.

Bursitis - ischial (Weaver's bottom)

An inflammation of the bursa separating the gluteus medius from the ischial tuberosity.

Cause:

Injury or irritation to the bursa by prolonged sitting on a hard surface.

Signs and Symptoms:

The pain is localized to the groin region and is worsened on passively extending the hip or by active flexion. Both movements put pressure on the bursa. The

Notes

See Bursitis.

pain may radiate to the L2, L3 segments ie. to the front of thigh and knee joint and lower lumbar region.

Risk Factors:

Occupations involving repeated, full extension or flexion of the knee predispose to this condition.

Caution and Recommendations to Therapists:

See Bursitis.

References

Adams JC. Hamblen DL. Outline of orthopaedics. 11th ed. London: Churchill Livingstone; 1990. p. 98.

Musculoskeletal system	# Bursitis - olecranon (Student's elbow)
	An inflammation of the olecranon bursa

Notes

See Bursitis.

Cause:

Injury or irritation to the bursa by repetitive flexion and extension of the elbow.

Signs and Symptoms:

The pain is localized to the posterior aspect of the elbow region and is worsened on extension or active flexion of the elbow. Both movements put pressure on the bursa.

Risk Factors:

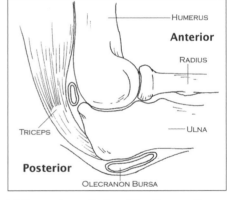

Occupations involving repeated, full extension or flexion of the elbow predispose to this condition. If it is acutely inflamed, infection has to be ruled out.

Caution and Recommendations to Therapists:

See Bursitis.

References

Adams JC. Hamblen DL. Outline of orthopaedics. 11th ed. London: Churchill Livingstone; 1990. p. 98.

Musculoskeletal system	# Bursitis - prepatellar (Housemaid's knee)
	Inflammation of the bursa over the patella.

Notes

See Bursitis.

Cause:

It is caused by trauma to or fall on the knee, or kneeling over prolonged periods of time.

Signs and Symptoms:

There is pain over the knee due to inflammation of the bursa between the patella and the skin or the bursa between the ligamentum patellae and the proximal part of the tibia. A localized, rounded swelling is seen over the patella (if prepatellar) or on either side of the ligamentum patellae. The knee joint may be stiff but there is no pain in the joint.

Risk Factors:

Recurrent stress over the knee predisposes to this condition.

Caution and Recommendations to Therapists:

Knee joint - Lateral view:
location of Bursae

Massage is indicated after the acute inflammation has subsided. All muscles of the thigh should be massaged. Friction strokes should used around the knee joint and the patella. Passive lateral movement of the patella helps to mobilize this joint (also see Bursitis).

References

Adams JC. Hamblen DL. Outline of orthopaedics. 11th ed. London: Churchill Livingstone; 1990. p. 98.

Bursitis - retrocalcaneal

An inflammation of the bursa located between the calcaneus and posterior surface of the Achilles tendon.

Musculoskeletal system

Cause:

It usually occurs after trauma to the region or in association with rheumatoid arthritis, gout and spondylitis.

Notes

See Bursitis.

Signs and Symptoms:

The pain is localized to the back of the heel. Swelling is seen on the medial and lateral side of the Achilles tendon.

Risk Factors:

See Cause.

Caution and Recommendations to Therapists:

See Bursitis.

References

Adams JC. Hamblen DL. Outline of orthopaedics. 11th ed. London: Churchill Livingstone; 1990. p. 98.

Bursitis - subdeltoid (Subacromial bursitis)

An inflammation of the subdeltoid bursa.

Cause:

It is usually caused by trauma to the shoulder by a fall or blow, or injury to the shoulder muscles. Infection can also cause this.

Signs and Symptoms:

There is localized pain in the shoulder. The pain is intense, dull or throbbing and increases when the arm is abducted. During abduction the acromion process presses on this bursa which is located between the deltoid muscle and the capsule of

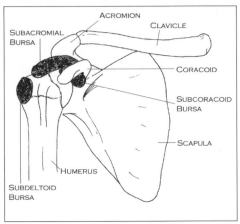

Shoulder joint - anterior view
showing location of bursae

the shoulder joint. There may be some warmth and swelling over the region. The movement of the shoulder is restricted because of the pain.

Risk Factors:

Stress and trauma to shoulder are predisposing factors.

Caution and Recommendations to Therapists:

In the acute stages apply cold pack over the affected area. Massage is contraindicated over the bursa. After a few days, massage can be given with the client in a seated position with the arm adducted and supported by a table or pillow. Start with effleurage and kneading strokes for the upper part of the chest and back. Then use light effleurage for shoulder and upper arm. Avoid areas of pain. Gentle friction is added after the pain subsides. Do not abduct the limb. In the subacute and chronic stage, passive movement should be encouraged. Heat packs may also help relieve pain. (Also see Bursitis).

References

Adams JC. Hamblen DL. Outline of orthopaedics. 11th ed. London: Churchill Livingstone; 1990. p. 98.

Bursitis - trochanteric

An inflammation of the trochanteric bursa.

Cause:

It is usually caused by a tear of the iliotibial band over the trochanter. This in turn produces irritation of the trochanteric bursa that lies around the insertion

Pathology A to Z -

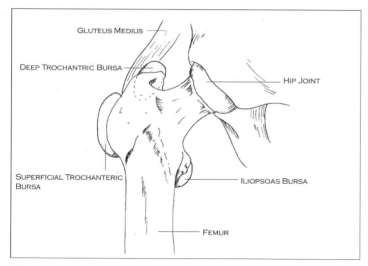

GLUTEUS MEDIUS

DEEP TROCHANTRIC BURSA

HIP JOINT

SUPERFICIAL TROCHANTERIC
BURSA

ILIOPSOAS BURSA

FEMUR

of the gluteus medius to the greater trochanter of the femur.

Signs and Symptoms:

There is pain in the lateral aspect of the hip and thigh. It may radiate to the back and is increased on climbing stairs, or when sitting cross-legged with the involved leg over the uninvolved one. The pain on sitting is brought about by the pressure put by the contracting gluteus maximus on the bursa. The pain is increased on lying on one side with pressure over the bursa. Passive abduction and external rotation of the leg also increases the pain. Pain is also produced by pressure on the bursa by a stretched gluteus maximus when the leg is adducted, flexed and internally rotated. However, there is no functional limitation of movement, pain or swelling in the joint. The posterolateral aspect of the greater trochanter is tender to touch.

Risk Factors:

A tight iliotibial band predisposes this condition.

Caution and Recommendations to Therapists:

Advice client to use pillows and support at night while sleeping, in order to reduce pressure over the bursa. Climbing stairs or long walks that can aggravate the pain should be avoided until the inflammation subsides. Use heat/cold packs to reduce pain and swelling. Later use friction massage over the bursa to reduce adhesions. Gently stretch the iliotibial band. Massage over the gluteal region to minimize spasm of the gluteus maximus (also see Bursitis).

References

Adams JC. Hamblen DL. Outline of orthopaedics. 11th ed. London: Churchill Livingstone; 1990. p. 98.

Callosities

Thickening of the skin due to repeated rubbing and/or pressure.

Cause:

Callosities are formed in areas, usually over bony prominences, in response to mechanical trauma. *Corn* or *clavus* is a more focal area of thickening that is seen in the foot. A *callus*, which is a more diffuse thickening, may be seen in areas as a response to chronic rubbing eg. as seen in the palms of a manual labourer.

Signs and Symptoms:

The skin appears thickened in the region. Corns may be painful.

Risk Factors:

See Cause.

Caution and Recommendations to Therapists:

Use of lubricant over the callosity while massaging can soften the tissue and facilitate reduction in size.

Notes

The key is to address the mechanical problem. Use of padding and wearing better fitting shoes are some of the measures that can be taken to prevent corn formation. The callosity can be pared off or keratolytics such as salicylic acid may be applied. In some cases surgery may be needed if there is an underlying bony spur. Generally, treatment is not needed for a callus. For more details see Appendix C: Keratolytics.

References

Mercier LR., editor. Practical orthopedics. 4th ed. New York: Mosby-Year book Inc; 1995. p. 251.

Cancer - bladder

An abnormal and uncontrolled growth of bladder tissue.

Cause:

The cause is unknown.

Signs and Symptoms:

It usually presents with blood in the urine. The person may have frequency, urgency and pain on passing urine. Secondary symptoms may arise if it has spread to the lungs, liver, lymph nodes and neighboring tissues.

Risk Factors:

It is more common in men over the age of 50. The excretion of cancer-producing chemicals in the urine have been implicated. Those working with aniline dyes as in cable or rubber industries are more prone. Bladder cancer is also common in chronic smokers. Bladder infections, bladder stones also increase the risk. A higher incidence is seen in those infected with the parasite Schistosoma (common in Egypt). Bladder cancer is more common in those ingesting painkillers containing phenacetin excessively.

Caution and Recommendations to Therapists:

Consult Physician as to the extent of the disease and the treatment that is being given. A light massage of short duration, avoiding the abdomen is recommended. See Appendix D for organizations and support groups.

Notes

This cancer is treated according to the extent and health of the person. Surgery is the most common form of treatment where the tumor is removed. The whole bladder and adjacent lymph nodes may be removed in some cases. Radiation and/or chemotherapy may also be used. In cases where the cancer is superficial, it may be treated by administration of drugs into the bladder. Laser therapy may also be used.

For more details see Appendix C: Radiation therapy; Cancer chemotherapy; Laser therapy.

References

Premkumar K. The massage connection: anatomy, physiology and pathology. Calgary: VanPub books; 1998. p. N8-N12.

Ferrell-Torry AT, Glick OJ. The use of therapeutic massage as a nursing intervention to modify anxiety and the perception of cancer pain. Cancer Nursing 1993; 16(2):93-101.

McNamara P. Massage for people with cancer. London: 1993. Wandsworth Cancer Support Center; 1993. .

Chamness A. Massage therapy and persons living with cancer. Massage Therapy Journal 32(3): 53-65.

MacDonald G. Massage for cancer patients: a review of nursing research. Massage Therapy Journal 34(3): 53-56.

Cancer - bone

Musculoskeletal system

An abnormal, uncontrolled proliferation of bone tissue.

Cause:

The cause is not known. There are many types of malignant bone tumors. Tumors may be primary or secondary. Primary tumors originate from bone tissue. Secondary or metastatic tumors are those that have spread to the bone from other tissues like the breast, lungs, prostate, kidney, thyroid etc. Secondary tumors are more common than primary tumors.

Many types of primary tumors are present. *Osteogenic sarcoma* is found in regions where rapid growth of bone occurs eg. distal femur, proximal end of tibia, proximal end of humerus. *Chondrosarcoma* - a malignant tumor of cartilage usually occurs in regions where muscles attach to bone and are more common in the trunk, pelvis, hip, knee and shoulder. *Ewing's sarcoma* - a highly malignant tumor, arises from immature bone marrow cells and occurs in the shaft of long bones or bones of the pelvis. Metastatic tumors are found in organs along specific vascular pathways.

Benign tumors may also develop in bone. These tumors are slow growing and do not spread to other organs. However, they may produce symptoms by obstruction to blood flow or pressure on surrounding tissue. They may also produce pathological fractures and deformities. The most common benign tumors are *osteochondromas, endochondromas, giant cell tumors, osteoid osteomas* and *nonossifying fibromas.*

Signs and Symptoms:

Bone tumors typically presents as bone pain. The pain comes on slowly and may be intermittent or constant, lasting for more than a week. The pain may be worse at night. Bone tumors may present as an abnormal swelling in the bone. Sometimes, a pathological fracture may be the first sign of the tumor. It is usually diagnosed by X rays, where the extent of involvement, tissue destruction and new bone formation is visualised. The tumor may restrict the range of motion of the adjacent joint. Other symptoms may be present if the tumor has metastasised to other organs.

In osteosarcoma the skin over the swelling appears shiny and stretched with prominent superficial veins.

Risk Factors:

Malignant bone tumors are rare before the age of 10. The incidence is higher in young adults. Osteogenic sarcoma is more common in males and in those with Paget's disease. Exposure to radiation increases the risk of osteogenic sarcoma. Chondrosarcoma is more common in middle or later life. Ewing's sarcoma is more common in males under the age of 30 years.

Caution and Recommendations to Therapists:

Advice clients with abnormal bone swelling to seek medical help. Clearance

Notes

Malignant bone tumors are usually treated with surgery where the tumor is removed along with a wide margin of normal tissue surrounding it. Amputation of the limb may be required. Radiation therapy may be used in conjunction to slow down the growth, prevent spread and decrease the pain. Immunotherapy and chemotherapy may be used in addition. The combination of therapy depends on the type of tumor and the extent of spread.

Benign tumors are treated by surgical removal of the abnormal mass. For more details see Appendix C: Radiation therapy; Immunotherapy; Cancer chemotherapy; Amputation.

References

Premkumar K. The massage connection: anatomy, physiology and pathology. Calgary: VanPub Books; 1998. p. N8-N12.

Ferrell-Torry AT, Glick OJ. The use of therapeutic massage as a nursing intervention to modify anxiety and the perception of cancer pain. Cancer Nursing 1993; 16(2):93-101.

McNamara P. Massage for people with cancer. London: Wandsworth Cancer Support Center; 1993.

Chamness A. Massage therapy and persons living with cancer. Massage Therapy Journal. 32(3): 53-65.

MacDonald G. Massage for cancer patients: a review of nursing research. Massage Therapy Journal 34(3): 53-56.

from the Physician is required before massage, as presentation and spread vary with the type of bone tumor. In those under treatment, avoid areas of radiation. If on chemotherapy, remember that the immunity will be lowered and ensure that the client is not exposed to infectious agents in your clinic. Refer to the section on Amputation for those who have undergone surgical excision. See Appendix D for organizations and support groups.

Cancer - breast

Reproductive system

A malignant growth affecting the breasts of women (rarely men may be affected).

Notes

It is the most common malignancy that affects women. It is also the most treatable of all malignancies.

Breast cancers are of many types and are classified according to the location and appearance under the microscope. The mode of spread, outcome and treatment varies with the type of cancer and the stage it is in. It spreads directly to adjacent structures, via the lymphatics to lymph nodes, or through the blood stream to distant sites such as the lungs, liver, bones and brain.

It is treated according to the stage. Surgery, chemotherapy, radiotherapy and/or hormonal therapy (use of tamoxifen; removal or destruction of the ovaries by surgery/radiation; use of progestin in postmenopausal women) are some of the treatment options available.

Regular breast self examination should be done by all women - especially those above the age of 35 or who are at risk. Mammography - an X-ray technique that can visualize abnormally dense breast tissue should be done after the age of 35 and repeated every two years - if above the age of 40 or every year above 50 years of age.

For more details see Appendix C: Cancer chemotherapy; Hormone therapy/ replacement; Radiation therapy; Mammography.

References

Premkumar K. The massage connection: anatomy, physiology and pathology. Calgary: VanPub books; 1998. p. N8-N12.

Ferrell-Torry AT, Glick OJ. The use of therapeutic massage as a nursing intervention to modify anxiety and the perception of cancer pain. Cancer Nursing 1993; 16(2):93-101

Cause:

The cause is not known. A relationship between levels of estrogen and breast cancer has been shown.

Signs and Symptoms:

Usually there is no symptom. Most breast cancers are detected by the person herself noticing a hard lump. Breast cancer can also present as abnormal fluid discharge from the nipples, retraction of the nipples or as ulcers. Sometimes it presents as redness and increased temperature of the breast. The cancer can spread via the lymphatic system to the axillary and cervical lymph nodes. Spread to the axillary lymph nodes can cause edema of the arm. Through the blood, the cancer can spread to the lungs, bone, liver and surrounding sites.

Risk Factors:

It is more common in women between the ages of 35 and 54. Incidence is higher in those with a family history of breast cancer, who have attained menarche at an early age, who have had a late menopause, have long menstrual cycles, those who have never been pregnant or have had late pregnancies, those with cancers of ovary or uterus and those exposed to ionizing radiation. Incidence may be higher in those using oral contraceptives for over 4 years before the first pregnancy. Also, the risk has been shown to be higher in those using oral contraceptives for over 10 years. Those who have become pregnant at an early age - earlier than age 20, history of multiple pregnancies, those of Asian or Indian origin are at lower risk.

Male breast cancer, though rare is possible. Predisposing factors include history of breast cancer in the family, exposure to radiation etc.

Caution and Recommendations to Therapists:

Refer client to Physician if a hard mass is felt in the axilla or in upper part of chest. In general, the benefit of massage in reducing stress levels in these individuals is undisputed. Massage may boost the general immunity of the client and thereby facilitate the body's own defense against cancer. Although the role of massage in spreading cancer to other areas is controversial, spread of cancer is also determined by the type of breast cancer (some types spread rapidly while others are very slow growing). Consult Physician regarding extent of disease in those clients who have just been diagnosed to have breast cancer

Clients who have had surgery that involved removal of the axillary lymph nodes are likely to have edema of the arm. Elevate the edematous arm above heart level throughout the massage. Gently massage arm with strokes directed towards the axilla. Manual lymph drainage is beneficial. However, this technique requires special training. Advice clients to open and close the hand tightly six to eight times every few hours. The contraction of the muscles helps venous and lymphatic flow. If the client is on radiation therapy, avoid areas of radiation. If on chemotherapy, they are more prone to infections due to reduced immunity. Avoid massaging such individuals if you have even a mild form of any infection. Ensure that these clients are scheduled at a time when they are unlikely to come in contact with other infected individuals.

Encourage all women clients to perform regular breast self-examinations.See Appendix D for organizations and support groups.

Chamness A. Breast cancer and massage therapy. Massage Therapy Journal 1996; Winter: 44-46.

Curties, D. Could massage therapy promote cancer metastasis? Journal of Soft tissue Manipulation 1994; April-May.

McNamara P. Massage for people with cancer. London: Wandsworth Cancer Support Center; 1993.

Chamness A. Massage therapy and persons living with cancer. Massage Therapy Journal 32(3): 53-65.

MacDonald G. Massage for cancer patients: a review of nursing research. Massage therapy Journal.34(3): 53-56.

Cancer - cervix

Reproductive system

An abnormal and uncontrolled growth of the tissue in the cervix.

Cause:

It is a result of slow changes of the normal cervical tissue into an abnormal type, on being exposed to cancer-producing agents.

Signs and Symptoms:

It is asymptomatic in the early stages. Later there may be foul-smelling, blood-stained discharge through the vagina. Low back pain, loss of weight, unexplained anemia and pain during intercourse are other symptoms.

Risk Factors:

It is common in women who have had sexual intercourse. It is more frequent in those who have had their first intercourse at an early age, who have several partners, and have had sexually transmitted disease before. There is an association between herpes simplex viral infection and cervical cancer. There is a higher incidence in those with a family history of cancer. Smoking has also been shown to increase the risk. People whose immunity is lowered, as in patients with AIDS, transplant patients etc seem to be more susceptible to the disease.

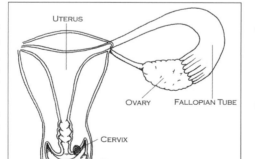

UTERUS
OVARY   FALLOPIAN TUBE
CERVIX
VAGINA

Notes

Cervical cancer can be detected at an early stage by regular Pap (Papanicolaou) smear tests. This test examines the cervical tissue to detect abnormal cell types. Annual Pap smear examination is recommended for those at risk. If the smear is abnormal, the cervix is visualized and a biopsy may be taken. The treatment varies according to the stage. At an early stage, just the abnormal area may be removed or destroyed. In others, radiation and/or surgery may be resorted to. Depending on the extent, just the uterus or uterus along with the fallopian tubes, ovaries and pelvic lymph nodes and upper part of the vagina may be removed. The survival rate over 5 years averages about 66%. If diagnosed early, it may be as high as 80-100%.

For more details see Appendix C: Radiation therapy; Pap smear.

References

Premkumar K. The massage connection: anatomy, physiology and pathology. Calgary: VanPub books; 1998. p. N8-N12.

Ferrell-Torry AT, Glick OJ. The use of therapeutic massage as a nursing intervention to modify anxiety and the perception of cancer pain. Cancer Nursing 1993; 16(2):93-101.

McNamara P. Massage for people with cancer. London: Wandsworth Cancer Support Center; 1993.

Chamness A. Massage therapy and persons living with cancer. Massage Therapy Journal 32(3): 53-65.

MacDonald G. Massage for cancer patients: a review of nursing research. Massage therapy Journal 34(3): 53-56.

Caution and Recommendations to Therapists:

Consult physician as to the extent of cancer and type of treatment. If the client is on radiation, remember that the general immunity may be depressed and exposure to any kind of infection should be avoided.

Encourage women clients to have Pap smear done annually, if at risk. See Appendix D for organizations and support groups.

Gastrointestinal system

Cancer - colon

An abnormal, uncontrolled growth of the colonic tissue.

Notes

This condition is treated surgically, with removal of the affected part and local lymph nodes (if it has spread) and colostomy (colon opened onto the surface of the abdomen). Chemotherapy and radiation are other options adopted. For more details see Appendix C: Colostomy; Cancer Chemotherapy; Radiation therapy.

Cause:

The exact cause is not known.

Signs and Symptoms:

In the early stages, the signs and symptoms are vague and related to the location of the cancer. Initially, there is change in bowel habits in a person with regular bowel movements. A dull abdominal pain may or may not be present. General symptoms include loss of weight, fatigue, anemia and weakness. If the tumor is on the right side of the abdomen ie. in the cecum or ascending colon, symptoms of obstruction appear slowly as tumors in this region generally tend to spread along the walls of the gut without narrowing the lumen of the gut. Also, the contents of the intestines are more fluid here. If on the left side - descending colon, sigmoid colon or rectum, the signs of obstruction appear early in the disease since the contents are more solid. There is constipation or diarrhoea, with passage of pencil-shaped or ribbon-like stools. The blood in the stools may be red if the tumor is located close to the anus. The stools appear black and tarry if the bleeding is from a tumor located closer to the small intestines.

Risk Factors:

It is common over the age of 40 and affects both men and women. The incidence is related to the diet, with a higher incidence in individuals whose dietary intake is low in fibre contet and high in animal fat. Colon cancer is one of the complications of ulcerative colitis. There is a greater risk in people with a family history of colorectal cancer. History of polyps in the intestines also increases the risk.

References

Premkumar K. The massage connection: anatomy, physiology and pathology. Calgary: VanPub books; 1998. p. N8-N12.

Ferrell-Torry AT, Glick OJ. The use of therapeutic massage as a nursing intervention to modify anxiety and the perception of cancer pain. Cancer Nursing 1993; 16(2):93-101.

McNamara P. Massage for people with cancer. 1993. Wandsworth Cancer Support Center. London.

Chamness A. Massage therapy and persons living with cancer. Massage Therapy Journal 32(3): 53-65.

MacDonald G. Massage for cancer patients: a review of nursing research. Massage Therapy Journal 34(3): 53-56.

Caution and Recommendations to Therapists:

Massage is contraindicated in the abdominal region if a person has been diagnosed with this condition. Consult Physician regarding spread of disease and type of treatment if the client is under treatment. Abdominal massage is not contraindicated for those treated with colostomy. Adjust pressure and strokes on an individual basis. The immunity is reduced in those on chemotherapy or radiation. Do not schedule such clients if you are harboring even a mild form of infection such as a cold. See Appendix D for organizations and support groups.

Cancer - gallbladder

An abnormal and uncontrolled growth of tissue in the gallbladder.

Cause:

Chronic irritation of the mucosa of the gall bladder can eventually lead to cancer.

Signs and Symptoms:

Indigestion and colicky pain may be present especially after a fatty meal. The pain is located in the right upper quadrant of the abdomen and may be referred to the back, the right shoulder, right scapula or between the scapula. Jaundice, weight loss and/or a palpable mass in the upper quadrant are other symptoms that may be seen. Often the cancer is diagnosed unexpectedly during gallbladder surgery or laparoscopy.

Risk Factors:

Blockage to the flow of bile as in gallstones, obstruction by enlarged lymph nodes or tumors in neighboring areas can predispose to this condition. It is more common in females.

Caution and Recommendations to Therapists:

Consult Physician as to the extent of the disease. Avoid massage to the right upper quadrant. See Appendix D for organizations and support groups.

Notes

Surgery is the treatment of choice. In most cases, the cancer has spread to adjacent areas directly, via blood, or lymphatics by the time symptoms appear. As a result, in more that 75% of cases, surgery is not possible. The response to chemotherapy and radiation is not very good. The 5-year survival rate is about 3%

For more details see Appendix C: Cancer chemotherapy; Radiation therapy; Cholecystectomy.

References

Premkumar K. The massage connection: anatomy, physiology and pathology. Calgary: VanPub books; 1998. p. N8-N12.

Ferrell-Torry AT, Glick OJ. The use of therapeutic massage as a nursing intervention to modify anxiety and the perception of cancer pain. Cancer Nursing. 1993; 16(2): 93-101.

McNamara P. Massage for people with cancer. London: Wandsworth Cancer Support Center; 1993.

Chamness A. Massage therapy and persons living with cancer. Massage Therapy Journal 32(3): 53-65.

MacDonald G Massage for cancer patients: a review of nursing research. Massage Therapy Journal 34(3): 53-56.

Cancer - kidney

An abnormal and uncontrolled proliferation of kidney tissue.

Cause:

The cause is not known. Cancer of the kidney is classified according to the type of cells found in the tumor.

Signs and Symptoms:

There are no symptoms initially. Symptoms of a swelling in the abdomen or blood in the urine denote advanced disease. Anemia, weight loss and loss of appetite are other general symptoms that may be noticed.

Risk Factors:

Nephroblastoma or *Wilms' tumor* - a form of cancer with muscle, bone and epithelial tissue is more common in children. *Hypernephroma, renal adenocarcinoma* or *renal cell carcinoma* is more common in men over the age of 60. Smoking, exposure to cadmium and presence of kidney stones are predisposing factors.

Notes

Surgery is the preferred form of treatment. In advanced cases, chemotherapy is resorted to. For more details see Appendix C: Cancer chemotherapy.

References

Premkumar K. The massage connection: anatomy, physiology and pathology. Calgary: VanPub books; 1998. p. N8-N12.

Ferrell-Torry AT, Glick OJ. The use of therapeutic massage as a nursing intervention to modify anxiety and the perception of cancer pain. Cancer Nursing 1993;16(2): 93-101.

McNamara P. Massage for people with cancer. London: Wandsworth Cancer Support Center; 1993.

Chamness A. Massage therapy and persons living with cancer. Massage Therapy Journal 32(3): 53-65.

MacDonald G. Massage for cancer patients: a review of nursing research. Massage Therapy Journal 34(3): 53-56.

Caution and Recommendations to Therapists:

Encourage clients to see a physician if they complain of blood in urine. Consult Physician regarding the extent of disease if cancer is diagnosed. Massage helps reduce leg cramps that are common in these individuals. A light, soothing massage is beneficial. If the person is on chemotherapy the immunity will be reduced. Do not treat if you are harboring any infection. Cross fibre friction can be used over surgical scars to reduce adhesions, if the person has had surgery. See Appendix D for organizations and support groups.

Cancer - liver (Hepatocarcinoma)

Gastrointestinal system

An abnormal, uncontrolled growth of tissue in the liver that can invade surrounding areas.

Notes

The prognosis for this cancer is very poor as it progresses very rapidly. The five-year survival rate is 1% and most people with liver cancer die within 6 months. Surgical resection, if possible is the only chance of cure. Liver transplantation, immunotherapy and gene therapy, among others are other treatment options being evaluated.

For more details see Appendix C: Immunotherapy; Organ transplantation.

References

Premkumar K. The massage connection: anatomy, physiology and pathology. Calgary: VanPub books; 1998. p. N8-N12.

Ferrell-Torry AT, Glick OJ. The use of therapeutic massage as a nursing intervention to modify anxiety and the perception of cancer pain. Cancer Nursing 1993; 16(2): 93-101.

McNamara P. Massage for people with cancer. London: Wandsworth Cancer Support Center; 1993.

Chamness A. Massage therapy and persons living with cancer. Massage Therapy Journal 32(3): 53-65.

MacDonald G. Massage for cancer patients: a review of nursing research. Massage Therapy Journal 34(3): 53-56.

Cause:

The more common type of liver cancer is that which has spread from other areas of the body - *metastatic carcinoma*. Spread is common from those areas from which blood flows through the liver. Cancer can also arise from the liver tissue - primary cancer.

Signs and Symptoms:

Liver cancer may present as a swelling in the right upper quadrant assocated with jaundice or fluid in the abdomen (ascites). Other general symptoms of weight loss, weakness and loss of appetite may be present.

Risk Factors:

Chronic hepatitis B or C virus infection, chronic alcoholism, cirrhosis and potential toxic agents in the diet predispose to this type of cancer.

Caution and Recommendations to Therapists:

Usually, the cancer is well advanced when diagnosed, whether arising primarily from the liver or secondary to cancer elsewhere in the body. Consult the Physician as to the extent of the disease. Avoid massaging the abdominal area and alter the areas of massage on an individual basis. In any event, keep the duration of massage short. The aim is to alleviate stress and reduce pain. Essential oils of rose or neroli of 1% dilution are recommended for their calming effect. However, avoid use of oil, essential oils and lotions before chemotherapy and radiotherapy. If the client is on chemotherapy or radiation, remember that the immunity will be lowered and avoid massage if harboring any infection. See Appendix D for organizations and support groups.

Cancer - lung (Bronchogenic carcinoma)

A malignant growth in the walls or epithelium of the bronchi.

Cause:

It may be caused by chronic inhalation of cancer-producing air and industrial pollutants such as cigarette smoke (actively or passively), asbestos fibres, uranium, arsenic, nickel, iron oxides, chromium, radioactive dust, and coal dust.

Signs and Symptoms:

Usually there are no symptoms initially and it is often detected only in the advanced stages. Late symptoms include chronic cough, hoarseness of voice, difficulty in breathing, chest pain, blood in sputum, weight loss, and weakness.

Risk Factors:

It is more common in men. Smokers are most susceptible - especially chronic smokers who have started smoking before the age of 15, those who smoke a whole pack or more per day and those who have been smoking for over 20 years. It is also associated with the depth of inhalation and nicotine content of cigarettes.

People exposed to asbestos and other industrial pollutants listed under cause, are also prone. Individuals with family history of lung cancer are more predisposed.

Caution and Recommendations to Therapists:

Encourage clients to stop smoking if smokers. Keep brochures on dangers of smoking in your clinic. Have addresses and telephone numbers of local 'Quit Smoking Clinics' handy. In general, the benefit of massage in reducing stress levels in these individuals is undisputed. However, massage may help spread the cancer to other regions especially if it has already spread to lymph nodes or other neighboring structures. Consult Physician as to the stage of disease in individual clients.

If a client is on radiation therapy, avoid massaging the skin over radiation areas. Clients on chemotherapy are more prone to any type of infection. Avoid massaging such individuals if you have even a mild form of any infection. Ensure that such clients are scheduled at a time when they are unlikely to come in contact with other infected individuals. See Appendix D for organizations and support groups.

Notes

Prevention by anti-smoking efforts still remains the best option. Treatment used depends on the type of lung cancer and how much it has spread. In early stages, resection of the whole/part of the lung is carried out. Radiotherapy and chemotherapy are other forms of treatment that may be used. For more details see Appendix C: Radiation therapy; Chemotherapy.

References

Premkumar K. The massage connection: anatomy, physiology and pathology. Calgary: VanPub books; 1998. p. N8-N12.

Ferrell-Torry AT, Glick OJ. The use of therapeutic massage as a nursing intervention to modify anxiety and the perception of cancer pain. Cancer Nursing. 1993; 16(2): 93-101.

McNamara P. Massage for people with cancer. London: Wandsworth Cancer Support Center; 1993. London.

Chamness A. Massage therapy and persons living with cancer. Massage Therapy Journal 32(3): 53-65.

MacDonald G. Massage for cancer patients: a review of nursing research. Massage Therapy Journal 34(3): 53-56.

Cancer - oral

An uncontrolled growth of abnormal tissue in the mouth.

Cause:

It may be caused by chronic irritation of the mucosa of the oral cavity as in tobacco chewing. Recurrent or chronic ulcers of the mouth can lead to this type of cancer.

Notes

The patients are usually treated with surgery and/or radiation. Surgery can result in changes in appearance, difficulty in chewing and communicating, adding to the psychological trauma. Radiation can be followed by poor wound healing, ulcers in the mouth, dryness of mouth, difficulty in swallowing etc. Prognosis worsens as the location of the cancer gets closer to the pharynx. For more details see Appendix C: Radiation therapy.

References

Premkumar K. The massage connection: anatomy, physiology and pathology. Calgary: VanPub books; 1998. p. N8-N12.

Ferrell-Torry AT, Glick OJ. The use of therapeutic massage as a nursing intervention to modify anxiety and the perception of cancer pain. Cancer Nursing. 1993; 16(2): 93-101.

McNamara P. Massage for people with cancer. London: Wandsworth Cancer Support Center; 1993.

Chamness A. Massage therapy and persons living with cancer. Massage Therapy Journal 32(3): 53-65.

MacDonald G. Massage for cancer patients: a review of nursing research. Massage Therapy Journal 34(3): 53-56.

Signs and Symptoms:

Oral cancer may appear as a non-healing, slowly growing red ulcer or as a growth. Usually it is painful and firm to touch. All chronic ulcers that fail to heal in 1 to 2 weeks have to be investigated.

Risk Factors:

The incidence is higher in men. Chronic smoking, tobacco chewing, chewing of betel nut (more common in India), alcoholism, iron deficiency and deficiency of vitamins predispose to this condition. Infection due to herpes simplex and pailloma virus has also been implicated.

Caution and Recommendations to Therapists:

It can spread to the lymph nodes in the neck. The nodes are felt as hard, rounded or irregular swelling. These clients are treated with radiation or surgery. Radiation lowers the immunity in the local area and these individuals are prone to thrush and dental caries. Avoid massage to face and neck. Encourage client to stop smoking and drinking. See Appendix D for organizations and support groups.

Reproductive system	# Cancer - ovaries
	An abnormal and uncontrolled growth of tissues in the ovary.

Notes

Since it is usually detected in an advanced stage, mortality rate of this disease is very high. It is treated with a combination of surgery, radiation/ chemotherapy depending on the stage and type of tumor. For more details see Appendix C: Radiation therapy; Cancer chemotherapy.

References

Premkumar K. The massage connection: anatomy, physiology and pathology. Calgary: VanPub books; 1998. p. N8-N12.

Ferrell-Torry AT, Glick OJ. The use of therapeutic massage as a nursing intervention to modify anxiety and the perception of cancer pain. Cancer Nursing. 1993; 16(2): 93-101.

McNamara P. Massage for people with cancer. London: Wandsworth Cancer Support Center; 1993.

Chamness A. Massage therapy and persons living with cancer. Massage Therapy Journal 32(3): 53-65.

MacDonald G. Massage for cancer patients: a review of nursing research. Massage Therapy Journal 34(3): 53-56.

Cause:

The cause is not known.

Signs and Symptoms:

It is asymptomatic. Diagnosis is usually made after the cancer has spread extensively. The symptoms are vague and usually associated with gastrointestinal symptoms such as bloating of the abdomen, mild abdominal pain and excessive passage of gas. There may be fluid in the peritoneal cavity (ascites) in late stages. The fluid can be so extensive that a ripple can be felt on shaking the abdomen.

Risk Factors:

It is more common in women between the ages of 65-84. Those with no or few children are at higher risk. Suppression of ovulation over a long-term (as in prolonged use of oral contraceptives) seems to provide some protection against ovarian cancer.

Caution and Recommendations to Therapists:

Consult Physician regarding the extent of the disease and the type of treatment used. Avoid abdominal massage. The immunity is suppressed in clients on radiation or chemotherapy. Do not massage such clients when you harbor a cold or any mild infection. See Appendix D for organizations and support groups.

Cancer - pancreas

An abnormal and uncontrolled growth of pancreatic tissue.

Cause:

The cause is unknown.

Signs and Symptoms:

The person presents with severe weight loss and pain in the lower back. The pain increases a few hours after taking food, is worsened on lying down and improves on bending forward. If the tumor is growing around the bile duct, obstruction may result in jaundice and diarrhoea. The gallbladder may be palpable. The accumulation of bilirbin under the skin causes severe itching. The jaundice may be so severe that the skin may turn green or black as the bilirubin changes in structure. The reduction of bile slows down the absorption and digestion of fat causing clay-colored, foul-smelling stools. The cancer spreads directly and rapidly to the surrounding tissues including the lymph nodes and the liver. Kidneys, spleen and blood vessels may also be involved. The symptoms vary according to the tissues affected.

Risk Factors:

It is more common in men between the ages of 35 and 70. The incidence is higher in the United States, Canada, Sweden and Israel. Smoking, ingestion of food high in fat and protein, high intake of food additives and exposure to industrial chemicals such as urea and benzidine are predisposing factors. The incidence is also higher in alcoholics and those with chronic pancreatitis and diabetes mellitus.

Caution and Recommendations to Therapists:

The cancer spreads rapidly and massage may help spread the cancer further. However, often this cancer is diagnosed only in an advanced stage when the condition cannot be worsened. Consult physician as to th extent of the cancer. Avoid the abdominal area if massaging an individual in an advanced stage. See Appendix D for organizations and support groups.

Notes

Treatment options include surgery, if confined to a localized area. Radiation and chemotherapy may also be used. However, prognosis is poor for those with this disease. For more details see Appendix C: Radiation therapy; Cancer chemotherapy.

References

Premkumar K. The massage connection: anatomy, physiology and pathology. Calgary: VanPub books; 1998. p. N8-N12.

Ferrell-Torry AT, Glick OJ. The use of therapeutic massage as a nursing intervention to modify anxiety and the perception of cancer pain. Cancer Nursing. 1993; 16(2): 93-101.

McNamara P. Massage for people with cancer. London: Wandsworth Cancer Support Center; 1993.

Chamness A. Massage therapy and persons living with cancer. Massage Therapy Journal 32(3): 53-65.

MacDonald G. Massage for cancer patients: a review of nursing research. Massage therapy Journal 34(3): 53-56.

Cancer - prostate

It is an abnormal and uncontrolled growth of the prostatic tissue.

Cause:

The prostate is a gland that surrounds the male urethra and secretes a milky white fluid that helps to maintain the pH of the semen and movement of the sperms. The gland is surrounded by smooth muscles that contract during orgasm and expel the ejaculate.

Notes

Prostatic cancer is treated with surgery, radiotherapy or hormonal therapy depending on the stage of the disease. Drugs that reduce the effect of testosterone (eg. estrogens) are given to reduce symptoms and growth of the cancer. A person on hormonal therapy may have enlargement of breasts and change in voice. For more details see Appendix C: Radiation therapy; Hormone therapy/replacement.

The cause is not known. Genetic predisposition, high testosterone levels and environmental factors may be responsible.

Signs and Symptoms:

Usually no symptoms are seen. If the cancer is located close to the urethra, there may be frequency of micturition, urgency, difficulty in voiding, blood in urine (hematuria) or blood in the ejaculate. Cancer of the prostate is often diagnosed by rectal examination, where the prostate feels nodular and hard. Prostate cancer spreads usually to the bones and produces bony pain, or causes fractures in the bone after trivial injury. In the advanced stage, as in all cancers, the person looses weight and is anemc.

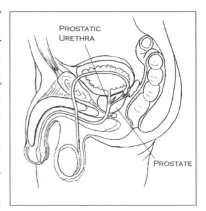

PROSTATIC URETHRA

PROSTATE

Risk Factors:

The incidence increases with age. It is more common in African-American males. Due to the variation in incidence between races, environmental factors have been implicated. People working in occupations like welding, electroplating, or production of alkaline batteries, which exposes them to cadmium have been found to be at increased risk.

Caution and Recommendations to Therapists:

Consult Physician to determine the stage of the disease. No evidence is still available to prove or disprove that massage can spread cancer. Remember that the prostate can be accessed only through the rectum and a Massage Therapist has no scope of giving clients a prostatic massage. See Appendix D for organizations and support groups.

References

Premkumar K. The massage connection: anatomy, physiology and pathology. Calgary: VanPub books; 1998. p. N8-N12.

Ferrell-Torry AT, Glick OJ. The use of therapeutic massage as a nursing intervention to modify anxiety and the perception of cancer pain. Cancer Nursing. 1993; 16(2): 93-101.

McNamara P. Massage for people with cancer. London: Wandsworth Cancer Support Center; 1993.

Chamness A. Massage therapy and persons living with cancer. Massage Therapy Journal 32(3): 53-65.

MacDonald G. Massage for cancer patients: a review of nursing research. Massage Therapy Journal 34(3): 53-56.

Cancer - skin

Integumentary system

A malignant change in the skin which may be slow growing (basal cell epithelioma) or rapidly growing with potential to spread (squamous cell carcinoma and malignant melanoma).

Notes

Treatment options include surgery, local application of creams or solutions, chemotherapy and radiation. The incidence of skin cancer can be markedly reduced by client and physician education. It has to be

Cause:

Prolonged exposure to the sun and radiation exposure are the most common causes of the malignant change in the cells of the epidermis. Chronic skin irritation and exposure to carcinogens such as tar or oil can cause squamous cell carcinoma.

Pathology A to Z -

Signs and Symptoms:

Basal cell epithelioma is of different types and can occur as pinkish, smooth swellings with blood vessels over the lesion. It can later ulcerate. Sometimes it appears as thickened areas of skin in the chest and back that are lightly pigmented. *Squamous cell carcinoma* appears as a palpable swelling that grows slowly. *Melanomas* are common in the head, neck and leg areas and usually arise from preexisting pigmented areas such as a mole (nevus). It appears as irregular growths that may be blue, red, white or pigmented. See Appendix A: pages 353 &357 (Solar damaged skin).

Risk Factors:

Outdoor employment, residence in sunny, warm climates, fair skin, presence of large nevi (moles) and family history increase the risk of contracting this condition. Skin cancer is more common in areas of the body exposed to the sun and is more common in the right side in England and left side in the United States, possibly in relation to the side more exposed to the sun during driving! Exposure to arsenic eg. through well water or certain medications increase the risk. There is a higher incidence in people whose immunity has been suppressed as in those with AIDS or who have undergone transplantation.

Caution and Recommendations to Therapists:

Bring to the attention of regular clients, if you notice changes in color, size, shape or texture of preexisting moles and advise medical help. Consult Physician regarding indication of massage in those who have been diagnosed with skin cancer as the mode of spread and treatment varies according to the type and stage of cancer. The immunity is lowered in those on chemotherapy or radiation therapy making the client susceptible to infection. Remember that the skin over the site where radiation is given is easily damaged. See Appendix D for organizations and support groups.

emphasised that damage from ultra violet radiation begins early in life though the cancer develops later in life. Use of sunscreen and avoidance of direct exposure to the sun between 10 A.M to 2 P.M and prudent use of tanning salons is recommended.

For more details see Appendix C: Sunscreen; Cancer chemotherapy; Radiation therapy.

References

Premkumar K. The massage connection: anatomy, physiology and pathology. Calgary: VanPub books; 1998. p. N8-N12.

Ferrell-Torry AT, Glick OJ. The use of therapeutic massage as a nursing intervention to modify anxiety and the perception of cancer pain. Cancer Nursing. 1993; 16(2): 93-101.

McNamara P. Massage for people with cancer. London: Wandsworth Cancer Support Center; 1993.

Chamness A. Massage therapy and persons living with cancer. Massage Therapy Journal 32(3): 53-65.

MacDonald G. Massage for cancer patients: a review of nursing research. Massage Therapy Journal 34(3): 53-56.

Cancer - stomach

Gastrointestinal system

An abnormal uncontrolled growth in the stomach.

Cause:

The cause is unknown.

Signs and Symptoms:

In the early stages, the person has chronic pain or discomfort in the upper part of the abdomen. Since the symptoms are vague, this cancer is often not diagnosed till it has spread considerably. There is weight loss, anemia, easy fatigue and loss of appetite. Vomiting is common and often the contents have blood in it. A mass may be felt in the upper abdomen.

Risk Factors:

Smoking and alcoholism have been associated with a higher incidence of this

Notes

It is usually treated by surgery with removal of part/whole stomach (gastrectomy) and resection of adjacent lymph nodes. Chemotherapy and radiation may also be used. For more details see Appendix C: Cancer chemotherapy; Radiation therapy; Gastrectomy.

References

Premkumar K. The massage connection: anatomy, physiology and pathology. Calgary: VanPub books; 1998. p. N8-N12.

Ferrell-Torry AT, Glick OJ. The use of therapeutic massage as a nursing intervention to modify anxiety and the perception of cancer pain. Cancer Nursing. 1993; 16(2): 93-101.

McNamara P. Massage for people with cancer. London: Wandsworth Cancer Support Center; 1993.

Chamness A. Massage therapy and persons living with cancer. Massage Therapy Journal 32(3): 53-65.

MacDonald G. Massage for cancer patients: a review of nursing research. Massage Therapy Journal 34(3): 53-56.

cancer. Genetic factors are also implicated - it is more common in people of type A blood group (mucous secretion may vary between people of different blood groups) and in those with a family history of cancer. Specific diet and method of cooking (smoking, pickling and salting the food) also predispose to the disease. It is believed that long-term ingestion of high concentrations of nitrates present in dried, smoked or salted foods and their conversion to carcinogenic nitrites by bacteria may predispose to cancer in the region.

Caution and Recommendations to Therapists:

Consult Physician regarding the spread of cancer and type of treatment given. Avoid abdominal massage. The immunity is lowered in those on chemotherapy or radiation therapy making the client susceptible to infection. Remember that the skin over the site where radiation is given is easily damaged. See Appendix D for organizations and support groups.

Reproductive system

Cancer - testis

An abnormal and uncontrolled growth of the testicular tissue.

Notes

The 5 year survival rate for testicular cancer that has been detected early is very good (about 90%). The tumor spreads through the lymphatics to the abdominal lymph nodes. The prognosis is good even for tumors that have spread to other areas. It is treated by surgery with additional radiotherapy or chemotherapy according to the extent of spread. For more details see Appendix C: Radiation therapy; Cancer chemotherapy.

References

Premkumar K. The massage connection: anatomy, physiology and pathology. Calgary: VanPub books; 1998. p. N8-N12.

Ferrell-Torry AT, Glick OJ. The use of therapeutic massage as a nursing intervention to modify anxiety and the perception of cancer pain. Cancer Nursing. 1993; 16(2): 93-101.

McNamara P. Massage for people with cancer. London: Wandsworth Cancer Support Center; 1993.

Chamness A. Massage therapy and persons living with cancer. Massage Therapy Journal 32(3): 53-65.

MacDonald G. Massage for cancer patients: a review of nursing research. Massage Therapy Journal 34(3): 53-56.

Cause:

The cause is unknown.

Signs and Symptoms:

Slight enlargement of the testis is the first symptom. It may be accompanied by pain, discomfort and heaviness of the scrotum. Soon there is a rapid enlargement of the testis.

Risk Factors:

It is more common between 15 and 35 years of age. Those with cryptorchidism (undescended testis) are more susceptible. The incidence is found to be higher in those men whose mother had had estrogen therapy at the time of pregnancy. Trauma to and infection of the testis increase the risk.

Caution and Recommendations to Therapists:

Consult Physician as to the extent of the disease. If confined only to the testis, a light, soothing whole body massage is recommended. If the cancer has spread get clearance from the treating Physician. See Appendix D for organizations and support groups.

Integumentary system

Candidiasis (Moniliasis; Thrush)

A superficial fungal infection.

Notes

Antifungal creams/solution are used locally. In the case of vaginal infections,

Cause:

It is caused by a yeast-like fungus - *Candida albicans*. The fungus infects the nails, skin or mucous membrane of vagina (*moniliasis*), mouth (*thrush*) or other parts of the gastrointestinal tract. Rarely, it affects the brain, kidneys, and other structures. The fungi are a part of the normal flora, which take over when the conditions of the body permit multiplication, as in AIDS, cancer, aging etc.

antifungal vaginal tablets may be inserted along with the use of lotion or cream.

For more details see Appendix C: Antimicribial - antifungal agent; Suppository.

Signs and Symptoms:

The skin may be red and scaly with white-colored secretions. A rash may also be seen. Lesions are commonly seen below the breast, between fingers, axillae, groin and umbilicus. There may be reddening, swelling and darkening of the nail bed. In oral infections, cream-colored patches may be seen on the tongue, mouth or pharynx. There may also be itchiness associated with a white or yellow discharge. Men may experience soreness of the glans penis.

Risk Factors:

Individuals with diabetes mellitus, those on drugs that suppress the immunity or on heavy antibiotic treatment and those undergoing radiation therapy are more susceptible.

Caution and Recommendations to Therapists:

The fungi are present in healthy people without causing symptoms. Although it can be transmitted by close intimate contact, it requires a favorable environment for its growth. The bodily secretions of the client may harbor the pathogen. Observe strict hygienic procedures at all times. Do not massage if client describes a condition resembling candidiasis or any other sexually transmitted disease unless it has been completely treated. Refer to Appendix B:Strategies for infection prevention and safe practice. Also see Appendix D for organizations and support groups.

References

Morello JA, Mizer HE, Wilson ME, Granato PA. Microbiology in patient care. 6th ed. New York: McGraw-Hill; 1998. p. 313-314.

Carbohydrate intolerance

Gastrointestinal system

A condition where there is difficulty in digestion of a specific type of carbohydrate.

Cause:

It is caused by lack of the enzyme required for digesting a specific type of carbohydrate. *Lactose intolerance* is the most common type.

Notes

Dietary adjustment is the best mode of treatment.

Signs and Symptoms:

The person has diarrhea, bloating, increased gas formation and abdominal pain on ingesting food that contains the carbohydrate that cannot be absorbed. In the case of lactose intolerance, food such as milk, yogurt, ice cream etc.

Risk Factors:

There is usually a genetic predisposition.

References

Isselbacher KJ. Galactosemia, galactokinase deficiency, and other rare disorders of carbohydrate metabolism. In: Isselbacher KJ et al. Harrison's principles of internal medicine. 13th ed. London: McGraw-Hill Co; 1994. p. 2131-2132.

Caution and Recommendations to Therapists:

Massage over the abdomen can help release the gas that produces the bloating.

However, if the client has diarrhea, massage may increase the motility. In this case, avoid abdominal massage. If the client is asymptomatic at the time of massage, no restrictions apply.

Encourage client to follow the dietary changes advised by the Physician. See Appendix D for organizations and support groups.

Integumentary system

Carbunculitis (Carbuncle; Carbunculosis)

A bacterial infection of the skin affecting several hair follicles.

Cause:

Notes

It is a contagious condition requiring oral antibiotic treatment. For more details see Appendix C: Antimicrobial - antibacterial agents.

It is usually caused by the *staphylococci* or *streptococci bacilli*.

Signs and Symptoms:

It appears as a single or cluster of pustules that have spread beneath the epidermis. There is redness, swelling and pus in a large area of skin. See Appendix A: page 350.

Risk Factors:

Carbuncles are commonly seen in patients with diabetes or lowered immunity.

Caution and Recommendations to Therapists:

It is contagious. Cover the lesion with a piece of gauze and avoid massaging the area with carbunculosis. Avoid the lymph nodes draining the area, which will often be painfully enlarged. Wash linen, towels etc. that has come in contact with the client in hot soapy water. Since it responds to antibiotics it may be better to postpone massage till the condition is completely treated. Advice client not to share towels, face cloth etc. with family members to prevent spread of disease. Refer to Appendix B: Strategies for infection prevention and safe practice.

References

Morello JA, Mizer HE, Wilson ME, Granato PA. Microbiology in patient care. 6ᵗʰ ed. New York: McGraw-Hill; 1998. p. 430.

Gastrointestinal system

Carcinoid tumors

Abnormal growths of neuroendocrine cells commonly found in the gastrointestinal tract.

Cause:

Notes

Treatment depends on the severity of the symptoms. Various drugs such as antidiarrheals, antihistamines, bronchodilators etc are used to produce symptomatic relief. Since most of these tumors spread to other regions, surgery is not curative in these cases. If the tumor is small and confined to one region, surgery may be done. The prognosis depends on the site and stage of the disease.

Neuroendocrine cells are embryologically related to melanocytes and cells of the adrenal medulla.

The cause for this abnormal multiplication of neuroendocrine cells is not known. The tumors may be found anywhere from the stomach to the rectum. Rarely, they may be found in the pancreas, ovary, thymus or the pulmonary bronchi.

Signs and Symptoms:

The signs and symptoms depend on the location. Usually, they present as

Pathology A to Z -

gastrointestinal bleeding, abdominal pain or as intestinal obstruction. The tumour may spread to surrounding areas and produce symptoms.

The neuroendocrine cells secrete a variety of hormones. Serotonin, histamine, adrenaline, enkephalins and endorphins, among others, are examples of the hormones secreted. The effects of the secretions typically produce flushing, diarrhea, valvular heart disease, wheezing and periodic hypotension. This is often referred to as the *carcinoid syndrome.*

Risk Factors:

It is more common in people with pernicious anemia or certain types of thyroiditis.

Caution and Recommendations to Therapists:

Get a detailed history of symptoms in the client and the medications taken. Avoid abdominal massage. Be informed about the side effects of the medication taken.

For more details see Appendix C: Antihistamines; Vasodilators; Antidiarrhoeal drugs.

References

Kaplan LM. Endocrine tumors of the gastrointestinal tract and pancreas. In: Isselbacher KJ et al. Harrison's principles of internal medicine. 13th ed. London: McGraw-Hill Co; 1994. p. 1535-1537.

Cardiomyopathies

Cardiovascular system

Diseases of the heart that primarily affect the cardiac muscle.

Cause:

There are many causes of cardiomyopathy. The cause of the condition is classified as *primary* or *secondary.* A primary type is where the cause is not known. A secondary type is that due to some other associated disease such as infection (eg. bacterial myocarditis, viral myocarditis), electrolyte or nutritional deficiency (eg. thiamine deficiency), connective tissue disorders (eg. systemic lupus erythematosus, rheumatoid arthritis), amyloidosis, chronic alcoholism, muscular dystrophy, drug reaction etc. It may be due to familial diseases in some people.

Signs and Symptoms:

Cardiomyopathies present in different ways according to the type of pathology in the muscle. Some cardiomyopathies result in dilation (*congestive cardiomyopathy*) of the heart while others produce decrease in size (*restrictive cardiomyopathy*). Others may cause hypertrophy of the muscle.

In the dilated type the ventricle has difficulty in pumping the blood that reaches it with resultant backing up of blood and symptoms of congestive cardiac failure. Difficulty in breathing, fatigue, edema and palpitations are some of the symptoms.

In the restrictive type, there is difficulty in ventricular filling. Here too, there is backing up of blood in the venous vessels and edema, ascites and liver enlargement are common symptoms.

Notes

The prognosis is usually poor for people with dilated type of cardiomyopathy. Rarely, there may be spontaneous improvement. Anticoagulants may be given to reduce the incidence of embolus. Symptomatic treatment for congestive cardiac failure may be given. In severe cases, cardiac transplant may be considered. Treatment is symptomatic for other types. Since sudden death is common and usually occurs after strenuous exercise, undue physical exertion should be avoided.

For more details see Appendix C: Anticoagulants; Organ transplantation.

Many patients with *hypertrophic cardiomyopathy* do not have symptoms. Fatigue, angina pectoris and fainting spells are some of the symptoms that may be seen.

Risk Factors:

See Cause.

References

Wynne J, Braunwald E. The cardiomyopathies and myocarditides. In: Isselbacher KJ et al. Harrison's principles of internal medicine. 13th ed. London: McGraw-Hill Co; 1994. p. 1088-1093.

Caution and Recommendations to Therapists:

The client may be more comfortable in a half-lying or seated position for the massage. Enquire if the client is on anticoagulants. If yes, s/he is prone to bleeding. See Appendix D for organizations and support groups.

Carpal tunnel syndrome

Musculoskeletal, Nervous systems

The collection of signs and symptoms produced by compression of the median nerve in the wrist.

Cause:

In the hand, the median nerve supplies the muscles of the thenar eminence, and the first two lumbricals. Sensations are carried by it from the lateral three and a half fingers and distal part of the palm.

Notes

Carpal tunnel syndrome is treated by rest, splinting, and injection of corticosteroids. In some cases, surgery may be required to relieve the pressure on the nerve. For more details see Appendix C: Antiinflammatories - steroidal drugs.

Any condition that reduces the size of the tunnel formed by the transverse carpal ligament and the carpal bones can cause this syndrome. Reduction in size of the tunnel affects the functioning of the flexor tendons and the median nerve as they pass through it.

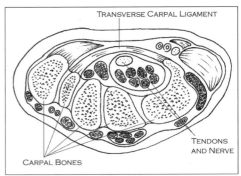

Section of hand at the wrist

The size of the tunnel can be reduced by bony or ligamentous changes, increase in the volume of contents as in inflammation of the tendons, edema or tumors. Systemic diseases like rheumatoid arthritis, hyperthyroidism, acromegaly and diabetes mellitus can also produce this condition. Other causes are pregnancy, use of contraceptive pills and wrist injury. Entrapment or injury of the median nerve in the elbow or shoulder (following whiplash injuries), displaced fracture of the distal radius, swelling of the common flexor sheath, dislocation of the carpal bone and vascular deficiency of the median nerve at the carpal tunnel are other causes.

Signs and Symptoms:

Pain in the wrist and hand, numbness of the thumb, pointer, middle finger and half of the ring finger, atrophy and weakness of the thenar muscles are some of the symptoms seen. Pain and reduced sensations are more at night. There is a tingling sensation radiating along the palm if the wrist is tapped (*Tinel's sign*). If the wrist is flexed over a minute or so, the patient feels numbness along the distribution of the median nerve (*Phalen test*). There may be clumsiness of movements that require fine coordination.

Risk Factors:

There is a higher risk in occupations requiring repetitive strains of the wrist by flexion, extension, pronation, supination, gripping, pinching movements and overwork of the muscles of the arm eg. massage therapists, secretaries, and pianists. Sewing, driving, operating computers, cash registers, playing squash, golf etc. are all activities that may predispose to this condition. Carpel tunnel syndrome is more common in women.

Caution and Recommendations to Therapists:

Since this is one of the occupational hazards, the Therapist should take precautions to prevent its onset by massaging the forearms and hands regularly. Practice stretching and range of motion exercises for the hands, shoulders and neck. Strengthen the forearm and hand muscles using isometric and isotonic exercises. Special exercise equipment is now available in the market. Maintenance of correct posture in occupations that strain the wrist can prevent carpal tunnel syndrome.

In a client, if the cause of the condition is due to endocrine or other systemic disease symptoms should disappear if the primary disease is treated by a Physician.

Avoid local massage over the wrist if there is acute inflammation n the region. In chronic conditions, lymphatic drainage techniques and elevation of the limb can reduce the local edema. The limb should be elevated above the level of the heart 5-10 minutes before massage. Deep, moist heat can help soften and allow stretch of collagen fibres that produce adhesions. Movement of the hand under warm water is another form of treatment. Techniques to stretch the flexor retinaculum should also be employed. Use cross fibre friction to loosen scar tissue and adherent fibres. Remember to keep the tendons taut while using this technique. Passively move the elbow, wrist and finger joints to maintain range of motion.

The neck, shoulders and arms should be thoroughly massaged. Ensure that the tissue is not damaged inadvertently by vigorously massaging regions with reduced sensation.

Help the client identify and avoid risk factors. Encourage clients to do remedial exercises such as passive stretching of flexors and extensors of wrist and fingers. Help the client correct postural dysfunctions, if any. The muscles of the shoulders have to be assessed and worked on as well.

Inially, half hour sessions twice a week for three weeks is recommended. See Appendix D for organizations and support groups.

References

Hackwood RA. Conservative treatment plan for carpal tunnel syndrome. BC Massage Practitioner 1997; Fall 17 (1): 19-22.

Hackwood R Understanding carpal tunnel syndrome. BC Massage Practitioner 16 (4) 1997; 17-22.

Crouch T, Madder M. Carpal tunnel syndrome and overuse injuries. Berkeley: North Atlantic books; 1992.

Cataract

Opacity of the lens of the eye.

Notes

No significant effect is produced by the use of drugs. Once the cataract has become mature, only surgical removal of the lens is beneficial. Many types of surgery exist for treating cataract.

Cause:

Cataract can be developmental or acquired. Viral infections in the mother such as German measles, maternal malnutrition and reduced availability of oxygen to the developing fetus are some causes. Acquired cataract is due to degeneration of the lens. The most common cause is aging (senile cataract). Vitamin B12 deficiency, administration of certain toxic substances (eg. naphthalene, thallium etc), hypocalcemia, prolonged use of corticosteroids, trauma, diabetes mellitus and exposure to radiation are some of the causes. Sometimes, inflammatory or degenerative disease of other parts of the eye can result in cataract by altering the availability of nutrition to the lens.

Signs and Symptoms:

The person complains of seeing spots before the eye. Objects may appear double or treble and colored halos may be seen. As the cataract progresses, the person has difficulty in vision.

Risk Factors:

The onset of senile cataract may be influenced by hereditary factors.

References

Miller SH. Parsons' diseases of the eye. 18th ed. New York: Churchill Livingstone; 1990.

Caution and Recommendations to Therapists:

Establish proper communication with those who have difficulty with vision and remember to explain in detail what you plan to do during the session and watch more carefully for verbal and non-verbal feedback.

Cellulitis

A superficial bacterial infection of the skin.

Notes

It is treated with oral antibiotics. For more details see Appendix C: Antimicrobial - antibacterial agents.

Cause:

It is usually caused by the *streptococci bacilli.*

Signs and Symptoms:

It presents as pain, redness and swelling of extensive areas of the skin along with enlargement of the lymph nodes draining the area. The bacteria secrete enzymes which breakdown the fibrin networks that confine the inflammation to one area. It may be associated with generalized symptoms like fever and body pain ie. flu-like symptoms.

Risk Factors:

It is more common in those with lowered immunity, diabetes, or after surgery.

Caution and Recommendations to Therapists:

Due to the pain and swelling, clients will not seek massage. If it is localized to a small area, avoid massage in and around the area, to prevent spread. Advice clients to seek medical help and take the full course of the prescribed antibiotic treatment. See Appendix D for organizations and support groups.

References

Morello JA, Mizer HE, Wilson ME, Granato PA. Microbiology in patient care. 6th ed. New York: McGraw-Hill; 1998. p. 514.

Cerebral palsy

A group of disorders that is non-progressive, affecting the nerves and muscles in children.

Nervous system

Cause:

Cerebral Palsy is caused by damage to the central nervous system of the baby during pregnancy, delivery or soon after birth. The damage could be due to bleeding, lack of oxygen or other injuries to the brain.

Signs and Symptoms:

The signs and symptoms depend on the area of the brain affected. A child may or may not have mental retardation. The speech is impaired in most individuals and there may be difficulty in swallowing. The muscles may be increased in tone - spastic, making coordinated movement difficult. The muscles are hyperexcitable and even small movements, touch, stretch of muscle, pain or emotional stress can increase the spasticity. Due to the spasticity, the posture is abnormal. The spasticity of muscles is altered with changes in posture. For example, if the head is moved to one side, the flexor muscles of the opposite side increase in tone. The gait is also affected. Some may have abnormal involuntary movements of the limbs that may be exaggerated on voluntarily performing a task. Associated weakness of muscles may be present. Seizures, problems with hearing and vision may be seen.

Notes

This condition cannot be cured but can be supported by a concerted effort of Doctors, Nurses, Physiotherapists, Massage Therapist and the family. The aim is to reduce stress, reduce spasticity, prevent contractures, improve the posture, improve circulation to skin and muscles that are unused and provide emotional support.

Risk Factors:

It is common in premature babies, and babies small in size for gestational age. The incidence is higher in Caucasian male babies. During pregnancy, rubella infection, diabetes, toxemia and malnutrition in the mother can increase the risk. At the time of delivery, damage may be caused by forceps delivery, breech delivery, abnormal placement of the placenta in the uterus, prolapse of the cord etc. - all conditions that result in reduced oxygen availability to the baby. Soon after delivery, brain infection, trauma to head etc. can predispose to cerebral palsy.

Caution and Recommendations to Therapists:

This condition cannot be cured but can be supported by a concerted effort of Doctors, Nurses, Physiotherapist, Massage Therapist and the family. Though these individuals are physically and mentally challenged, it is important for the Therapist to consider them as a person first and the impairment should take the backseat.

References

Fritz S. Mosby's fundamentals of therapeutic massage. St. Louis: Mosby - yearbook Inc; 1995. p. 339-342.

The aim is to reduce stress, reduce spasticity, prevent contractures, improve the posture, improve circulation to skin and muscles that are unused and provide an emotional support. Since any form of stress increases the symptom, a relaxing massage helps reduce the spasms and involuntary movements. Passive movements and range of motion exercises of joints prevent contractures of muscles. Use transverse friction strokes around joints. Do not use force to stretch muscles that are in spasm.

Since most individuals are confined to bed or wheel chair they are prone for decubitus (stress) ulcers and edema in the dependent parts such as the legs or sacral region. The poor circulation in these areas makes the skin very fragile with a tendency to breakdown with minimal pressure. Avoid massaging areas with ulcers and bring it to the notice of the caregivers. Some clients may have reduced sensations. Also, due to mental retardation or speech disorder they may be unable to give adequate feedback about pressure and pain. Use only mild to moderate pressure throughout. Schedule massages once a week or once in two weeks. To reduce spasticity, use rhythmic, repetitive strokes with each session. Initially each session should last for 15-20 minutes. Tapotement of the antagonist muscles help reduce the spasm in the agonist muscle eg. tapotement to flexors can reduce the spasticity of the extensors. See Appendix D for organizations and support groups.

Reproductive system

Cervicitis

An inflammation of the cervix.

Cause:

It is due to an infection by fungus, bacteria or virus.

Signs and Symptoms:

The symptoms are usually low back pain, excessive white discharge, painful intercourse and dysmenorrhea (painful menstruation).

Risk Factors:

Cervicitis may be a sequelae to infections of the uterus or vagina.

Caution and Recommendations to Therapists:

Massage over the low back and lower abdomen may help relieve some of the pain. A comfortable position is for the client to lie face down, with the head turned to one side, and with the heels rolled apart. A pillow may be placed under the abdomen and another under the lower leg so that the hip and knee joints are slightly flexed.

Notes

It is treated by minor surgical techniques that destroy the superficial layer of the affected tissue. Antibiotics may also be given. For more details see Appendix C: Antimicrobial - antibacterial agents.

References

Berek JS, editor. Novak's gynecology. 12th ed. Philadelphia: Williams & Wilkins; 1996. p. 346,435.

Chagas' disease (American trypanosomiasis)

An infection caused by the parasite Trypanosoma cruzi.

Cause:

The parasite is transmitted from one host to another by infected insects or reduviid bugs that suck blood from animals or humans. The organisms multiply in the insect and are discharged in the feces. The next animal/human is infected when the feces containing the organisms enter the body via breaks in the mucous membrane, skin or through the conjunctiva. The organisms may be transmitted when infected blood is used for transfusion.

Signs and Symptoms:

A firm, inflamed lesion known as *chagoma* is seen at the site of entry within one week of infection. The draining lymph nodes may be enlarged. If the conjunctiva is infected, there is painless edema of the eyelid and surrounding tissue of that eye. Fever and loss of appetite may occur. The acute symptoms disappear spontaneously. The symptoms of chronic infection appear only years after the initial infection. The organism is disseminated throughout the body via the lymphatics and blood and inflammatory reactions occur in various organs. The heart is the most commonly affected organ. Enlargement, thinning of the walls, arrhythmias, formation of aneurysm and thrombi are some of the problems seen. When the gastrointestinal tract is affected, there is dilatation of the esophagus and colon. The individual may present with difficulty in swallowing (dysphagia), chest pain and regurgitation of food. Aspiration of food into the respiratory tract may occur during sleep with resultant lung infection. Those with enlarged colon may complain of abdominal pain and suffer from chronic constipation.

Risk Factors:

The organism is found in the Americas. There is a higher incidence in Latin America as the bugs find residence in the wood and stone houses more commonly seen there.

Caution and Recommendations to Therapists:

Though this condition is an infection it is not easily transferred from one person to another by direct contact. A detailed history and signs and symptoms have to be obtained and an individualized treatment planned.

Ensure that the clinic is 'insect proof'. See Appendix D for organizations and support groups. Also see Appendix B: Strategies for infection prevention and safe practice.

Notes

The disease is treated with specific drugs such as nitfurtimox, but the treatment is unsatisfactory and does not produce a cure. Vaccines are not available. Prevention is best. Spraying of insecticides, use of mosquito nets and insect repellents, improvement in housing and proper screening of blood before transfusion are some of the measures that can be taken to prevent the disease.

For more details see Appendix C: Blood transfusion.

References

Kirchoff LV. Chagas' disease. In: Isselbacher KJ et al. Harrison's principles of internal medicine. 13th ed. London: McGraw-Hill Co; 1994. p. 899-901.

Chicken pox (Varicella)

A viral infection which produces skin rashes.

Cause:

It is caused by the chickenpox virus. Chickenpox is highly contagious and the virus is transmitted by direct contact, airborne or droplet respiratory secretions. The incubation period ranges from 2-3 weeks.

Notes

Usually no treatment is indicated. Lotions or medication to reduce itching may be prescribed.

The chickenpox virus can remain dormant in the dorsal root ganglia of the spinal sensory nerves and years later get reactivated to present as shingles/herpes zoster (see herpes zoster). Vaccines are available against chickenpox.

For more details see Appendix C: Immunization.

Signs and Symptoms:

Usually, there is no flu-like symptoms preceding the rash. The rashes appear as fluid-filled vesicles in any part of the body. The rashes develop first on the trunk and then spread to the face and extremities. Fresh crops of vesicles occur over the next 3-5 days. The vesicles slowly become pustules (filled with pus) and finally crusts are formed.

Healing of individual lesions occur in a week. Itching is more during the stage of healing. Mild fever, muscle pain and irritability may be present. In those who are immunocompromised the symptoms are severe and may be fatal.

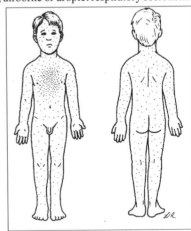

Section of hand at the wrist

Risk Factors:

Exposure to an infected individual increases the risk. Patients are infectious from approximately 48 hours prior to the appearance of the rash until all vesicles are crusted. Infection occurs 10-14 days after exposure to another individual with chicken pox or herpes zoster (See Appendix A: Figure 9). Children between the ages of 5 and 9 are most commonly affected.

Caution and Recommendations to Therapists:

Individuals are infective until the crusts are formed on the lesions. Those who are exposed to the disease should refrain from work from days 10-21 after exposure. See Appendix D for organizations and support groups. Also see Appendix B: Strategies for infection prevention and safe practice.

References

Morello JA, Mizer HE, Wilson ME, Granato PA. Microbiology in patient care. 6th ed. New York: McGraw-Hill; 1998. p. 291-292.

Chilblains (Pernio)

A condition where cyanosis and swelling occurs a few hours after exposure to cold.

Cause:

Notes

Use of warm clothing and effective heating are some of the preventive measures used. The drug nifedipine has been found to be

The exact cause is not known. Inflammation in and around blood vessels has been shown to occur.

Signs and Symptoms:

Swelling, itching, blue discoloration (cyanosis) and raised red or purple plaques are seen in the areas exposed to cold. A burning sensation may be felt. The lesions may form blisters and ulcerate. The hands, face, ears, legs and toes are usually affected. The lesion develops within 12 to 24 hours of exposure and resolves within 2-3 weeks.

Risk Factors:

It is more common in women. The incidence is higher in northern Europe probably due to the damp and cold climate.

Caution and Recommendations to Therapists:

Avoid areas of chilblains. Do not use cold packs as it may aggravate the condition.

beneficial. Ulcers should be kept clean and sterile to prevent superinfection.

References

Craeger MA, Dzau VJ. Vascular diseases of the extremities. In: Isselbacher KJ et al. Harrison's principles of internal medicine. 13th ed. London: McGraw-Hill Co; 1994. p. 1140.

Cholecystitis

Gastrointestinal system

An inflammation of the gall bladder.

Cause:

Partial or complete blockage of the bile duct and flow of bile cause this condition. The chemical irritation of the concentrated bile produces an inflammatory reaction in the gall bladder. Infection from the gut may spread to the area resulting in further damage. The gall bladder dilates and swells. Death of tissue can cause gangrene and perforation of the gall bladder with spillage of bile into the peritoneal cavity and further complications.

Signs and Symptoms:

Indigestion and colicky pain may be present especially after a fatty meal. The pain is located in the right upper quadrant of the abdomen and may be referred to the back, the right shoulder, right scapula or between the scapula. If perforation has occurred, the muscles in the upper right quadrant go into a spasm and the area is tender to touch. Vomiting may be present. The inflammation causes fever in the individual.

Risk Factors:

Blockage to the flow of bile as in gallstones, obstruction by enlarged lymph nodes or tumors in neighboring areas can predispose to this condition.

Caution and Recommendations to Therapists:

Encourage the client to reduce weight and be active. Avoid massage to the right upper quadrant of the abdomen. See Appendix D for organizations and support groups.

Notes

Cholecystectomy - removal of the gall bladder is the treatment of choice. Since the function of the gall bladder is only to collect, concentrate and store bile, surgical removal of the gall bladder does not compromise normal digestion and function.

For more details see Appendix C: Cholecystectomy.

References

Nahrwold DL. Acute cholecystitis. In: Sabiston DC, editor. Textbook of Surgery-the biological basis of modern surgical practice. 14th ed. WB Saunders Co; 1991. p. 1050-1063.

Cholera

A bacterial infection that results in acute diarrheal disease.

Cause:

The infection is caused by the organism *Vibrio cholerae*. The infection can be spread by eating contaminated shellfish or drinking water contaminated with infected human feces. It may also spread by eating contaminated food at home or restaurants. The organism requires salt for multiplication and thrives in coastal water or in tidal rivers and bays, especially at higher temperatures (summer months).

The ingested organism resides in the small intestines. The toxins produced change the activity of the intestinal cells causing sodium chloride (salt) to enter the lumen. The salt passively draws water into the lumen ultimately resulting in watery diarrhoea.

Signs and Symptoms:

There is an acute onset of painless, watery diarrhoea. The diarrheal content is slightly cloudy due to flecks of mucus and is typically described as *'rice water' stools* as it resembles the water in which rice has been washed. The diarrhoea begins within 24 to 48 hours after infection. It may be accompanied with vomiting. If the fluid and electrolytes are not promptly replaced the person becomes dehydrated very quickly and goes into shock. Electrolyte imbalances present as muscle cramps. Hypotension, weakness, thirst, rapid pulse, lax and wrinkled skin, reduced urine and sunken eyes are some of the signs of dehydration.

Risk Factors:

See Cause. For some unknown reason, people of blood type O are more susceptible and those of type AB the least.

Caution and Recommendations to Therapists:

The client is too ill to seek a Therapist. Refer to Appendix B: Strategies for infection prevention and safe practice, to prevent spread of infectious diseases in your clinic. Also see Appendix D for organizations and support groups.

References

Morello JA, Mizer HE, Wilson ME, Granato PA. Microbiology in patient care. 6th ed. New York: McGraw-Hill; 1998. p. 340-342.

Chondromalacia

Softening of the articular cartilage of joints.

Cause:

Chondromalacia is more common in the knee joint, with softening of the undersurface of the patella. It may be due to overuse of the joints as happens in professional athletes or caused by recurrent subluxation of the patella.

Signs and Symptoms:

The patient complains of pain especially when using the joint. In the case of the knee joint, pain is more on climbing stairs or on bending the knee. There may be weakness of the joint.

Risk Factors:

It is more common in young adults.

Caution and Recommendations to Therapists:

In the acute phase encourage client to rest. Application of compression and ice is helpful. In subacute and chronic stages, massage to the quadriceps from origin to insertion may help reduce the stiffness and pain by increasing blood flow and lymph drainage. Work in conjunction with a Physiotherapist to increase the strength and stability of the quadriceps muscle.

the patella may have to be removed by surgery or shaved using instruments inserted through an arthroscope.

For more details see Appendix C: Arthroscopy.

References
Mercier LR, editor. Practical orthopedics. 4th ed. New York: Mosby-Year book Inc. 1995. p. 219-221, 304-305.

Chronic Fatigue Syndrome (Chronic Fatigue &
Immune Dysfunction Syndrome; CFIDS; Chronic Epstein-Barr virus infection; Myalgic encephalomyelitis; Yuppie flu)

Nervous, Musculoskeletal systems

A chronic illness characterized by persistent or relapsing, debilitating fatigue.

Cause:

The cause is unknown. Earlier it was thought that it was caused by an infection by the *Epstein-Barr virus*. Now it is believed that the high level of antibodies to the virus is because of the disease. It may be associated with a reaction to a viral infection in those with an abnormal immune response. Age, genetic predisposition, gender, stress, environment and previous illness influence this abnormal immune response.

Signs and Symptoms:

It is characterized by prolonged extreme fatigue. Specific criteria have been formulated by the Centers for Disease Control to diagnose the disease. A person should have 2 *major criteria*, at least 8 of the 11 *symptom criteria*, or 6 of the symptom criteria along with 2 *physical criteria*.

Major criteria - a) new onset of persistent or recurrent fatigue in a person without a history of similar symptoms. The fatigue is not resolved by bed rest and impairs the normal daily activity of a person by 50% for 6 months. b) there is no sign of any other disorder on examination and laboratory investigations.

Symptom criteria - a) extreme fatigue especially after what was considered as a minimal exercise by the person when not having these symptoms b) mild fever c) painful lymph nodes d) muscle weakness e) muscle pain f) sleep disturbances g) headache h) fleeting pain in the joints that migrates from one joint to another, without joint swelling or signs of inflammation i) forgetfulness, irritability, confusion, depression, photophobia, difficulty thinking, inability to concentrate.

Notes

As yet, there is no treatment available to cure the condition. Treatment is only supportive in the form of antidepressants, painkillers, massage etc. Moderate, graded exercise regimen should be advised.

For more details see Appendix C: Antidepressants; Painkillers.

Physical criteria - a) low-grade fever b) sore throat c) palpable or painful lymph nodes. These findings should be recorded at least twice, one month apart.

Risk Factors:

It is more common in women below the age of 45.

Caution and Recommendations to Therapists:

The symptoms vary from individual to individual and in the same individual from day to day. Hence a proper history is warranted on every occasion. The techniques should be modified accordingly. In general, a gentle, whole body relaxation massage of short duration is recommended. The feedback may be inadequate if the client is on painkillers and tissue damage may be done inadvertently by the Therapist, so use only gentle pressure. Massage has been shown to relieve pain and discomfort and to improve sleep in these clients. Refer client to a local support group if available. See Appendix D for organizations and support groups.

References

LeBrun H. In the treatment of Chronic Fatigue Syndrome. Massage & Bodywork. 1998; Winter: p106-109, 111.

Information for clients and doctors about chronic fatigue syndrome. The chronic fatigue clinic, Harborview medical Center, Seattle, Washington, 1997.

The facts about chronic fatigue syndrome. US Department of health and human services, Public Health Service, Center for Disease Control and Prevention, National Center for Infectious Disease. Atlanta, Georgia. March 1995.

Gastrointestinal system	# Cirrhosis
	A chronic disease of the liver.

Cause:

There are many causes of cirrhosis (Greek: *kirrhos* - yellowish-orange; *osis* - condition). The most common cause is damage to the liver in chronic alcoholism. It can also be a complication of viral hepatitis. Prolonged obstruction to the flow of bile, toxic reaction to certain drugs, prolonged congestion of blood in the liver due to right heart failure and autoimmune reaction are other causes. Rarely, no known cause is found.

There is destruction, death and regeneration of the hepatic tissue with distortion of the normal architecture. The process results in extensive fibrosis and impairment to blood and lymph drainage with loss of normal function.

Signs and Symptoms:

General symptoms include weight loss, weakness and loss of appetite. Jaundice is usually present. The liver and spleen may be enlarged and can be palpated as a swelling in the right and left upper quadrant of the abdomen respectively. The distortion of the architecture of the liver results in damming up of blood and increased pressure in the veins of the abdomen. This causes fluid to move out of the capillaries into the peritoneal cavity (ascites). The fluid accumulation can be so extensive that ripples can be felt and heard if the abdomen is shaken. The damming also forces the blood to find alternative routes to reach the right heart. One of the routes is through the anastomoses in the esophagus. Thus in people with cirrhosis and high blood pressure in the portal veins (*portal hypertension*) there is danger of the dilated esophageal blood vessels rupturing

Notes

Treatment is largely supportive. Dietary alterations with daily multivitamin supplements and at least 1g of protein per kg body weight and 2000-3000 kcal per day should be advocated. Fat-soluble vitamins should be given as injections periodically. Alcohol should be forbidden. All medicines should be administered with care - especially those degraded by the liver, to avoid drug toxicity. Complications such as ascites and portal hypertension may require specific treatment. Hepatic transplantation may be considered for those with advanced disease.

For more details see Appendix C: Organ transplantation.

and causing fatal hemorrhage. Dilated blood vessels are also seen around the umbilicus and anal region (see Appendix A: page 357: Spider nevi).

The build up of toxins in the blood affects the nervous system producing lethargy, mental changes and finally coma. The toxins (ketones) cause a musty smell to the breath.

The alteration in the metabolism of steroidal hormones produces menstrual irregularities in women and development of breast (*gynecomastia*), loss of chest and axillary hair in men.

The deposition of bilirubin under the skin causes the yellow coloration, severe itching and dryness of skin (see Jaundice). Hepatic failure can also produce edema due to the lack of the protein albumin. The white blood cells are decreased in number making the individual prone to infection.

The impairment of liver function is reflected in various other ways. The lack of clotting factors causes easy bruisability and bleeding tendencies. See Appendix A: page 355: Purpura. Reduction in bile formation affects the digestion and absorption of fat and fat-soluble vitamins A, D, E and K.

Risk Factors:

See Cause. The amount and duration of consumption of alcohol is an important determinant of liver injury.

Caution and Recommendations to Therapists:

Obtain a detailed history from the client and call the Physician, if necessary, as to the infectivity. If the cirrhosis is due to viral hepatitis, the person may be in a carrier state and can transmit hepatitis (refer to hepatitis). A gentle full body massage avoiding the abdominal area may be beneficial. Do not try to reduce the edema that may be present in the legs and other areas. The massage oil may help reduce the itching and dryness of the skin. Remember that sensations especially in the distal ends of the limbs may be altered in people with cirrhosis and feedback is likely to be inadequate. These individuals also have a bleeding tendency and bruise easily. Hence use only gentle pressure. They are prone to infection due to the reduction in white blood cells. Do not massage if you are harboring any kind of infection. See Appendix D for organizations and support groups.

References

Podolsky DK, Isselbacher KJ. Alcohol-related liver disease and cirrhosis. In: Isselbacher KJ et al. Harrison's principles of internal medicine. 13th ed. London: McGraw-Hill Co; 1994. p. 1483-1495.

Clubfoot (Talipes equinovarus)

A congenital disorder of the foot giving it a club-like appearance. The talus is deformed and the Achilles tendon is shortened.

Musculoskeletal system

Cause:

Clubfoot may be due to genetic abnormalities. Environmental factors in utero especially in the 9th and 10th week of pregnancy or muscle abnormalities can also cause this condition. It may be seen secondary to poliomyelitis, cerebral palsy and paralysis.

Notes

Clubfoot is easily diagnosed and is treated with corrective shoes or by surgery.

Signs and Symptoms:

The deformity varies in severity, with the worst form being to the extent of the toe touching the ankle. The talus is deformed and the calf muscles are shortened with contractures at the site of deformity. It is a painless condition.

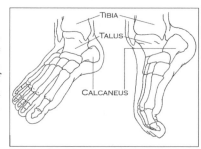

Risk Factors:

It is more common in boys. Family history of clubfoot may be a predisposing factor. It may be associated with other birth defects like spina bifida and myelomeningocele.

Caution and Recommendations to Therapists:

References
Adams JC. Hamblen DL. Outline of orthopaedics. 11th ed. London: Churchill Livingstone; 1990. p. 263-368.

Do not force the foot into a normal position. Relaxation massage with friction movements in the affected foot is beneficial. Thoroughly massage other muscles of the body that are stressed by compensating for the deformity. Work in conjunction with Physiotherapist.

Nervous system

Coma

A state of unconsciousness where the person cannot be aroused by stimulation and there is no purposeful attempt by the person to avoid painful stimuli.

Notes

Acute respiratory and cardiovascular problems should be attended to at once. Measures to prevent further central nervous system damage are also taken. Tracheal intubation and/or use of mechanical ventilation may be required. Also, an intravenous access has to be established. The cause of the coma has to be identified by taking a thorough history from family and observers and by physical examination.

The prognosis varies with the age, type of disease etc. A 'Glasgow Coma Scale' has been devised to predict (to some extent) the prognosis of clients in coma.

For more details see Appendix C: Intubation; Mechanical ventilation.

References

Wine ZK. Russian Medical Massage: coma. Massage 1994; 60 (August): 90,92.

Ropper AH, Martin JB. Coma and other disorders of consciousness. In: Isselbacher KJ et al. Harrison's principles of internal medicine. 13th ed. London: McGraw-Hill Co; 1994. p. 146-153.

Ivan L, Bruce D. Coma. Springfield: Ill, Charles C Thomas; 1982.

Cause:

The reticular activating system (located in the brainstem) and its connections to the cerebral hemispheres are responsible for wakefulness and any condition that depresses the functioning of these regions can result in coma. Coma may be due to damage to the cerebrum or suppression of its function by lack of oxygen (hypoxia), hypoglycemia, epilepsy, diabetic ketoacidosis, drugs and toxins or due to brainstem lesions.

Signs and Symptoms:

The person does not respond to various stimuli.

Risk Factors:

See Cause.

Caution and Recommendations to Therapists:

Gentle touch may serve as a sensory stimulant in these clients. Due to the immobility, muscles may be atrophied and joints stiff. They are also prone to bedsores. Since the cause of the coma varies and treatment options vary with the cause, the Physician should be consulted. It is important to obtain written consent from guardians / care givers.

Pathology A to Z -

Common cold (Rhinitis)

An acute inflammation of the upper respiratory tract due to viral infection.

Cause:

It is usually caused by a virus. Rarely, mycoplasma may produce this condition. There are hundreds of viruses like rhinovirus, adenovirus, coxsackievirus, echovirus etc. that can produce this condition. It is transmitted from person to person by airborne respiratory droplets, contact with contaminated objects like cups, doorknobs and hand-to-hand contact. A person is infective for 2-3 days after the onset of symptoms.

Signs and Symptoms:

The incubation period is from 1- 4 days. It presents as sore throat, congestion of nose, watery eyes, headache and dry cough. It may be associated with fever, body ache, lethargy and joint pains. The major symptoms subside after 2-3 days but the stuffiness of the nose may persist for a week. Rarely, complications like sinusitis, otitis media (ear infection), pharyngitis and lower respiratory tract infection occur.

Risk Factors:

People with lowered immunity are more prone to frequent colds.

Caution and Recommendations to Therapists:

A cold may resemble more serious illness like measles and rubella (German Measles). If the body temperature is above 100 degrees centigrade accompanied by exudate from the throat or tender enlarged lymph glands it is unlikely to be a common cold. Educate clients on using other remedies like steam vaporizers and heating pads for relief of pain and stuffiness. Do not massage immuno-compromised or susceptible individuals when you have a cold. Wash hands frequently, cover coughs and sneezes. Avoid sharing of towels and drinks. Consider wearing a mask if it is necessary to massage a client while having a cold. Ideally, the Therapist should cancel appointments and take bed rest until no longer infective. See Appendix B: Strategies for infection prevention and safe practice.

Notes:

Antibiotics are not indicated for common cold. Usually, common cold is mild and self-limited. Analgesics and nasal decongestants may be beneficial.

For more details see Appendix C: Antimicrobial - antibacterial; Painkillers; Nose drops/Nasal decongestants.

References

Maran AGD, editor. Logan Turner's diseases of the nose, throat and ear. 10th ed. London: Wright; 1988. p. 34-36.

Li J. Prevention and treatment of rhinitis and common cold by self-massage. Journal of Traditional Chinese Medicine 1992; 12(4): 290-291.

Concussion

An immediate, transient loss of consciousness often associated with loss of memory for a short period.

Cause:

It usually follows a sudden, blunt impact to the skull that results in sudden movement of the brain inside the skull.

Signs and Symptoms:

Some people may have a short convulsion or autonomic response such as hypotension, slowing of the heart rate and sluggish pupillary reaction. A brief

Notes

The person has to be closely monitored to rule out more severe injury.

a Handbook for Massage Therapists

period of loss of consciousness and memory may follow. Memory may be lost for more recent events (moments before impact or spans a few weeks before that) and the extent of memory loss depends on the severity of the injury.

Headaches, faintness, nausea, difficulty concentrating and blurring of vision are some of the common symptoms. The headache may last for a few days. The patient is fully alert and attentive.

Risk Factors:

Use of seatbelt and helmets can reduce the incidence of head injury and concussion.

Caution and Recommendations to Therapists:

Avoid massage until the cause of the concussion has been found and clearance has been obtained from a treating physician.

References

Ropper A. Trauma of the head and spine. In: Isselbacher KJ et al. Harrison's principles of internal medicine. 13th ed. London: McGraw-Hill Co; 1994. p. 2321-2322.

Cardiovascular system	# Congenital heart disease

A defect in the formation of the heart that usually decreases its efficiency.

Cause:

Notes

Depending on its severity, treatment varies. Usually it is corrected by surgery.

The cause of the congenital heart disease is often unknown. Defects in the formation of the heart may be associated with other genetic disorders eg. Down's syndrome. Some types of heart defects are more prevalent in premature infants. Rarely, defects may be a result of ingestion of certain drugs (eg. thalidomide), or exposure of the fetus to high levels of alcohol (as in infants born to alcoholic mothers) or viral infections in the mother during the early stages of pregnancy.

The defects may be in the form of nonclosure of opening between the right and left ventricle - *ventricular septal defects;*

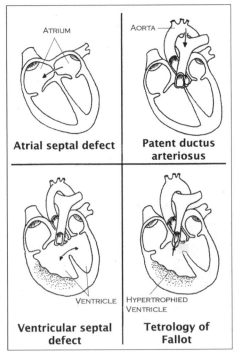

Atrial septal defect

Patent ductus arteriosus

Ventricular septal defect

Tetrology of Fallot

Pathology A to Z -

nonclosure of the opening between the right and left atrium - *atrial septal defect*, narrowing of the aorta - *coarctation of the aorta*; narrowing of the pulmonary artery - *pulmonary stenosis*; nonclosure of the communication between the pulmonary artery and the aorta that exists in the fetus until delivery - *patent ductus arteriosus*; or a combination of defects - *Tetralogy of Fallot* (ventricular hypertrophy, pulmonary stenosis, ventricular septal defect and over riding of the aorta).

Signs and Symptoms:

The symptoms vary according to the type and severity of the defect. If the defect is mild, the person is asymptomatic. Heart murmurs (abnormal sounds in the heart) may be heard. In some, there may be difficulty in breathing on exertion and the person has cyanosis (ble coloration due to increased deoxygenated blood) at rest or on exertion. Palpitations may be present. If oxygenation of blood is inadequate, normal growth is affected. Slowly, as the demand on the heart is increased, the heart begins to fail - heart failure. The blood that returns to the heart is not pumped out efficiently, and the damming up of blood in the venous circulation leads to development of edema in the liver and the legs. If the left ventricle begins to fail, edema can develop in the lungs (see heart failure).

Risk Factors:

Exposure of a pregnant woman to radiation, certain viral infection, drugs or alcohol in the early months of pregnancy may cause heart defects in the fetus. Premature infants are more prone to certain types of heart problems.

Caution and Recommendations to Therapists:

Take a proper history regarding symptoms, signs and medical/surgical treatment. It is wise to get clearance from the treating Physician if the client exhibits symptoms of heart failure. The duration and frequency of massage have to be decided on an individual basis. In general, a full body relaxation massage in a comfortable position (often seated position is most comfortable), for a short duration is recommended. Support the body using pillows under the knee, arms and legs. See Appendix D for organizations and support groups.

References

Friedman WF, Child JS. Congenital heart disease in the adult. In: Isselbacher KJ et al. Harrison's principles of internal medicine. 13th ed. London: McGraw-Hill Co; 1994. p. 1037-1046.
Friedman WF. Congenital heart disease in infancy and childhood. In: Braunwald E, editor. Heart disease. 4th ed. Phuladelphia: Saunders; 1992. p. 887.

Conjunctivitis

Integumentary, Nervous systems

An inflammation of the conjunctiva (the mucosa lining the external surface of the eye).

Cause:

Conjunctivitis or pink eye may be caused by many factors. Often it is an infection. The infection may be viral or bacterial. In some it may be due to sexually transmitted infections like gonorrhea and Chlamydial infection. The infection spreads by contact with the secretions from the eye of the infected

Notes

Conjunctivitis is treated with antibiotic eye ointments/ drops if due to infection. Drops to reduce inflammation are given for conditions due to other causes.

For more details see Appendix C: Antimicrobial - antibacterial agents; Eye drops.

person. Conjunctivitis may also be due to a reaction to chemicals instilled into the eye for other reasons.

Signs and Symptoms:

There is itching, redness, watering and sometimes a pus-like discharge from the eye. The eyelids may stick to each other because of the secretions.

Risk Factors:

Direct contact with the secretions of the infected individual increases the risk.

Caution and Recommendations to Therapists:

Do not massage an individual with conjunctivitis of infective origin until all symptoms have gone. Encourage the client to see an Ophthalmologist if they exhibit symptoms of conjunctivitis. See Appendix D for organizations and support groups. Also see Appendix B: Strategies for infection prevention and safe practice.

References

Miller SH. Parsons' diseases of the eye. 18th edition. New York: Churchill Livingstone; 1990. p. 128-141.

Constipation

Gastrointestinal system

A condition where there is difficulty in passing stools or incomplete/infrequent passage of stools. It has been defined as a frequency of defecation of less than three times per week.

Cause:

There are many causes of constipation (Latin: *constipare - to crowd together*). They include direct obstruction of the lumen as seen in tumors, diverticulitis or intestinal obstruction. Other causes include failure to respond to the urge to defecate, diet with reduced fibre intake, reduced fluid intake and drugs that slow down the motility of the gut. The desire to defecate may be inhibited by painful conditions like hemorrhoids or fissures. Constipation may be made worse by chronic illnesses that result in reduced physical activity.

It may be caused by alteration in the motility of the colon by disruption of its' parasympathetic innervation as seen in spinal cord injuries of the lumbosacral region, multiple sclerosis and lesions of the central nervous system (eg. Parkinsonism, stroke). In a condition called *Hirschsprung's disease*, the nerve plexus in the distal colon is absent resulting in contraction in this region and difficulty in passing stools.

People with diabetes or who are hypothyroid may have mild constipation. It is also common during pregnancy as the altered estrogen and progesterone levels affect the motility of the gut.

In many cases, no cause can be identified.

Signs and Symptoms:

Feeling of abdominal fullness, back pain, excessive straining, a sense of incomplete evacuation and loss of appetite are some of the symptoms that accompany the infrequent passage of stools.

Notes

Treatment of constipation should be individualized, taking into account the age of the person, duration of constipation, predisposing factors etc. Initially, it is treated by increasing dietary fiber intake.

Different types of laxatives may be used. However, prolonged use of laxatives should be discouraged. Bulk-forming laxatives are similar to fibers in that they work by increasing the weight of stools. Emollient laxatives, eg. mineral oils work by softening the stools. Hyperosmolar solutions work by moving water into the colon by osmosis and increasing the bulk and softening the stools. Stimulant laxatives like castor oil stimulate the colon and increase intestinal motility. Biofeedback techniques may be effective in people who have inadequate contraction of the muscles of the pelvic floor.

For more details see Appendix C: Biofeedback; Laxatives.

Risk Factors:

Sedentary lifestyle, prolonged bed rest, ingestion of drugs like diuretics, calcium, iron, aluminium hydroxide (antacids), laxatives, codeine, antidepressants and drugs that mimic the action of the sympathetic nervous system are all predisposing factors. It is more common in the elderly. Also see Cause.

Caution and Recommendations to Therapists:

If the onset of constipation is sudden, with associated colicky pain, it is likely to be due to some form of intestinal obstruction. Massage is contraindicated in such situations. A full body massage with special abdominal techniques is beneficial to those with constipation due to other causes.

Massage reduces stress and inhibits the sympathetic system. For abdominal massage, position the client supine, with the knee and hip flexed. Pillows can be used under the knee for support. Standing to the right of the client, begin with vibration over the four quadrants of the abdomen. Then use overhanded effleurage. The strokes should be in a clockwise direction along the movement of the feces. In order to loosen the impacted feces, use kneading strokes in the lower left quadrant - ie. over the descending and sigmoid colon followed by the left upper quadrant ie. over the splenic flexure of the colon, then the right upper quadrant ie. over the hepatic flexure of the colon, and finally the right lower quadrant ie. over the caecum. This sequence of kneading helps to soften the faeces in the end closest to the anus first and then works backwards. Follow this up by firm strokes in the clockwise direction. In addition, stretching of the colon can be done by stabilizing one end with firm pressure with the fingertips.

While stretching the descending colon, fix its lower end just medial to the left anterior superior iliac spine; for transverse colon, fix the splenic flexure - below the ribs on the left; for the ascending colon, fix the hepatic flexure below the right costal margin. Repeat effleurage in a clockwise direction. In the prone position, massage the muscles in the lumbar, gluteal and sacral region. Depending on the client, a four-week schedule at a frequency of twice a week for two weeks followed by once a week is recommended. Encourage client to alter dietary habits and consume more fluids, fruits, vegetables and whole grain cereal. Recommend regular exercise training. See Appendix D for organizations and support groups.

References

Friedman LS, Isselbacher KJ. Diarrhea and constipation. In: Isselbacher KJ et al. Harrison's principles of internal medicine. 13th ed. London: McGraw-Hill Co; 1994. p. 219-221.

Contact dermatitis

Integumentary system

An inflammation of the skin due to irritants or allergens.

Cause:

It is an inflammation resulting from disruption of the natural physiological barrier property of the stratum corneum and stratum granulosum of the skin against entry by foreign matter or organisms. The removal of the fat in the stratum corneum by various external processes reduces the ability of this layer

Notes

Contact dermatitis is not contagious. The contactant that produced the reaction has to be identified by detailed history and avoided. Antihistamines are given to reduce itching. Lotions containing corticosteroids are used to reduce the inflammatory reaction. In severe cases, oral steroids may be given.

For more details see Appendix C: Antihistamines; Antiinflammatories - steroidal drugs.

to retain water. It also makes it ineffective as a barrier. In the specific type of contact dermatitis, the irritant is carried through the skin to the local lymph nodes where proliferation of lymphocytes that react specific to the chemical occurs. Thus in subsequent exposures to the chemical, the individual develops a reaction.

Signs and Symptoms:

There may be mild redness, edema and severe itching on exposure to the chemical. It may progress to vesicles or bullae. In chronic stages with prolonged exposure to the irritant or allergen, there is dryness, scaling and thickening of the skin. See Appendix A: page 350. Secondary bacterial infections may occur in the region.

Risk Factors:

A history of allergy increases the risk.

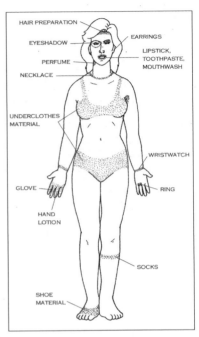

Common locations and possible causes of contact dermatitis

Repeated washing of hands with soap, detergents, exposure to specific chemicals in predisposed individuals can increase the risk. The allergens may include fats such as coconut oil, olive oil, palm oil, fish and whale oil, fat soluble chemicals, perfume, seed oil, oil of bergamot, bitter almond oil, eucalyptus oil, geranium oil, lavender oil, peppermint oil, rosemary oil, linseed oil, musk, rubber, metals, metal salts, turpentine, gloves, foot wear, oak, pine (reaction to the resin or turpentine used for treating the wood) etc.

Caution and Recommendations to Therapists:

Always get a thorough history of previous dermatitis and allergies. Keep accurate records of the list of chemicals the client is allergic to. In new clients with a history of allergy or dermatitis, test a small area of skin with a drop of oil that is going to be used and watch for itching, redness and swelling. Wash area immediately and thoroughly if a reaction is seen. Keep antipyretic creams (reduces itching) handy in case it sets off a reaction. Avoid using oils with aroma in such clients unless sure that it will not produce a reaction. If the reaction is severe, the client may require antihistaminics or even oral steroids. Refer immediately to physician. See Appendix D for organizations and support groups.

References

Fitzpatrick TB et al, editors. Dermatology in general medicine. 3rd ed. New York: McGraw-Hill; 1987.

Pathology A to Z -

Contusion

An injury to the surface of the brain that may follow head injury.

Cause:

Contusion to the surface of the brain follows head injury that causes the brain to move within the skull and impact on the inner surfaces of the skull. The brain directly beneath the point of impact may be injured (*coup injury*) or the region in the opposite side of the impact may be injured (*contrecoup injury*) due to the slow movement of the brain relative to the skull.

There is mild hemorrhage and edema on the surface of the injured brain and can be visualised on CT scan.

Signs and Symptoms:

The signs depend on the location and extent of the injury. Dizziness, vomiting, unsteadiness and blurring of vision may be accompanied by delirium. Severe memory loss, speech disorders, drowsiness, stroke, convulsions and coma are some other presentations.

Risk Factors:

Use of seatbelt and helmets have reduced the incidence of such forms of head injury.

Caution and Recommendations to Therapists:

Massage is contraindicated until all complications are ruled out and the Physician gives clearance.

Notes

The client has to be hospitalised and carefully investigated and monitored to rule out hematoma, hemorrhage, skull fracture and other forms of severe injury. Glucocorticoids may be given to reduce edema. For more details see Appendix C: Antiinflammatories - steroidal drugs.

References

Ropper A. Trauma of the head and spine. In: Isselbacher KJ et al, editors. Harrison's principles of internal medicine. 13th ed. London: McGraw-Hill Co; 1994. p. 2322.

Coxa Plana

(Legg-Calvé-Perthes disease; Juvenile osteochondrosis)

A condition that produces necrosis and flattening of the head of femur.

Cause:

The necrosis is due to the interruption of blood supply to the head of femur by unknown causes. The necrosis is followed by new blood supply to the area with resorption of dead bone and regeneration of new bone. Due to the pressure on the weakened bone, deformity of the head of femur develops.

Signs and Symptoms:

The patient presents with pain in the thigh and hip, and a limp that slowly increases in severity. The pain may radiate to the knee and is aggravated by activity and reduced by rest. Due to the deformity of the femoral head, there is muscle spasm and atrophy of thigh muscles. Progressive shortening of the leg occurs with difficulty in abduction and internal rotation (rotation towards the center of body) of the hip. The deformity may be unilateral or bilateral.

Notes

The aim is to protect the femoral head from abnormal forces. The treatment involves bed rest for 1-2 weeks, splinting of the limb using braces or casts in a slightly abducted and internally rotated position. In severe cases, surgery may be required.

Initially, gait training with crutches may be required. Exercises to improve range of motion of the hip, knee and ankle are helpful after complete healing has occurred.

For more details see Appendix C: Plaster cast.

a Handbook for Massage Therapists

Risk Factors:

It is more common in boys, aged 3-12. There is a familial predisposition to this condition.

Caution and Recommendations to Therapists:

Massage the whole body avoiding use of oil near plaster casts. The oil hastens skin break down and softens the cast. Massage without oil, in and under the edges of the cast to improve circulation in skin. Passively move all joints especially around the cast. After removal of cast, massage all muscles deeply. Use oil liberally over skin that was previously covered by cast.

Work in conjunction with the Physiotherapist to help strengthen the muscles that have atrophied due to disuse. Some of the principles used by Physiotherapists early in reeducation are: use of warmth to increase blood flow; stabilization of the bones of origin of the affected muscles and joints lying distal to those over which the muscles work; application of pressure by the assistant in the direction of the movement; stretch of the muscle (this stimulates muscle spindles and elicits the stretch reflex) to produce reflex contraction; application of resistance to muscles of the opposite side that produce fixator action – this causes irradiation of impulses to the affected side. Normally, irradiation happens in the body in order to maintain balance. Later, methods are used to specifically strengthen the affected groups of muscles using graded increase in resistance.

References

Adams JC. Hamblen DL. Outline of orthopaedics. 11th ed. London: Churchill Livingstone; 1990. p. 304-308.

Nervous system

Creutzfeldt-Jakob disease (Mad cow disease)
A transmissible disorder that results in degeneration of nervous tissue.

Cause:

Notes

There is no specific treatment available. It is important to keep abreast with the outcome of scientific research in this area, as there may be breakthrough in finding the cause, mode of spread and treatment in the near future.

It is believed to be caused by the transmission of an infectious, protein particle (*prion*) that is encoded by a gene present in chromosome 20. Modified forms of this protein have been isolated from the brains of animals and humans who had the disease. How this protein is modified and replicated is not known.

Most often the cases are sporadic. In some the condition may be familial. The disease is not contagious. Person-to-person spread can occur when tissue (eg. cornea) from infected individuals is used for transplant. A few cases have been reported where instruments used for neurosurgery had not been properly decontaminated. Rarely, use of pituitary hormones obtained from cadavers has resulted in the disease.

Signs and Symptoms:

It may present as a progressive mental impairment. Memory loss, impaired judgement, mood changes, hallucinations are some symptoms. Motor function may be disturbed and tremors, clumsiness and abnormal movements may be seen. Symptoms of Parkinson's disease may be present.

Risk Factors:

See Cause.

Caution and Recommendations to Therapists:

This rare condition, though infectious, does not spread from person to person by direct contact. The motor function of the client has to be assessed carefully and treatment individualized. See Appendix D for organizations and support groups. Also see Appendix B: Strategies for infection prevention and safe practice.

References

Tyler KL. Viral and prion diseases of the nervous system. In: Isselbacher KJ et al, editors. Harrison's principles of internal medicine. 13th ed. London: McGraw-Hill Co; 1994. p. 2309-2312.

Cryptorchidism (Undescended testis)

A condition where one or both testes fail to descend into the scrotum from the abdominal cavity but remain in the abdomen, inguinal canal or other areas.

Reproductive system

Cause:

Lack of adequate levels of hormones - from the mother or in the fetus, has been implicated.

Signs and Symptoms:

There is an absence of testis in the scrotum. Occasionally, the testis may be felt as a swelling in the inguinal region.

Risk Factors:

It could be genetic. It is more common in premature infants.

Caution and Recommendations to Therapists:

The undescended testis may be located in the inguinal canal and appear as a soft swelling in the lower abdominal area. Avoid massage over area if the testis is present there.

Notes

In the fetus, the testis develops in the abdomen and descends into the scrotum in the eighth or ninth month of pregnancy. The lower temperature of the scrotum is necessary for proper formation of sperms. Undescended testis can therefore lead to sterility. The incidence of cancer of the testis is also higher in this condition. Hormonal (testosterone) treatment is given and/or surgery may be done to locate the testis in a position where cancerous changes can be detected.

For more details see Appendix C: Hormone therapy / replacement.

References

Weinerth JL. The male genital system. In: Sabiston DC, editor. Textbook of Surgery- the biological basis of modern surgical practice. 14th ed. Philadelphia: WB Saunders Co; 1991. p. 1461.

Cubital tunnel syndrome

Entrapment of the ulnar nerve in the tunnel formed by the aponeurosis of the flexor carpi ulnaris near its insertion, close to the medial epicondyle of humerus.

Nervous system

Cause:

Stretching or compression of the ulnar nerve due to overuse of elbow, prolonged flexion of elbow or adhesions may cause this condition.

Signs and Symptoms:

Pain, paresthesia and /or numbness in the area distributed by the ulnar nerve ie. medial one and a half fingers are the predominant symptoms. The patient complains of a dull ache after using the hand. The pain may radiate above and

Notes

Rest and support, use of antiinflammatory drugs and in severe cases, surgical intervention are some of the treatment options. For more details see Appendix C: Antiinflammatories - steroidal drugs; Antiinflammatories - non steroidal drugs.

below the elbow. The muscles supplied by the ulnar nerve viz. hypothenar muscles and adductor of the thumb may appear wasted. The ulnar nerve may be thickened and can be felt in the medial aspect of elbow. Tingling sensations may be produced on applying mild pressure to the nerve in this area.

Risk Factors:

It is common in people in occupations that involve leaning on the elbow, in manual laborers and individuals involved in throwing sports. Those with a wide carrying angle (*cubitus valgus deformity* - a wide angle between the upper arm and forearm) are also prone.

Caution and Recommendations to Therapists:

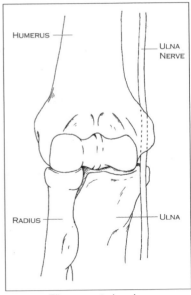

Elbow - anterior view

The client should be advised to avoid activities that may aggravate the symptoms. Encourage clients to wear elbow pads. Avoid local massage if the region is acutely inflamed. Passively move the elbow joint to maintain range of motion. Deep massage to the hypothenar and thenar muscles of the hand can help increase blood flow and reduce atrophy. With the client positioned on his/her back and then on the front, the neck, shoulder and rest of the upper arm should be worked on as well. Special attention should be given to the flexor carpi ulnaris muscle from insertion to origin, with the elbow extended, avoiding direct massage over the ulnar nerve in the cubital tunnel.

The soft tissue may be stretched gently in a direction perpendicular to the direction of the ulnar nerve, without applying pressure on the nerve. Passively stretch the flexor carpi ulnaris muscle by extending the elbow and with the wrist joint in an adducted and extended position. Specific work should be done on the other synergistic muscles such as flexor carpi radialis, flexor digitorum superficialis and palmaris longus and flexor digitorum profundus muscles. Do not massage vigorously in areas where the sensation is compromised.

Stretching exercises concentrating on the extrinsic flexor and extensor muscles along with the intrinsic muscles innervated by the ulnar nerve are helpful. Sometimes, the normal longitudinal movement of the ulnar nerve may be limited by adhesions. In these cases, movement of the ulnar nerve may be facilitated by regular repetitions of flexion and extension of the elbow. The wrist should be extended, forearm supinated and shoulders depressed and abducted at the start of the repetitions. Client education should include improvement in posture and strengthening of muscles that stabilise the upper arm (eg. Scapular stabilizers, pectoralis minor).

References

Hall C M. Brody LT. Therapeutic exercise moving toward function. Philadelphia: Lippincott Williams & Wilkins; 1999. p. 646-647.

Pathology A to Z -

Cushing's syndrome

A spectrum of abnormalities produced by excess adrenocortical hormones.

Endocrine system

Cause:

The adrenal cortex is the outer portion of the adrenal gland, situated superior to both kidneys. The secretion is regulated by the adrenocorticotrophic hormone of the anterior pituitary.

Since the secretion of cortisol from the adrenal cortex is regulated by adrenocorticotrophic hormone (ACTH) from the anterior pituitary, excess secretion is most often due to increased levels of ACTH. Tumors in the adrenal cortex can also produce symptoms. Sometimes symptoms are seen in individuals who are on prolonged steroid therapy for other diseases.

Signs and Symptoms:

The symptoms of Cushing's syndrome are observed in multiple body systems. Diabetes mellitus is one of the endocrine problems produced. The muscles are weak and the bones fracture easily (osteoporosis). The skin is weak, bruises easily and purple-colored stretch marks are seen especially in the abdomen. This is due to the rupture and weakening of collagen fibres in the dermis. There is a classical accumulation of fat above the clavicle and upper part of the back giving a "buffalo" hump appearance. The face becomes rounded ("moon" face) and fat tends to accumulate in the trunk rather than the limbs ("truncal" obesity). There is a tendency to form peptic ulcers.

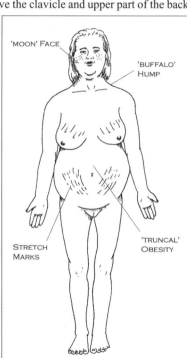

'MOON' FACE

'BUFFALO' HUMP

STRETCH MARKS

'TRUNCAL' OBESITY

The person is irritable and emotionally labile. The retention of water and sodium causes the blood pressure to be increased. Cortisol decreases the function of white blood cells - especially lymphocytes, thus making the person very vulnerable to infection. Since the corticosteroids resemble the androgens (male reproductive hormone), in females, there is a tendency for growth of beard, moustache and enlargement of the clitoris. The menstrual cycles are also abnormal.

Risk Factors:

See Cause.

Notes:

Treatment varies according to the cause. Tumors are surgically removed. If it results from pituitary overactivity, the pituitary gland may be irradiated. For more details see Appendix C: Radiation therapy.

Caution and Recommendations to Therapists:

Very light pressure should be used due to the tendency of the bones to fracture. Also, the skin is fragile and tends to bruise easily. Do not massage if harboring any infection, as the client's immunity is low. The Therapist should take into consideration the other complications of the condition that may be present in the client and side effects of medications being taken. Encourage client to take proper medications.

References

Williams GH, Dluhy RG. Diseases of the adrenal cortex. In: Isselbacher KJ et al, editors. Harrison's principles of internal medicine. 13th ed. London: McGraw-Hill Co; 1994. p. 1960-1963.

Cyanosis

Cardiovascular system

Bluish discoloration of the skin/mucous membrane due to increased amount of deoxygenated hemoglobin in the blood.

Notes

The cause of the cyanosis has to be determined and treated.

Cause:

Cyanosis can be classified as *central* or *peripheral*. Central cyanosis is due to larger quantities of reduced hemoglobin in the arterial blood. Conditions causing central cyanosis include congenital heart defects that result in mixing up of venous and arterial blood in the heart. Any condition (eg. lung disease, ascent to high altitude) that results in less oxygen reaching the pulmonary blood vessels also result in central cyanosis. Abnormalities of hemoglobin (eg. methemoglobinemia) are other conditions that produce this type of cyanosis.

Peripheral cyanosis is due to slowing of blood flow in one area and greater extraction of oxygen from the blood in the region. Cold exposure, shock, cardiac failure and obstruction of blood vessels are some of the causes.

Signs and Symptoms:

Usually the lips, fingertips and nail beds, ears and tongue have a bluish tinge. The degree of cyanosis depends on various factors such as thickness of the skin, color of skin, the state of the capillaries of the skin, presence of anemia etc.

Risk Factors:

See Cause.

Caution and Recommendations to Therapists:

It is important for the Therapist to know the cause of the cyanosis. If the cyanosis is due to reduced blood flow to the periphery due to changes in temperature, warmth and massage may help improve circulation and bring the blood flow back to normal. Even here, massage may be detrimental if tissue damage has occurred as a result of extreme cold exposure. It is best to obtain clearance from the treating Physician and individualizing the treatment plan according to the cause of cyanosis.

References

Ganong WF. Review of medical physiology. 15th ed. California; Appleton & Lange; 1991. p. 635.

Cystic fibrosis (Mucoviscidosis)

A chronic genetic disease that affects the function of exocrine glands (sweat glands, pancreas etc.).

Cause:

It is due to the defect in a gene that codes for a protein that involves the transport of chloride across epithelial membranes. The lack of the protein makes the mucus secretions of the bronchus, pancreas and other mucus glands to become viscid. The viscid mucus blocks the ducts of glands, thus producing the symptoms and resulting in other complications. The gene is transmitted as a recessive trait, affecting both sexes equally.

Signs and Symptoms:

The symptoms may develop soon after birth or very slowly. There is excessive loss of sodium and chloride in the sweat making the child susceptible to electrolyte imbalance. The viscid mucus causes obstruction and narrowing of the bronchi. There is difficulty in breathing, associated with wheezing, and dry cough. The chest tends to be barrel-shaped due to the retention of air. The person is very susceptible to respiratory infections. The reduced oxygenation of the hemoglobin makes the mucous membrane appear blue (cyanosis).

The increased viscosity of the mucous secretions not only affects the respiratory tract, but also causes symptoms of intestinal obstruction. There may be distention of the abdomen, vomiting, and constipation. The narrowing/blockage of the pancreatic duct can result in difficulty in digestion and absorption of proteins and fat (see malabsorption syndrome) and associated symptoms. Difficulty in fat absorption also reduces the uptake of the fat-soluble vitamins A, D, E and K. The endocrine function of the pancreas may be affected leading to Diabetes Mellitus. Other complications include obstruction of the bile duct leading to jaundice and liver dysfunction.

Risk Factors:

Family history of cystic fibrosis increases the risk.

Caution and Recommendations to Therapists:

The aim should be to help drain the viscid mucus from the lungs and to increase blood flow and venous/lymphatic drainage in the fatigued respiratory muscles. Before treatment, increase the humidity and warmth in the clinic. This helps to loosen the thick mucus. Steam inhalation is very beneficial. If possible, position the client with the head end lower than the leg to use the effect of gravity on drainage. However, the client may be most comfortable in a half-lying position – a position that does not restrict breathing. Support the flexed knee, flexed and slightly abducted arm and the neck with pillows.

Massage the respiratory muscles and back using broad strokes. The intercostals may be stretched by placing the fingers (2nd-3rd or 2nd-4th fingers) in the intercostal spaces and rhythmically applying inward pressure during expiration.

Notes

The aim is to facilitate clearance of secretions, control infection, prevent intestinal obstruction and provide adequate nutrition. Antibiotics are used to prevent and treat infections. Bronchodilators may be given to reduce constriction of bronchi. Replacement of pancreatic enzymes via capsules and administration of fat-soluble vitamins are other options.

For more details see Appendix C: Antimicrobial - antibacterial; Bronchodilators; Oxygen therapy.

References

Boucher RC. Cystic fibrosis. In: Isselbacher KJ et al, editors. Harrison's principles of internal medicine. 13th ed. London: McGraw-Hill Co; 1994. p. 1194-1197.

Use repetitive vibratory strokes on the chest. Cupping, tapping and hacking strokes should be used all over the chest to loosen the thick mucus. A cup may have to be provided for the sputum. Handle the container with gloves and ensure that the cup and the contents are disposed in a leak proof bag. If not too uncomfortable, change the position of the client to facilitate drainage through the different bronchi.

These clients are prone to respiratory infections. Ensure that they do not come in contact with any form of infection in the clinic. The susceptibility to infection increases the risk of tuberculosis in these clients. Ensure that you are not put at risk inadvertently. You may have to check with the Physician regarding infectivity of the client if TB has been diagnosed. Refer client to local support groups and for genetic counseling. (see Appendix D)

Renal system

Cystitis

An inflammation of the urinary bladder.

Notes

The predisposing conditions are treated along with the use of antibiotics to control infection. For more details see Appendix C: Antimicrobial - antibacterial agents.

Cause:

It is usually caused by infection of the bladder lining.

Signs and Symptoms:

Pain just above the pubic bone, lower back or inner thigh, blood in urine, urgency and frequency of urination are common symptoms. Fever with chills is usually present.

Risk Factors:

It is more common in women - due to the shortness of the urethra and close proximity to the anus, which harbors bacteria. Stagnation of urine in the bladder due to spinal cord injuries or obstruction to flow of urine as in urethral strictures is a risk factor. Prostatic hyperplasia in men that narrows the urethral lumen also predisposes to this.

Bladder stones may be a complication of cystitis.

Caution and Recommendations to Therapists:

Encourage the client to take the full course of antibiotics and increase fluid intake. A full body massage avoiding the abdominal area may be beneficial. See Appendix B: Strategies for infection prevention and safe practice.

References

Chisholm, GD Williams DI, editors. Scientific Foundations: Urology. 2nd ed. London: William Heinemann Medical books; 1982.

Integumentary system

Dandruff (Seborrheic dermatitis)

A chronic inflammation of the skin involving the seborrheic areas of the skin.

Notes

Shampooing is the best form of treatment. Frequent shampooing even with

Cause:

The cause is not known. There is some evidence that there could be some form of fungal (*Pityrosporum ovale*) involvement. Various bacteria have also been

Pathology A to Z -

implicated. Some believe that it is due to rapid proliferation of cells located superficially.

Signs and Symptoms:

The dry form of seborrheic dermatitis is known as dandruff. Here small dry to thick powdery scales are produced. There is no redness. In the oily form, the scales are greasy and form crusts over red, inflamed skin. There may be some oozing and formation of pustules. The lesions are found in the scalp, eyebrows, between the eyebrows, eyelid margins, cheeks, in the folds between the lips and nose, and around the ear. Sometimes, the lesions may be found in the body creases like the axillae, under the breasts, groin area and in the gluteal cleft. See Appendix A: page 356.

In infants, greasy scales and crusts on a red base may be seen in the scalp and is often referred to as 'cradle cap'.

Risk Factors:

It is more common in males and is more severe in winter. For unknown reasons, the incidence is higher in people with Parkinson's disease.

Caution and Recommendations to Therapists:

The flakes, if extensive may be a cause for annoyance, but they are nor infective. If the skin is inflamed and pustules are present, avoid the area.

unmedicated shampoo is beneficial. Various antidandruff shampoos are available in the market.

Daily or twice weekly regimens are necessary. Since the scalp is being treated, it is important to leave the shampoo on for at least 5 minutes. For more severe cases, corticosteroid lotions may be used. Some forms of lotions have to be left on the scalp overnight and rinsed the next morning.

Steroid lotions are available for treatment of lesions located in areas other than the scalp. Infants require special consideration and irritating substances have to be avoided.

For more details see Appendix C: Antimicrobial - antibacterial agents.

References

Fitzpatrick TB et al. editors. Dermatology in general medicine. 3rd ed. New York: McGraw-Hill; 1987.

Decubitus ulcers (Bed sores; Pressure ulcers; Pressure sores)

Integumentary system

Ulcers of the skin and underlying structures due to excessive pressure.

Cause:

The ulcers are produced in areas that are exposed to external pressures, friction, or shearing forces that impair blood flow and lymphatic drainage. The forces compress, tear or injure blood vessels. It is usually seen over bony prominences but can occur in any part of the body. The five classical areas of the body that are most susceptible to decubitus ulcers are the bony prominences of the sacrum, greater trochanter, ischial tuberosity, tuberosity of the calcaneus and lateral malleolus.

In a normal person, the body position is frequently shifted to reduce constant pressure over a particular area. In people with reduced sensations or in those who are bedridden, body position changes are infrequent and pressure ulcers are common. It is also seen in nursing home situations where the bed is elevated in one end. This causes shearing forces on the skin as the bone and fascia slide over skin that is fixed against the bed linen. Shearing forces are also caused when a patient with reduced sensations is dragged off the bed rather than lifted.

Signs and Symptoms:

In the initial stages, the susceptible area is red with a superficial ulcer or blister. If the deeper areas are affected, the ulcer has a deep crater-like appearance.

Notes

The incidence of pressure ulcers can be reduced by a) lifting or rolling clients across the bed instead of dragging them, b) reducing the exposure of the skin to urine, feces, sweat or drainage from wounds, c) eliminating shearing forces created by the action of gravity that results from raising the head end of the bed.

Pressure ulcers are avoided by constant inspection of skin, protection against mechanical forces, and frequent changes of position in susceptible individuals. Special pressure relief aids such as gel flotation pads, water mattresses, turning beds etc. are available. Local or systemic antibiotics are used to prevent superinfections. Use of growth factors is of benefit. Surgical treatment includes cleaning of wound with removal of dead tissue and the use of flaps/skin grafts in severe cases.

For more details see Appendix C: Skin grafts; Antimicrobial - antibacterial agents.

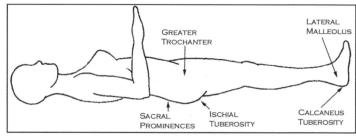

Classical areas susceptible to ulcers

Infection may result in foul smelling discharges from the ulcer. In severe cases, the underlying muscle, fat and tendons may be exposed. In very severe cases, damage to muscle, bone and supporting tissue occurs.

Risk Factors:

Quadriplegics, paraplegics, comatose individuals, those with reduced mobility, those malnourished (leading to weight loss and reduction of subcutaneous and muscle tissue) are at risk. It is more common in the elderly due to the frail skin.

Caution and Recommendations to Therapists:

Do not massage over and around the area. Recent research has shown that massage decreases skin blood flow and increases the risk of deep tissue injury in such conditions. Perform active and passive range of motion exercises in bed-ridden individuals. Do not use excessive pressure and force while massaging individuals who are prone for pressure ulcers. If erythema \ blisters \ ulcers are noticed while massaging susceptible individuals, bring to the notice of nurses or others caring for the individual. Since massage tends to lower the blood pressure, clients with severe orthostatic hypotension, or who have been on prolonged bed rest, have to be warned against changing positions abruptly. See Appendix D for organizations and support groups.

References

Porth CM. Alterations in blood flow.In: Porth CM, editor. Pathophysiology concepts of altered health states. 4th ed. Philadelphia: JB Lippincott Co; 1994. p. 373-376.

Nervous system

Delirium

An acute confusional state.

Cause:

Notes

The person has to be thoroughly investigated to identify the cause. If the person is agitated and violent a tranquilizer may be required. The cause of the condition has to be treated while the individual is kept hydrated and proper nutrition given.

For more details see Appendix C: Tranquillizers.

There are various causes of delirium. Problems the affect the reticular activating system, thalamus and the cerebral hemispheres can cause depression of consciousness and confusion. For example, focal changes in the brain produced by brain tumors, hematoma, hydrocephalus or diffuse changes such as tumor metastasis and multiple areas of brain tissue death can produce this. Many systemic diseases can cause this condition too. Inadequate supply of oxygen (hypoxia), hypoglycemia, deficiency of other factors required for metabolic processes (vitamins like thiamine, B12 and nicotinic acid, hormones such as thyroid, parathyroid), electrolyte imbalances, circulating toxins, high fever and dehydration can all produce delirium.

Pathology A to Z -

In vulnerable individuals like the elderly, more than one mechanism can cause delirium.

Signs and Symptoms:

The onset is acute and the symptoms are transient lasting for hours to weeks. The confusional state may fluctuate over time and sleep-wake cycles are disrupted. All aspects of the intellectual function are impaired as neurons are affected diffusely. There is clouding of consciousness with impaired alertness, attention and awareness. Impairment of memory may present as poor recent memory, disorientation of time and place. Cognitive impairment may present as difficulty in doing tasks like simple calculations, and those requiring logic. Speech may be rambling or incoherent and errors in writing may be elicited. The person may hallucinate and disturbances in emotions may occur. The person may be hyperactive and restless and involuntary movements may be present. The condition may be associated with autonomic impairment.

Risk Factors:

See Cause.

Caution and Recommendations to Therapists:

Obtaining an informed consent is of importance before massaging those who are psychologically challenged. If it cannot be obtained, massage should not be given. More research is required to find out the effects of massage on mentally challenged individuals. The Therapist may require more training and knowledge of specific mental conditions to modify treatment plan according to individual clients.

References

Brown MM, Hachinski VC. Acute confusional states, amnesia, and dementia. In: Isselbacher KJ et al, editors. Harrison's principles of internal medicine. 13th ed. London: McGraw-Hill Co; 1994. p. 139-141.

Dementia

An acquired syndrome affecting the brain diffusely, with impairment of cognitive function.

Nervous system

Cause:

It is a syndrome with many causes. It may result from Alzheimer's disease. Diseases affecting the basal ganglia, thalamus and white matter in the brain (eg. multiple sclerosis) can cause this condition. Chronic infection like syphilis, Creutzfeldt-Jakob disease, chronic subdural hematoma, some forms of hydrocephalus, late stages of Parkinson's disease, hypothyroidism, brain damage due to head injury, hypoxia, hypoglycemia, chronic alcoholism and encephalitis are other causes. Some psychiatric illnesses may mimic dementia (pseudodementia).

Signs and Symptoms:

The onset of the condition is insidious and symptoms may persist for months to years. Unlike delirium, sleep-wake cycles are not disrupted and consciousness level and attention is normal. The person may be disoriented with impairment

Notes

It is important to identify the cause of dementia as many have treatable neurologic or systemic illness, psychiatric illness or contributing causes that can be controlled. For those where no treatable cause can be found support is required. As the severity increases, supervision may be required and the person may require help with daily activities. It is important to meet the needs of the relatives taking care of the individual, as the task is very demanding. Eventually, full-time nursing care may be required.

of long-term memory. Lack of interest and inhibition may be seen. Involuntary movements and autonomic changes are not common in this condition.

There is a decline in intellect, memory and personality with normal consciousness. The diagnosis is made if any three of the following: language, memory, emotion, personality, cognition and visuospatial skills are affected.

Risk Factors:

See Cause.

Caution and Recommendations to Therapists:

Obtaining an informed consent is of importance before massaging those who are psychologically challenged. If it cannot be obtained, massage should not be given. A medical clearance may be necessary. More research is required to find out the effects of massage on mentally challenged individuals. The Therapist may require more training and knowledge of specific mental conditions to modify treatment plan according to individual clients.

Massage is unlikely to cause any harm and may be given within the comfort levels of the client.

References

Brown MM, Hachinski VC. Acute confusional states, amnesia, and dementia. In: Isselbacher KJ et al, editors. Harrison's principles of internal medicine. 13th ed. London: McGraw-Hill Co; 1994. p. 142-146.

Diabetes insipidus

Endocrine system

An endocrine disorder of the posterior pituitary affecting the metabolism of water in the body.

Notes

It is treated with hormonal replacement therapy and surgery if due to a tumor. The hormones are taken as injections or as a nasal spray. For more details see Appendix C: Hormone therapy / replacement.

Cause:

This condition is produced when the secretion of antidiuretic hormone (ADH; vasopressin) is deficient. It is usually caused by a tumor in the pituitary, after neurosurgery, trauma to the head or fracture of the skull. Rarely, it may be a complication of infection.

Signs and Symptoms:

Since the antidiuretic hormone regulates the permeability of the kidney tubules and thereby the volume of water that is excreted, its' lack results in excessive loss of fluid in the urine. The person has polyuria (excess urination) and polydipsia (drinking excessive volumes of water). The volume of urine excreted per day may be as high as 30 liters as compared to 1 liter by a normal person. It is accompanied by excessive thirst. The person appears dehydrated with loss of elasticity of the skin, dry mouth and mucous membranes, constipation, muscle weakness and dizziness.

Risk Factors:

See Cause.

Caution and Recommendations to Therapists:

Encourage client to continue hormone replacement therapy. Ensure that the client has the prescribed medicines handy when scheduled for a massage. You may have to provide water to the client during the session. Keep record of the address of treating Physician and other contacts. Massage should be for shorter durations. Watch for postural hypotension and advice client to get off table slowly after massage.

References

Ganong WF. Review of medical physiology. 15th ed. California; Appleton & Lange; 1991. p.227-228.

Diabetes mellitus

A chronic disease of the endocrine part of the pancreas with inadequate secretion of insulin.

Endocrine system

Cause:

Diabetes may be due to impaired release of insulin by the pancreas, presence of inadequate or abnormal insulin receptors on the cells, or the rapid destruction of insulin even before it can carry out its action. Diabetes is classified as *Insulin-dependent* (*Type I; juvenile-onset diabetes*) and *non-insulin-dependent* (*Type II; maturity onset diabetes*) forms. Other forms of diabetes are those that develop only during pregnancy - *gestational diabetes* and diabetes produced by other conditions eg. Cushing's syndrome. Certain drugs that result in loss of potassium in the urine can cause diabetes, as potassium is required for the normal release of insulin. Steroids, oral contraceptives, drugs that mimic the effect of the sympathetic system, certain antiepileptic drugs and diuretics can produce diabetes.

Type I diabetes is thought to be caused by genetic predisposition. A triggering agent in the environment such as a virus or chemical toxin, stimulates the immune system to attack the beta cells of the pancreas that produce insulin.

Type II diabetes is more common in people who are overweight and in the older age group. Here, the cause of diabetes has been attributed to decreased number or defective receptors for insulin in fat cells. Also, the release of insulin from the pancreas is inadequate. There is an association between incidence of diabetes and family history.

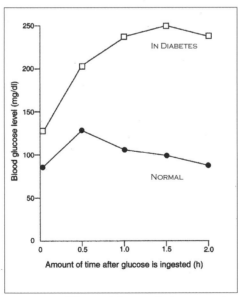

Glucose tolerance test

Notes:

Insulin is required for transport of glucose into skeletal muscle and fat tissue. It also helps store glucose as glycogen. Insulin decreases the breakdown of fat. For protein metabolism, insulin is required for the transport of amino acids into cells. It also increases the synthesis and conservation of proteins. Inadequate insulin results in high glucose levels in the blood. Normally, the plasma glucose level while fasting (overnight) is less than 140mg/dl. High fasting levels of glucose on at least two separate occasions and levels greater than 200mg/dl at two hours (and one occasion within two hours) after ingestion of 75gms of glucose (glucose tolerance test) are used as criteria for diagnosis of diabetes mellitus.

The goal of treatment is to maintain blood glucose levels as close to normal as possible, in order to prevent complications. It is important for the person to accept that it is a chronic disease and requires lifelong change in life style.

Diabetes is treated with dietary changes, exercise and/or antidiabetic drugs. Dietary tables taking into account the age, body build and activity of the individual are available. Antidiabetic drugs work by stimulating the beta cells to secrete insulin and are of use in Type II diabetes. If severe, or Type I, insulin injections are given. A variety of insulins are available, including types where it can be infused subcutaneously on a continuous basis. Hypoglycemia can be a side effect especially in those using insulin for treatment.

Pancreas transplantation is one of the newer techniques available. The possibility of utilizing genetically engineered cells that produce insulin is being researched.

For more details see Appendix C: Antidiabetics; Organ transplantation ; Hormone therapy / replacement.

Signs and Symptoms:

The onset is abrupt in Type I diabetes, while slow in Type II. Typically, diabetes is characterized by excessive urination, thirst and hunger: the three poly's - polyuria, polydipsia and polyphagia respectively. The high level of glucose in the blood is responsible for these symptoms. Loss of glucose in the urine forcibly increases the excretion of water by osmosis. The loss of glucose and water causes the hunger and thirst. There is weight loss in spite of the increased appetite.

The high glucose levels have detrimental effects on almost all systems. Eyesight is affected due to bleeding in the retina. There is loss of sensation in the periphery especially the hands and feet (glove and stocking effect). The effect on the autonomic nervous system results in postural hypotension, diarrhea and impotence. The high level of cholesterol in the blood speeds up the formation of atherosclerosis with its' associated complication of thrombosis and emboli. The person is dehydrated, weak and fatigued. A diabetic is prone to infection and wounds take longer to heal.

Risk Factors:

See Cause.

Caution and Recommendations to Therapists:

Take a detailed history and determine if the diabetes is Type I or Type II. Type I is more serious than Type II in terms of management. Although not documented yet, experience has shown that massage is beneficial to diabetics and may have an effect on daily insulin requirements. A relaxing and gentle massage is recommended. Ensure that these individuals are not exposed to infections (even mild) in the clinic. The feedback may be inadequate in those with decreased sensation, so the pressure of strokes should be monitored carefully.

Avoid working in and around diabetic ulcers, if present. Insulin injection sites should be avoided too as massage may speed up absorption of insulin into the blood and cause hypoglycemia. Often, cell death (fat necrosis) occurs at the site of injection.

Ensure that glucose as well as necessary medications are available with the client when coming for treatment. Encourage client to loose weight and participate in exercise programs, if obese. Refer to local support groups. Emphasize the need for regular and frequent glucose level monitoring. Keep a record of the address of treating Physician as well as a contact person.

The person may have acute complications like hypoglycemia while in the clinic. Hypoglycemia presents as dizziness, weakness, pallor, rapid heart rate and excessive sweating. Fruit juice, hard candy, honey or any other carbohydrate should be given immediately before calling for help.

See Appendix D for organizations and support groups.

References

Ganong WF. Review of medical physiology. 15th ed. California; Appleton & Lange; 1991. p. 318-319, 332-333.

Diarrhea

A frequent passage of loose, watery stools. It is formally defined as an increase in daily stool weight above 200 g.

Cause:

Diarrhea (*Greek*-to flow) is considered to be *acute* if it lasts less than 7-14 days and *chronic* when lasting 2-3 weeks.

There are many causes of diarrhea. The most common cause is infectious agents. Large volume diarrhea is produced when substances in the lumen of the bowel draw water from the interstitial tissue by osmosis. Such a diarrhea is seen in lactase deficiency, high intake of magnesium containing antacids, or when the motility of the gut is rapid. It may also be caused by infections that stimulate the mucosa to secrete water (eg. cholera). Infections can also destroy the mucosa and allow loss of water into the lumen eg. *Hamburger disease.*

Normal stool:

weight: <200 g
water content: 60-85%
frequency: 3/week - 3/day

Diarrhea can also be caused by inflammatory conditions of the bowel like Ulcerative colitis and Crohn's disease. In the latter, the volume is usually small, with blood and mucus. Bacterial infection is another cause of small volume diarrhea.

Signs and Symptoms:

It is characterized by frequent passage of watery stools. There may be colicky pain in the abdomen. The loss of fluid leads to dehydration where the skin is dry and loose, mouth parched and the eyes sunken. The person feels tired, weak and faint. Nausea and vomiting are other symptoms.

Risk Factors:

Infectious diarrhea is transmitted by fecal contamination of water or contact with clothes or other articles soiled by a person with diarrhea, food poisoning, presence of bacteria in uncooked meat or sexual activity with an infected individual. Inadequate sewage disposal and water supplies, lack of refrigeration, overcrowding, lack of personal hygiene and lack of education are all contributing factors.

Intravenous drug users, homosexuals and prostitutes are groups of people particularly prone to diarrhea.

Caution and Recommendations to Therapists:

Avoid massage in individuals with an acute onset of diarrhea until all symptoms have abated as this type is most often due to infection. This is to prevent inadvertent spread of infection to you and other clients. Therapists should refrain from work till all symptoms have subsided if they have diarrhea due to infection. In chronic diarrhea, ie. diarrhea lasting for more than three weeks, the

Notes

Treatment includes rest, oral/intravenous fluid and electrolyte replacement. Antibiotics may be used in specific types of infectious diarrhea. Drugs that reduce motility of intestines may be used in situations where there is no accompanying fever or blood/pus in stools (ie. diarrhea not caused by infectious agents).

The cause of chronic diarrhea has to be identified and treated accordingly. For more details see Appendix C: Antimicrobial - antibacterial agents; Antidiarrhoeal drugs.

References

Friedman LS, Isselbacher KJ. Diarrhea and constipation. In: Isselbacher KJ et al, editors. Harrison's principles of internal medicine. 13th ed. London: McGraw-Hill Co; 1994. p. 219-221

cause is usually due to conditions like Inflammatory Bowel Disease. In such cases, massage can be given avoiding the abdominal area. See Appendix D for organizations and support groups. Also see Appendix B: Strategies for infection prevention and safe practice.

Diphtheria

Respiratory, Integumentary systems

A bacterial infection of the mucous membrane or skin caused by Corynebacterium diphtheriae.

Cause:

The inflammatory reaction of the body to the bacteria results in the formation of a membrane like tissue at the site of infection (pseudomembrane formation). Certain strains of bacteria produce toxins that cause inflammation and necrosis in cardiac tissue (myocarditis), nerves (polyneuritis) and other tissues.

Signs and Symptoms:

The signs and symptoms vary with the infective site and age of the individual. Infection is more common in the tonsils and pharynx, but it may occur in the nose, larynx, trachea and bronchi. Sore throat is the most common symptom. Fever, difficulty in swallowing (dysphagia), cough, hoarseness of voice are other symptoms. The spread of toxin to other tissues can result in tachycardia, pallor, listlessness etc.

In some patients, there is extensive pseudomembrane formation and they present with foul smelling breath, extensive swelling of the tonsils and adjacent regions, with painful, enlarged cervical lymph nodes. One of the serious complications of diphtheria is obstruction of the airways by the edema that occurs or blockage by the dislodged pseudomembrane. Obstruction is more common in children as the airway is smaller in size.

In the case of infection of the skin, it presents as punched out ulcers with a thick membrane of dead tissue. Myocarditis may present as various types of arrhythmias. If polyneuritis is present, paralysis of muscles in the pharynx and larynx may occur with difficulty in swallowing, speech etc. In severe cases, paralysis of other muscles may occur.

Risk Factors:

The course of infection and severity of symptoms is worse in unimmunized individuals.

Caution and Recommendations to Therapists:

Do not massage a client with diphtheria. If a Therapist has the condition, s/he should stay away from work until all symptoms have disappeared. Encourage clients to immunize their children.

Refer to Appendix B: Strategies for infection prevention and safe practice. Also see Appendix D for organizations and support groups.

Notes

It is treated with diphtheria antitoxins, which is administered as an injection. The patient has to be monitored for allergic reactions to the antitoxin. A course of antibiotics is given to kill the bacteria and prevent its spread to susceptible individuals. The patient has to be carefully monitored for airway obstruction and arrhythmias. Tracheostomy may have to be done if obstruction occurs.

It is important to keep close contacts under surveillance for 1 week and treatment with antibiotics and antitoxin may be required.

Diptheria can be prevented by immunization. Usually, the vaccine is given in combination with the tetanus and pertussis vaccine (DTP). It is given as four doses – the first at 6 weeks of age, second and third at 4-8 weeks interval and the fourth six months later. A booster dose is given when the child enters kindergarten.

For more details see Appendix C: Immunization ; Antimicrobial - antibacterial agent; Tracheostomy.

References

Morello JA, Mizer HE, Wilson ME, Granato PA. Microbiology in patient care. 6th ed. New York: McGraw-Hill; 1998. p. 257-260.

Disseminated Intravascular Coagulation (DIC)

Cardiovascular system

A type of bleeding disorder that results from consumption of clotting factors by coagulation induced inside blood vessels.

Cause:

In this condition coagulation (clotting) is induced inside the blood vessels and many small thrombi and emboli are formed. This in turn results in rapid depletion of factors required for the coagulation process and bleeding results.

There are many causes of DIC. Usually, it is associated with complications at the time of pregnancy. Abruptio placenta, abortion during the second trimester and retention of dead fetus in the uterus are common obstetrical causes. Some types of tumors, hemolysis, tissue damage due to burns, head injury and gunshot wounds can predispose to this condition. DIC can also be brought about by certain bacterial, viral, parasitic and fungal infections.

Signs and Symptoms:

The presentation varies with the stage and severity of the condition. Usually, bleeding occurs under the skin and mucous membrane. Bleeding may also occur in injured sites. Sometimes due to the blockage of blood flow by thrombi, changes similar to gangrene may be seen.

Risk Factors:

See Cause.

Caution and Recommendations to Therapists:

Massage is contraindicated. For clients recovering from this condition, medical clearance is required.

Notes

The hemorrhage due to the disease could be life threatening and should be treated promptly. The cause has to be quickly identified and treated. Fresh frozen plasma may have to be given to replace the coagulation factors that have been used up. Heparin may be used if thrombi formation is the major problem.

For more details see Appendix C: Blood transfusion ; Anticoagulants.

References

Handin RI. Disorders of Coagulation and Thrombosis. In: Isselbacher KJ et al, editors. Harrison's principles of internal medicine. 13th ed. London: McGraw-Hill Co; 1994. p. 1807-1808.

Diverticular disease (Diverticulosis; Diverticulitis)

Gastrointestinal system

A condition where the inner lining of the gastrointestinal tract protrudes or herniates through the muscular layer that surrounds it.

Cause:

The disease results from increased pressure in the lumen of the bowel, which push the inner lining through the muscular layer - especially in the weak areas. Potential weak areas are the locations where blood vessels enter the gut. It is most commonly seen in the sigmoid colon. Diverticulosis may be congenital or acquired.

Signs and Symptoms:

In the more common type Diverticulosis - where there is no inflammation, the

Notes

If asymptomatic, diverticular disease is left untreated. If symptoms are present, it is controlled by altering the diet, and by intake of stool softeners. If inflamed and infected, antibiotics and drugs to reduce spasm are given. If severe, surgery may be done and the portion of the gut affected is removed and joined with the normal gut, or the end of the colon is opened onto the surface of the abdominal wall - colostomy.

For more details see Appendix C: Colostomy; Laxatives; Antimicrobial - antibacterial agents.

person has no symptoms or has mild pain in the left, lower quadrant of the abdomen. The pain may be relieved by defecation. The person may also have alternating diarrhea and constipation. There may be blood in stools. In Diverticulitis - where the diverticula are inflamed, the symptoms include left lower abdominal pain, excess gas formation, nausea, low-grade fever and irregular bowel habits. Sometimes, the diverticula can form abscesses and rupture resulting in acute pain in the left lower abdomen along with spasm and rigidity of the abdominal muscles. The reaction to the fecal matter that has leaked into the abdominal cavity can cause peritonitis with high fever and chills and the person may go into shock.

If the condition is chronic, the inflammation and healing by fibrosis can cause the lumen to narrow and produce intestinal obstruction. Constipation, ribbonlike stools and abdominal distention are some of the symptoms of partial obstruction.

Risk Factors:

It is more common in the United States. It is seen in the older age group and about 50% of people over the age of 50 years are affected. Lack of fibre in the diet, sedentary life style and irregular bowel habits like neglecting the urge to defecate predispose to this condition.

Caution and Recommendations to Therapists:

A gentle abdominal massage in elderly individuals help regulate the bowel movement. Avoid increased pressure in the abdomen or rigorous massage of the abdomen in all clients in the geriatric age group even if there is a complaint of constipation, as diverticula, if present, can be ruptured. Encourage client to include vegetables, fruits, whole grain bread, wheat and bran in the diet and increase the intake of water.

Massage is contraindicated during the acute stage.

References

Porth CM, editor. Pathophysiology concepts of altered health states. 4ᵗʰ ed. Philadelphia: JB Lippincott Co; 1994. p. 830-832.

Nervous, Cardiovascular systems

Down's syndrome (Trisomy 21)

A disorder produced by the presence of three instead of two chromosomes 21.

Cause:

It is caused by the presence of three copies of chromosome 21 usually due to defects in the way the ovum or sperm divide. Rarely, there may be a family history.

Signs and Symptoms:

The child is mentally handicapped, with typical slanting, almond-shaped eyes, protruding tongue, small skull, mouth and chin. The development of teeth is slow. The bridge of the nose is flat. The person is of short stature, with short limbs, flat feet and hands. The tone of the muscles is decreased, and balance and

Notes

As in all genetic disorders prevention is the most effective way of dealing with the condition. Genetic screening and counseling are some of the preventive measures that can be taken.

For more details see Appendix C: Genetic testing / counselling.

coordination is poor. Pelvic bone abnormalities may be seen. There may be associated developmental defects of the heart.

Risk Factors:

The incidence is higher if the birth of the child occurs when the mother is older than 34, or the father older than 42. It may be inherited from the mother or father. Exposure to radiation and certain viruses also increase the chances of having a child with Down's syndrome.

Caution and Recommendations to Therapists:

Massage should be aimed to increase tone of muscles and improve balance and coordination. Encourage participation in suitable exercise programs. Refer parents to local support groups. Special training may be required by those considering regular treatment of such clients in order to understand the condition, the clients and the challenges they face. See Appendix D for organizations and support groups.

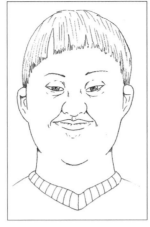

References

JD Wilson, Foster DW, editors. Williams Textbook of Endocrinology. 8th Ed. Philadelphia: WB Saunders Co; 1992.

German JL. Studying human chromosomes today. Am Sci. 1970; 58: 182.

Dupuytren's contracture

Musculoskeletal system

A deformity of the 4th and 5th fingers due to the shortening of the palmar fascia/aponeurosis.

Cause:

Most often the cause is not known. In some it may be caused by a hereditary factor.

Signs and Symptoms:

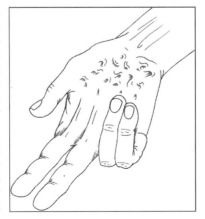

The palmar fascia/aponeurosis is a thin, tough membrane that stretches from the palmaris longus tendon at the front of the wrist and radiates to its insertion at the proximal and middle phalanges of the fingers. In this condition, the fascia thickens and shortens. It may feel nodular and thick.

At first there is a small, thickened nodule in the middle of the palm close to the ring finger. The thickening then spreads from this point eventually forming cord-like bands. The 4th and

Notes

Splinting of the hand or surgery may be done to release the contracture of the palmar fascia. In some clients, a similar contracture may be seen in the sole of the foot.

5th fingers remain flexed at the metacarpophalangeal and interphalangeal joints. The resultant restriction of movement in the small joints of the hand may lead to arthritis. Signs of inflammation may be present and pain may be felt on passively extending the fingers.

Risk Factors:

It is more common in men, the elderly, diabetics, alcoholics and epileptics. Dupuytren's contracture may be associated with occupations that require prolonged, forceful gripping of tools.

Caution and Recommendations to Therapists:

If signs of inflammation are present, ice application is of benefit. In subacute and chronic stages the aim is to maintain range of movement in the joints and to prevent adhesions and contractures. Deep moist heat helps to soften the connective tissue before treatment. Friction strokes followed by ice should be used to reduce adhesions. Use broad strokes to improve the circulation in the muscles of the forearm. The palms should be kneaded thoroughly to stretch the palmar fascia. The fingers should be stretched in a gentle, slow and sustained manner, holding the stretch for 15-30 seconds. Passively move all the small joints of the hand. Resistance exercises should be done to improve the strength of the muscles. Advice the client to stretch the finger many times during the day. This can be done easily, with the client standing and resting the palm on a table. The fingers are stretched and maintained in this position with the other hand. By moving the body over the arm, the wrist can be simultaneously extended.

References

Adams JC, Hamblen DL. Outline of Orthopaedics. 11th Ed. New York: Churchill Livingstone; 1990. p 265-268.

Hall CM. Brody LT. Therapeutic exercise moving toward function. Philadelphia: Lippincott Williams & Wilkins; 1999. p. 626-642.

Dysentery

Gastrointestinal system

A condition with inflammation of the intestine, especially the colon, that produces blood and mucus in stools.

Notes

A mild infection subsides with treatment in 10 days. Severe cases may last from 2-6 weeks. Treatment strategies include administration of antibiotics and maintenance of fluid and electrolyte balance. Drugs that slow down the motility of the gut should not be given, as it tends to retain the bacteria and toxins in the gut.

For more details see Appendix C: Antimicrobial - antibacterial; Antidiarrhoeal agent.

Cause:

The common causes of dysentery (Greek: *dys*-difficult; *enteron*-intestine) are infection by bacteria - Shigellosis (*Bacillary dysentery*) and protozoa (*Amebic dysentery*). The disease is spread by fecal-oral route and occurs by ingestion of contaminated food or water and contact with the contaminated articles used by an infected person. Houseflies can also spread it.

Chemical irritants can be a cause of dysentery in some.

Signs and Symptoms:

It presents as a sudden onset of diarrhea with blood and mucus in stools. The person strains to pass stools (tenesmus). There is nausea, vomiting and abdominal pain. Signs of dehydration - dry mouth, dry and loose skin, sunken eyes, lethargy, weakness and fainting with reduced passage of urine are seen. Fever may be present.

Risk Factors:

The incidence of shigellosis is higher in children, elderly and malnourished people and is common in confined populations like those in nursing homes and mental institutions. Outbreaks can also occur in hospitals.

Caution and Recommendations to Therapists:

Avoid massage until symptoms have subsided completely. This is to prevent inadvertent spread of infection to you and other clients. Be aware of outbreaks of dysentery in the local area. Stay away from work if you have dysentery, until two stool specimens have been shown to be negative for bacteria. In general, strict hygiene should be maintained. The importance of changing linen, washing hands thoroughly before and after treating clients, keeping nails short, maintenance of cleanliness and disinfection of the environment cannot be overemphasized (follow the Strategies for infection prevention and safe practice - Appendix -B). Also see Appendix D for organizations and support groups.

References

Morello JA, Mizer HE, Wilson ME, Granato PA. Microbiology in patient care. 6th ed. New York: McGraw-Hill; 1998. p. 382-383.

Dysmenorrhea

Reproductive system

The abdominal pain perceived during menstruation.

Cause:

The cause is not known in most cases of dysmenorrhea. In others, it may be due to other diseases like endometriosis, fibroids, pelvic inflammatory disease etc. Increased levels of prostaglandins in the uterus have been implicated.

Signs and Symptoms:

It is characterized by lower abdominal pain 1-2 days before or on the day of menstruation. The pain may be described as 'coming and going.' It is often accompanied by headache, nausea and vomiting. Irritability and dizziness may also be present.

Risk Factors:

See Cause.

Caution and Recommendations to Therapists:

A relaxing whole body with a focus on the lower back is recommended.

Notes

Primary dysmenorrhea with no physical cause is treated symptomatically with painkillers like aspirin, ibuprofen, indomethacin etc. Application of heat, exercise and reassurance may be beneficial. Sometimes hormonal therapy is used eg. use of oral contraceptives to prevent ovulation. Secondary causes should be ruled out in all cases of dysmenorrhea, and treatment directed towards the cause, if found.

For more details see Appendix C: Painkillers; Hormone therapy/ replacement; Contraceptives.

References

Readers digest family guide to Alternative medicine. New York: Readers Digest Association Ltd; 1991; 274-275.

Dysphagia

A sensation of obstruction as food passes through the mouth, pharynx and esophagus / difficulty in swallowing.

Notes

The person has to be thoroughly investigated and the cause identified and treated.

Cause:

Normally, the food is voluntarily pushed back into the pharynx by contraction of the skeletal muscles in the mouth and pharynx. In the pharynx, the presence of food stimulates nerve receptors that produce reflex (involuntary) contractions of the muscles to close the airway and transport the food down the esophagus by peristalsis. The lower esophageal sphincter relaxes to allow the bolus of food to enter the stomach. Any cause that affects the structures and nerves involved in swallowing can result in dysphagia.

Factors that cause dysphagia mechanically can be those located in the lumen (foreign body), those conditions that cause narrowing of the lumen such as inflammation, strictures (eg. congenital strictures; those due to ulceration; Crohn's disease etc), or pressure from outside the esophagus (eg. cervical spondylitis; enlarged thyroid gland; aortic aneurysm; tumors etc). Alternately, the neuromuscular structures may be affected. For example, paralysis of the muscles involved, lesions of the vagus and glossopharyngeal nerves that carry sensations and innervate some of the muscles, lesions of the swallowing center located in the brain etc. can all cause dysphagia.

Signs and Symptoms:

The person feels as if there is obstruction of the food passage. If the cause is mechanical, usually there is difficulty in swallowing solids and not liquids. If the duration of the condition is short, it may be due to inflammation. If the dysphagia progresses, invariably it is due to abnormal growths.

Risk Factors:

See Cause.

References

Goyal RK. Dysphagia. In: Isselbacher KJ et al, editors. Harrison's principles of internal medicine. 13th ed. London: McGraw-Hill Co; 1994. p. 206-208.

Caution and Recommendations to Therapists:

The cause of the dysphagia has to be identified. Encourage client to seek medical help. Massage may be given for general relaxation. The client may be more comfortable in a seated or half-lying position.

Dyspnea

An abnormal and uncomfortable awareness of breathing.

Cause:

Dyspnea occurs whenever the work of breathing is increased. It is produced when there is abnormal or excessive activation of the respiratory center in the brainstem. This may occur due to receptors located in the thorax, respiratory muscles, chest wall, excessive stimulation of chemoreceptors or stimulation from higher cortical areas in the brain.

The most common causes of dyspnea are obstructive diseases of the airways (eg. asthma, chronic bronchitis, bronchiectasis); diffuse lung diseases (eg. pneumoconiosis); pulmonary emboli and edema; heart disease (eg. congestive cardiac failure).

Signs and Symptoms:

Dyspnea may be described by the person in many ways. There may be complaints of tiredness or tightness in the chest, choking sensation, difficulty in getting enough air into the lungs etc. Some may complain of dyspnea only on lying down *(orthopnea)* while others may have periodic dyspnea at night *(paroxysmal nocturnal dyspnea)*.

Risk Factors:

See Cause.

Caution and Recommendations to Therapists:

The cause of the dyspnea has to be identified and treatment plan altered accordingly. In general, clients with dyspnea may feel comfortable in a seated or half-lying position. Keep the session short and focus on the respiratory muscles and other muscles of the thorax.

References

Ganong WF. Review of medical physiology. 15th ed. California; Appleton & Lange; 1991. p. 635.

Eating disorder - anorexia nervosa

A self-imposed starvation of the body.

Gastrointestinal, Nervous systems

Cause:

Notes

There is no specific treatment. Minimal benefit may be seen after psychiatric intervention and behaviour modification techniques. Support from Physicians and family is an important component. In severe cases, hospitalisation may be required.

The cause is not known. It is seen in people who have an irrational fear of gaining weight even though they are emaciated. It is also due to the slim body image being propagated by society as a sign of beauty.

Signs and Symptoms:

The person is usually emaciated and gives a history of inducing vomiting, exercising compulsively and using laxatives and other drugs to control appetite. Sleep alterations, changes in menstrual cycles and constipation are other associated features. The skeletal muscles are atrophied and there is a reduction of fatty tissue. The skin appears dry, blotchy and sallow. Constipation and cold intolerance may be present.

Many complications can occur due to malnutrition, dehydration and alteration in the electrolyte levels. The individual is also more susceptible to infection. The menstrual changes indicate alterations in hormonal levels that can lead to osteoporosis.

Risk Factors:

It is more common in young female adults from middle or upper class families. This disorder is often associated with depression. It may often coexist with bulimia.

Caution and Recommendations to Therapists:

Encourage clients who have symptoms of this condition to seek counseling and medical help as it can lead to dangerous medical complications and even death. Massage can do no harm and the Therapist has to decide on an individual basis. The person may have signs of malnutrition. The skin may be fragile and bruise easily. There may be a tendency to bleed as well. See Appendix D for resources.

References

Foster DW. Anorexia nervosa and bulimia. In: Isselbacher KJ et al, editors. Harrison's principles of internal medicine. 13ᵗʰ ed. London: McGraw-Hill Co; 1994. p. 452-455.

Newman MM, Halmi KA. The endocrinology of anorexia nervosa and bulimia nervosa. Endocrin Metab Clin North Am 1988; 17:195.

Gastrointestinal, Nervous systems

Eating disorder - bulimia

A disorder characterized by cycles of eating binges.

Notes

There is no specific treatment. Psychiatric therapy is usually required. Antidepressants may be of benefit.

Cause:

The cause is unknown. It is usually associated with depression. Many psychosocial factors like sexual abuse, cultural importance given to physical appearance have been associated.

Signs and Symptoms:

There is a history of eating excessively and compulsively. Often high calorie and carbohydrate foods are preferred. The individual may induce vomiting due to the feeling of guilt that follows.

Risk Factors:

See Cause. Parental obesity has been associated with this condition. It may often coexist with anorexia nervosa.

Caution and Recommendations to Therapists:

Due to the association of depression with this condition, it is important for clients to seek counseling and medical help as early as possible. Massage can do no harm and the Therapist has to decide on an individual basis. The person may have signs of malnutrition. The skin may be fragile and bruise easily. There may be a tendency to bleed as well. See Appendix D for resources.

References

Foster DW. Anorexia nervosa and bulimia. In: Isselbacher KJ et al editors. Harrison's principles of internal medicine. 13ᵗʰ ed. London: McGraw-Hill Co; 1994. p. 452-455.

Newman MM, Halmi KA. The endocrinology of anorexia nervosa and bulimia nervosa. Endocrin Metab Clin North Am 1988; 17:195.

Cardiovascular system

Ebola virus infection

An acute viral infection producing fever and hemorrhage.

Notes

The person has to be isolated until they are free of virus (usually about 21 days). Plasma containing antibodies specifically against the virus may be given to diminish

Cause:

The infection is caused by the Ebola virus (named after a river in Zaire where an epidemic occurred). The source of infection is suspected to be infected rodents. The virus has also been isolated from Asian macaques.

Signs and Symptoms:

The incubation period is from 4-6 days. There is a history of sudden onset of fever, headache, muscle pain, diarrhoea and abdominal pain. A dry cough may be present along with inflammation of the pharynx. A rash develops soon and bleeding may follow. Blood may be found in stools (malena) and vomitus (hematemesis). The person may bleed from the nose, gums and vagina. Death may follow within a few weeks due to severe blood loss and shock.

Risk Factors:

Those in close contact with an infected person are more at risk.

Caution and Recommendations to Therapists:

This is a rare condition. Be informed about cases in your locality and keep abreast with research and information related to this condition. See Appendix D for organizations and support groups. Also see Appendix B: Strategies for infection prevention and safe practice.

symptoms. However, the plasma is not freely available.

For more details see Appendix C: Antimicrobial - antiviral agents.

References

Morello JA, Mizer HE, Wilson ME, Granato PA. Microbiology in patient care. 6th ed. New York: McGraw-Hill; 1998. p. 440-441.

Ecthyma
Integumentary system

A bacterial infection involving the dermis and epidermis of the skin.

Cause:

It may be caused by *Streptococci*, *Staphylococci* or *Pseudomonas* bacteria. It usually follows a scratch or an insect bite, as a superinfection.

Signs and Symptoms:

It is a deep-seated infection with the formation of multiple, circular ulcers surrounded by reddened skin. It is painful and heals with scarring.

Risk Factors:

It is more common in patients with poor hygiene, malnutrition or trauma to the skin. There is a risk of ecthyma being spread to other parts of the body by contact with secretions from one site to another.

Caution and Recommendations to Therapists:

Since it is usually localized, cover with Band-Aid or bandage and avoid area while massaging. Disinfect table and wash linen thoroughly in hot soapy water. If associated with extensive folliculitis or impetigo, massage is contraindicated. Advice client to seek medical help. The lesion responds well to topical or oral antibiotics. See Appendix B: Strategies for infection prevention and safe practice.

Notes

It is treated with a full course of antibiotics. For more details see Appendix C: Antimicrobial - antibacterial agents.

References

Fitzpatrick TB et al, editors. Dermatology in general medicine. 3rd ed. New York: McGraw-Hill; 1987.

Ectopic pregnancy
Reproductive system

The implantation of the fetus outside the uterine cavity.

Cause:

Any condition that slows down or prevents the fertilized ovum from entering the uterine cavity can cause abnormal implantation.

Once ectopic pregnancy is diagnosed, it is treated surgically with the ligation of the tube if ruptured, or removal of the products if the tube is intact. In cases where the mass is unruptured and measures less than 4 cm it may be treated medically using methotrexate - a drug which affects DNA synthesis and multiplication of cells. For more details see Appendix C: Contraceptives.

Signs and Symptoms:

The most common site for ectopic pregnancy is the fallopian tube (*tubal pregnancy*). As the fetus grows it stretches and weakens the wall of the tube until it ruptures.

Ectopic pregnancy usually presents as a normal pregnancy accompanied by slight abdominal pain in the ectopic site. It is

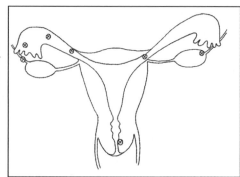

Common sites for ectopic pregnancy

usually diagnosed when it ruptures producing severe abdominal pain, with bleeding into the peritoneal cavity. The person may go into shock as a result of excessive bleeding.

Risk Factors:

Pelvic inflammatory disease, previous surgery to the fallopian tubes or any abdominal surgery that has resulted in adhesion formation in the reproductive organs increases the risk. Abnormal structure of the uterus, use of intrauterine devices for contraception are some of the other predisposing factors. Incidence of ectopic pregnancy is higher in a person with a previous history. However, the prognosis for future pregnancies is poor.

References

Fritz S. Mosby's fundamentals of therapeutic massage. New York: Mosby -Year book Inc; 1995. p. 145-146.

Waters B. Massage during pregnancy. Fuquay-Varina, NC: Research Triangle publishing; 1995.

Osporne-Sheets C. Pre- and Perinatal Massage Therapy. San Diego, CA: Body Therapy Associates; 1998.

Dodson MG. Bleeding in pregnancy. In: Aladjem S, editor. Obstetrical practice. London: CV Mosby Co; 1980. p. 451-458.

Caution and Recommendations to Therapists:

In general, do not massage the lower abdomen in a pregnant client in the first trimester. Avoid abdominal massage in a client who has been classified as high-risk pregnancy - this includes a pregnant client with a previous history of ectopic pregnancy. Always consult Obstetrician before massaging a pregnant client who is "high risk". Hypertension, diabetes, eclampsia, spontaneous abortions are some of the high-risk pregnancies. Also see under Abortion.

Lymphatic, Cardiovascular, Renal, Gastrointestinal systems

Edema (Oedema)

Collection of excess fluid in the interstitial compartment of the body.

Notes

The cause of the edema has to be identified and suitably treated. Diuretics may be used to treat some forms of edema. For more details see Appendix C: Diuretics.

Cause:

Edema is produced when the net capillary fluid pressure is higher than the pressure between the cells ie. the interstitial pressure. Such a situation arises when there is

a) obstruction or reduction of the venous drainage such as in varicose veins, right sided cardiac failure, venous thrombosis, obstruction to flow by an enlarged uterus or tumor, wearing tight garters, prolonged standing or the limb in a dependent position

b) capillary dilatation as in inflammation

c) lymphatic obstruction as in filariasis, removal of lymph nodes during treatment of cancers eg. removal of axillary lymph nodes for breast cancer can result in edema of the arm and

d) reduced plasma proteins as in severe malnutrition or malabsorption disorders, liver diseases and kidney failure.

Signs and Symptoms:

Most types of edema are pitting ie. when sustained pressure is applied over the area, indentations can be produced due to the movement of fluid away from the area under pressure. Pain and heaviness of the area may be felt. This is due to the fact that the excess fluid widens the distance between the blood vessels bringing nutrients and the cells. The stasis also results in the accumulaton of pain-producing waste products/toxins in the area.

It presents as localized or generalized swelling. *Ascites* - collection of excessive fluid in the peritoneal cavity and *hydrothorax* - excessive fluid in the pleural cavity are special forms of edema that may be present. *Anasarca* is a term given to gross, generalized edema that may be present.

Risk Factors:

See Cause.

Caution and Recommendations to Therapists:

A detailed history and a consultation with the attending Physician can help establish the cause. Generalized edema is usually due to chronic cardiac, kidney or liver problems. Massage may be detrimental to such clients. If the edema is due to causes other than cardiac, kidney or liver problems, massage may be beneficial.

In edema of the limbs after removal of lymph nodes, the limb is hard, tender and painful due to lymphatic congestion. The joints are stiff and the movements are painful. In the case of the arm, swelling may be seen in front of the chest or behind the shoulders. The purpose of massage in such clients is to help lymphatic drainage by forcing fluid back into the capillaries and relieving congestion, by increasing the pressure in the lymphatic vessels and assisting with the formation of new paths of drainage.

The client should be positioned with the edematous limb supported and elevated. Positioning the client in such a way for 10-15 minutes before treatment, uses gravity to help with the drainage. Use slow, deep effleurage and kneading strokes to the proximal areas and then the distal areas thus emptying the proximal lymph vessels before forcing the lymph from the distal vessels through them. Use friction movements around the joints. The client will have relief even though there is no visible reduction in the size of the limb. Make sure that the strokes follow the direction of movement of lymph in the area.

References

Guyton A. Textbook of medical physiology 8th edition. Philadelphia: WB Saunders; 1991. p.274-285, 398,801. WB Saunders. Philadelphia.

Harris R. Edema and its treatment in massage therapy. Journal of Soft Tissue Manipulation 1993; 1:4-6.

In the upper arms, strokes should be towards the axilla; in the chest, the movement should be towards the neck and axilla of the respective side; in the legs, towards the inguinal region. Use passive and active movements after the massage to assist both the venous and lymphatic flow. In clients with chronic edema, organization of the proteins in the interstitial region results in fibrosis and thickening of the skin and connective tissue. In such clients, adhesions have to be stretched. Use gentle friction movements here. If there are signs of increased pain and swelling stop treating and refer to Physician.

Ehlers-Danlos syndrome

Integumentary, Musculoskeletal systems

A group of disorders that are inherited that result in loose skin and hypermobile joints.

Cause:

It is due to abnormal structure of collagen.

Signs and Symptoms:

The disease has been classified into many subtypes according to the severity. The consistency of the skin varies according to the subtype from velvety skin, to skin that is easily stretched or scarred. There may be hyperpigmentation of the scars. Sometimes the skin is so thin that the underlying blood vessels can be seen. The joints may be so hypermobile that they get easily dislocated. Many associated lesions such as scoliosis and mitral valve prolapse may occur. The weakness of the blood vessels can predispose to aneurysms.

Risk Factors:

The disease is inherited.

Caution and Recommendations to Therapists:

Since the presentation varies according to the type of syndrome, a detailed history and physical examination is required. In any case, medical clearance should be obtained before massage. The Therapist has to be extremely careful, as they are prone to bruise very easily.

Notes

There is no specific treatment. Surgery may be done to tighten the ligaments in extremely lax joints.

For more details see Appendix C: Genetic testing/counselling.

References

Procop DJ, Kuivaniemi H, Tromp G. Heritable disorders of connective tissue. In: Isselbacher KJ et al, editors. Harrison's principles of internal medicine. 13th ed. London: McGraw-Hill Co; 1994. p. 2113-2115.

Emphysema

Respiratory system

A Chronic Obstructive Pulmonary Disease (COPD) where the alveolar septa are destroyed and the elastic recoil of the lungs are reduced due to recurrent inflammation.

Cause:

It occurs in combination with the other COPD - chronic bronchitis and the risk factors are the same as Bronchitis (see Bronchitis). Here, the recurrent inflammation results in release of protein-digesting enzymes from the immune

Notes

Like bronchitis, treatment involves cessation of smoking, prompt treatment of superinfections, exercise and nutrition. Symptoms may be reduced by the use of

cells causing damage to the supporting tissue as well as the alveolar wall. This in turn reduces the elasticity of the alveolar wall with difficulty in expiration. The destruction of the alveolar wall also reduces the surface area for exchange of gases leading to hypoxia (reduced availability of oxygen to tissues).

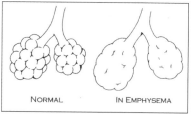

NORMAL   IN EMPHYSEMA

Bronchiole and alveoli

bronchodilator drugs. Postural drainage is beneficial. In severe cases, continuous oxygen therapy is warranted. Lung transplantation may be considered for some.

For more details see Appendix C: Bronchodilators; Antiasthmatics; Organ transplantation; Oxygen treatment.

Emphysema may be caused by congenital weakness or deficiency of elastic fibres in the walls of bronchioles and alveoli.

Signs and Symptoms:

The individual typically has a round, barrel-shaped chest (due to the large volume of residual air remaining in the lungs even after expiration). There is difficulty in breathing, chronic cough, weight loss, blue coloration of fingers, toes and mucous membrane (cyanosis). The blue coloration is due to the high levels of deoxygenated hemoglobin in the blood. The use of the accessory muscles of breathing can be seen.

Risk Factors:

See Bronchitis. Occupations that involve forceful expiration such as glass blowing, playing wind instruments predispose to this condition. Males are more often affected. Smoking, air pollution, infection, familial and genetic makeup are other predisposing factors.

Caution and Recommendations to Therapists:

The aim is to reduce the symptoms, help with the mobility of the thorax and facilitate drainage of mucus by dislodging them from the walls of the bronchi. Proper air circulation and filtration in the clinic helps these clients. Higher humidity and warmth also helps with the drainage of mucus. The client may be more comfortable seated or in a half-lying position. Let the client relax for about ten minutes in this position before massage. Steam inhalation at this point helps loosen the thick sputum, if present. Do a whole body relaxation massage and use vigorous chest clapping, hacking and vibrations for 10 to 20 minutes.

You may have to provide a sputum mug with disinfectant for the client. (Use proper precautions while handling and disposing the mug and contents). Massage the tired respiratory muscles and the accessory muscles that are used for respiration. This should include the pectorals, the latissimus dorsi, trapezius, sternocleidomastoid and scalene muscles. The intercostal muscles may be stretched using two fingers in the intercostal space and applying pressure downward during expiration. Encourage clients to breathe deeply with slow and full expiration throughout the massage treatment.

These clients are very prone to respiratory infection so massage should be avoided if the Therapist has even a mild form of respiratory infection. Schedule

References

Klimowitch P. Massage for sufferers of respiratory diseases. Massage Therapy Journal 1993; 32(2): 42-43.

Josephson GD et al. Airway obstruction. New modalities in treatment. Med Clin North Am 1993; 77: 539.

Reid LM. Chronic obstructive pulmonary diseases. In: Fishman AP, editor. Pulmonary diseases and disorders. 2nd ed. New York: McGraw-Hill Co; 1988. p. 1247-1272.

these clients for a time when they are unlikely to come in contact with others with infection. Encourage client to stop smoking if smokers. See Appendix D for organizations and support groups.

Encephalitis

An infection of the brain or spinal cord.

Cause:

Notes

Treatment is usually supportive. Painkillers, fluid and electrolyte maintenance, steroids and diuretics to reduce edema of the brain are some of the measures used. For more details see Appendix C: Painkillers; Antiinflammatories - steroidal drugs; Diuretics.

It is usually caused by a viral infection. The infection may be mosquito-borne, carried by ticks or spread by ingestion. Encephalitis can be caused by bacteria or fungi too. Other rare causes are toxic substances such as lead. It may also occur after vaccines for measles, mumps and rabies. Encephalitis usually occurs as an epidemic.

Signs and Symptoms:

It presents as headache, fever, vomiting and neck stiffness - similar to meningitis. In addition, there is always a neurological abnormality like disorientation, seizures, paralysis and coma.

Risk Factors:

See Cause.

Caution and Recommendations to Therapists:

References

Morello JA, Mizer HE, Wilson ME, Granato PA. Microbiology in patient care. 6th ed. New York: McGraw-Hill; 1998. p. 493-396.

Suspect encephalitis or meningitis in an individual with sudden onset of headache associated with fever and neck stiffness. Refer to Physician. Be fully informed about epidemics of encephalitis in your area. See Appendix D for organizations and support groups. Also see Appendix B: Strategies for infection prevention and safe practice.

Endometriosis

A condition where endometrial tissue (tissue from the inner lining of the uterus) is found in areas outside the uterus such as the ovaries, ligaments supporting the uterus, vagina, bladder, intestines etc.

Cause:

Notes

It is treated with hormones - estrogen or progesterone or a combination of both. Painkillers are also given. Laser surgery to destroy the tissue and reduce adhesions is also resorted to. In severe cases, more extensive surgery with removal of affected organs/lesions may be required.

The cause is not known. However, several explanations have been given. It is thought that backflow of the endometrial tissue through the fallopian tube during menstruation, and subsequent implantation and growth in surrounding areas in the pelvis may be the cause. Some believe that the endometrial tissue may be carried to other areas through the lymphatic system or blood. It may also be due to transformation of immature cells in other areas into endometrial tissue.

Pathology A to Z -

Signs and Symptoms:

For more details see Appendix C: Hormone therapy/replacement; Painkillers; Laser therapy.

The symptoms are vague and are usually produced by the cyclical changes that the endometrial tissue undergoes according to the changing hormonal levels in the blood. Lower abdominal pain is produced when the tissue bleeds into the pelvic cavity during menstruation. The resultant inflammation heals by fibrosis and causes adhesions between surrounding pelvic organs. There may be pain during menstruation and during intercourse. Endometriosis may be a cause of infertility.

Endometriosis may be found in many sites. Ovaries, pelvic peritoneum, fallopian tubes, pelvic lymph nodes are common sites. Rarely, endometrial tissue may be found in the rectosigmoid region, umbilicus, kidneys, lungs etc.

Risk Factors:

It is more common in women who have borne children at a late age. Those who started menstruating at an early age, have menstrual cycles shorter than 27 days with the menstrual flow lasting more than 7 days, or those with heavier flows are at risk.

Caution and Recommendations to Therapists:

The aim is to reduce the pain. Massage should be gentle and relaxing. Warm compresses to the low back and lower abdomen are recommended. Some advocate the use of essential oils such as lavender, chamomile or rose essential oil in a 5% dilution, to reduce spasm and pain. Oil may also be added to the water used for the warm compress.

Avoid deep abdominal work. Reflexive work may be beneficial.

References

Danford D. Obstetrics and Gynaecology. 3rd ed. New York: Harper & Row; 1977.

Endometritis

An inflammation of the endometrium - the inner lining of the uterus. Endometritis may be a misnomer for metritis, an infection of the uterus.

Reproductive system

Cause:

It is usually caused by bacterial infection.

Notes

It is treated with antibiotics that may be taken orally or given intravenously. For more details see Appendix C: Antimicrobial - antibacterial agents.

Signs and Symptoms:

Abnormal menstrual bleeding accompanied by lower abdominal pain and foul-smelling discharge are common symptoms. It is associated with fever and malaise.

Risk Factors:

Infection of the endometrium is more common soon after delivery, after an abortion, uterine surgery or insertion of intrauterine devices by improper techniques.

References

Danford D. Obstetrics and Gynaecology. 3rd ed. New York: Harper & Row; 1977

Caution and Recommendations to Therapists:

Avoid abdominal area during massage. Encourage the client to take the full course of antibiotic treatment prescribed by Physician.

Epilepsy (Seizures)

Nervous system

A group of disorders due to abnormalities of the electrical activities of the brain that makes an individual susceptible to recurrent, periodic changes in neurological function.

Cause:

Notes

The treatment is directed towards eliminating the cause, if found. Epilepsy can be controlled with a high degree of success with medication. Most women with epilepsy can have uneventful pregnancies; however, special attention has to be given to antiepileptic drug levels.

Each state or province has its own laws regarding driving and epilepsy. The client has to ensure that s/he is within the laws. In general, a person with epilepsy can drive after a seizure-free interval (range: 6 months to 3 years). A Physician may have to authenticate that the seizure is under control.

For more details see Appendix C: Antiepileptics.

Epilepsy results from abnormal neuronal discharge in the brain. Each episode is known as a *seizure*. The cause is unknown in most cases. But it may be caused by injury to the brain during birth, infectious diseases that affect the brain - meningitis or abscess in the brain, mercury, lead or carbon monoxide poisoning, brain tumors or head injury. It may also be associated with inherited disorders. A sudden drop in blood glucose levels may also produce epilepsy. In older individuals, it may follow hemorrhage, thrombosis or emboli in cerebral arteries.

Signs and Symptoms:

The signs and symptoms vary according to the type of seizure the person has and the area of the brain where the abnormal discharge occurs. Partial seizures may present as jerking movements and tingling sensations confined to one limb. The person does not loose consciousness. Epilepsy typically begins with an aura - the person may smell something pungent, feel nauseated, have an unusual taste, or have a purposeless behavior. In other types of epilepsy, there may be a change in consciousness with chewing or blinking movements or a blank stare lasting for a few seconds. There may be rhythmic involuntary movements of the limb.

During a generalized seizure, the person falls to the ground unconscious with a loud cry and becomes completely rigid - the tonic stage. This is followed by the clonic stage when the body alternately goes into violent spasm and relaxation for 2-5 minutes. Breathing is affected as the respiratory muscles go into spasm. The person then regains consciousness, with the muscles relaxed. Headache, confusion, weakness and fatigue may be present. Prolonged continuous seizures - a rare occurrence can be life-threatening.

Risk Factors:

See Cause. Head injury or family history of epilepsy are predisposing factors. Flashing lights, noise, pain, essential oils, perfumes or emotional stress may trigger an epileptic fit. In some women the seizures may have a relationship to hormonal changes that occur during the menstrual cycle, pregnancy or oral contraceptives.

Caution and Recommendations to Therapists:

Massage is not contraindicated in a client who has a history of epilepsy.

However, make a note in the client's record if they have a history of epilepsy and obtain the address of a contact person in case a fit occurs in the clinic. Since certain types of epilepsy can be triggered by specific smells - aromatherapy can serve as a trigger. Do not use techniques that are deep and vigorous in these clients - this may also trigger an attack in some.

If a client has an aura - a warning that an attack is underway, place the client flat on a couch or ground, well away from hard objects with a soft pillow behind the head. Place a soft object such as a rolled piece of linen between the teeth - to prevent the tongue from being bitten. Do not force anything into the mouth if the teeth are clenched. Turn the head sideways to maintain an open airway. Do not restrain the convulsive movements. Reassure client after an attack and ensure that the client is escorted home from the clinic. See Appendix D for organizations and support groups.

References

Curtis D. Massage therapy considerations in treating epileptic clients. Journal of Soft Tissue Manipulation 1997; 4(3): 5,6,8,10.

Aird RB, Masland RL, Woodbury DB. The epilepsies: a critical review. New York: Raven Press; 1984.

Erysipelas

Integumentary system

A bacterial infection of the skin.

Cause:

It is usually caused by streptococci bacilli.

Signs and Symptoms:

It appears as tender, red, swollen areas in the face, arms or legs with small and large fluid-filled vesicles and bullae. The edema in the skin, along with the hair follicles may give the appearance of orange skin (*peau d'orange*). The patient has flu-like symptoms. When the infection spreads deep into the dermis and subcutaneous fat it is termed cellulitis.

Risk Factors:

It is more common in those with diabetes or lowered immunity.

Caution and Recommendations to Therapists:

Due to the pain, swelling, clients will not seek massage. Avoid massage as it can spread the disease to surrounding areas. Advice immediate medical help. It can be treated with antibiotics. See Appendix B: Strategies for infection prevention and safe practice.

Notes

It is treated with antibiotics. For more details see Appendix C: Antimicrobial - antibacterial agents.

References

Fitzpatrick TB et al, editors. Dermatology in general medicine. 3rd ed. New York: McGraw-Hill; 1987.

Erythema multiforme

Integumentary system

A syndrome that causes recurrent, symmetrical skin lesions.

Cause:

It may be due to an immune reaction in the skin and mucous membrane to antigenic stimuli as it follows exposure to specific drugs such as penicillins, sulfonamides, nonsteroidal anti-inflammatory drugs etc or infection. There is inflammation in the epithelium and around the blood vessels.

Notes

It is treated symptomatically. Drugs for pain and itch are given. In severe cases, intravenous fluids, antibiotics (to prevent secondary infection) and moist dressings may be needed.

For more details see Appendix C: Painkillers; Antimicrobial - antibacterial agents.

Signs and Symptoms:

Symmetrically distributed, round, red lesions are seen. The lesions appear episodically and disappear within a few weeks. The lesion may appear as rings with edema and redness (erythema) in the periphery. The lesion may form a blister later. Usually the lesions are seen in the hands and feet and on the extensor surfaces of the leg and arm. See Appendix A: page 351. Rarely, mucous membranes may be involved (*Stevens-Johnson syndrome*). Itching and pain may be present. In severe cases there may be associated fever and body ache. There are many varieties of the condition.

Risk Factors:

Herpes simplex virus infections and certain drugs may predispose to the condition.

Caution and Recommendations to Therapists:

Do not massage if the client has fever. Avoid the areas with lesions. Elevation of the affected area may be beneficial. Even though the lesions may appear infectious, this condition is not infective. The client may be on painkillers, so adequate feedback may not be given during the massage. See Appendix B: Strategies for infection prevention and safe practice.

References

Fitzpatrick TB et al, editors. Dermatology in general medicine. 3rd ed. New York: McGraw-Hill; 1987.

Integumentary system

Erythrasma

A superficial bacterial infection of the skin.

Cause:

It is caused by the bacteria *Corynebacterium minutissimum.*

Notes

It is treated with local application or oral antibiotics. For more details see Appendix C: Antimicrobial - antibacterial agents.

Signs and Symptoms:

The infection may involve one of the body folds such as the groin, axilla or between the toes. A superficial rash consisting of redness, scales and hyper-pigmentation is seen. The rash is crossed by creases which run in directions different from the normal skin. It may sometimes itch. It is not painful.

Risk Factors:

Excessive sweating predisposes to this condition.

Caution and Recommendations to Therapists:

It is contagious. Avoid areas affected if confined to small region, or massage client after it is cured. It may require treatment for 3-6 weeks. See Appendix B: Strategies for infection prevention and safe practice.

References

Fitzpatrick TB et al, editors. Dermatology in general medicine. 3rd ed. New York: McGraw-Hill; 1987.

Esophageal stenosis (Esophageal stricture)

Narrowing of the esophagus.

Cause:

This is usually caused by chemical injury to the esophagus either accidentally or deliberately as in a suicide attempt. Soon after the ingestion, there is edema and inflammation followed by ulceration, tissue death and healing by scar tissue formation. Other causes of stricture could be due to cancerous growths or compression of the esophagus by an aortic aneurysm.

Signs and Symptoms:

In strictures due to chemical injury, soon after the ingestion, there may be intense chest pain and excessive salivation. If there is severe damage, there is vomiting of blood and esophageal tissue. Within weeks there is difficulty in swallowing due to the narrowing of the esophagus. In strictures caused by other factors, the difficulty in swallowing and chest pain may be slower in onset.

Risk Factors:

See Cause.

Caution and Recommendations to Therapists:

Consult Physician before massaging an individual with stenosis due to aortic aneurysm or malignant growth. The client may be more comfortable in a seated or half-lying position.

Notes

Strictures due to chemical ingestion are treated with corticosteroids to reduce scarring, and antibiotics to combat superinfection. Surgery may be required for severe damage.

For more details see Appendix C: Antimicrobial - antibacterial agents; Antiinflammatories - steroidal drugs.

References

Orringer MB. Disorders of esophageal motility. In: Sabiston DC, editor. Textbook of Surgery- the biological basis of modern surgical practice. 14th ed. London: WB Saunders Co; 1991. p. 663-678.

Esophageal varices

Presence of dilated and tortuous veins in the esophagus.

Cause:

The most common cause is diversion of venous blood that normally passes through the liver to the right side of the heart, into the esophageal veins. Conditions that alter the architecture of the liver result in damming up and increased pressure (*portal hypertension*) in the venous blood in the abdomen. The blood is therefore diverted through the esophageal veins into the thoracic cavity. Rarely, varicosities may be genetic.

Signs and Symptoms:

The person may show signs of liver failure like intolerance to fat intake, passage of foul-smelling, greasy stools and jaundice, among others. The abdomen is enlarged with accumulation of fluid in the peritoneal cavity (ascites). Enlarged dilated veins may be visible on the surface of the abdomen. The liver may be palpable as a swelling in the right upper quadrant of the abdomen. The person

Notes

One of the complications of this condition is rupture of the dilated veins with severe bleeding that may be fatal. The blood volume should be promptly brought back to near normal. Then measures are taken to prevent further and recurrent bleeding. Vasoconstrictors, ligation/sclerosing of blood vessels endoscopically are some forms of treatment. Balloon tamponade - a method where a multi-lumen tube is introduced into the stomach and esophagus and inflated, may be used if the bleeding is severe.

Long-term treatment includes surgery to create shunts between the portal and systemic circulation in order to reduce the pressure in the portal vessels.

For more details see Appendix C: Vasoconstrictors; Balloon tamponade; Shunts; Sclerosing agents.

may also vomit blood (hematemesis).

Risk Factors:

Cirrhosis of the liver is the most common cause. Alcoholism and liver damage predispose to this condition.

References

Rikkers LF. Surgical complications of cirrhosis and portal hypertension. In: Sabiston DC, editor. Textbook of Surgery-the biological basis of modern surgical practice. 14th ed. London: WB Saunders Co; 1991. p. 1019-1029.

Caution and Recommendations to Therapists:

Consult Physician. Avoid massaging the abdominal area. Since it is most often a complication of cirrhosis of the liver, the Therapist should be aware of the pathophysiology of cirrhosis and associated symptoms and signs. See Appendix D for organizations and support groups.

Nervous system

Fever

An increase in body temperature above normal limits.

Cause:

Notes

The cause of the fever has to be identified and treated. Antipyretics are usually given if the temperature is more than 41°C in children, pregnant women and those with heart, lungs and cerebral problems. There is no benefit in treating low-grade fever with antipyretics.

For more details see Appendix C: Antipyretics.

Normally, the body temperature is maintained by the thermoregulatory center located in the anterior hypothalamus. The center balances heat production and heat dissipation to maintain the body temperature between 36.8 ± 0.4 °C (98.2 ± 0.7°F). Usually, the temperature is lower at 6 AM and higher at 4 PM. The core temperature is generally about 0.6°C (1°F) higher. Substances that cause fever, called *pyrogens*, reach the hypothalamus and reset the temperature. The pyrogens may be microorganisms or substances they secrete. Pyrogens are produced inside the body too, especially by white blood cells. There are far too many causes of fever to list. The cause of the fever may not be identified in some cases and using specific criteria, they are classified as '*fever of unknown origin*' (*FUO*).

Signs and Symptoms:

The body temperature is higher than normal. The higher temperature setting of the hypothalamus results in stimulation of mechanisms that produce heat (shivering, chills) and mechanisms to conserve heat (seeking warm clothes etc). The pattern of fever may be indicative of certain conditions. *Intermittent fever* is when there is an exaggeration of the normal swings in the morning and evening. *Relapsing fever* is when there is normal temperatures between episodes of fever. The fever is described as *tertian* when the temperatures are high every third day (typical of a type of malaria) and *quartan* if the temperature is high every fourth day (typical of another type of malaria). *Remittent fever* is when the temperature is reducing every day but is higher than normal.

The advantage of fever is that the growth of many types of bacteria is inhibited by elevations of temperature. Also, the activity of neutrophils and lymphocytes is enhanced by fever. However, the metabolic rate increases in the individual and requirements of oxygen, fluid and calories increase. This may be a form of stress in individuals with heart problems. The fetus may be stressed if there is persistent fever in a pregnant woman. High fever may cause delirium. In children, high fever can cause seizures to occur.

Risk Factors:

Any condition that causes pyrogens to be released can produce fever.

Caution and Recommendations to Therapists:

Massage is contraindicated in a person with fever.

References

Gelfand JA, Dinarello CA, Wolff SM. Fever, including fever of unknown origin. In: Isselbacher KJ et al, editors. Harrison's principles of internal medicine. 13th ed. London: McGraw-Hill Co; 1994. p. 81-90.

Fibroadenoma - breast

Reproductive system

A benign, abnormal growth in the breast.

Cause:

The cause is not known.

Notes

It is not precancerous. The lump is surgically removed.

Signs and Symptoms:

It is felt as a painless, movable, firm, rubbery, round growth in the breast that slides under the fingers. It is usually single about 2-3 cm in diameter. The tumor does not change with the menstrual cycle and is very slow growing. It is often found by accident.

Risk Factors:

It is seen in women of the reproductive age group.

Caution and Recommendations to Therapists:

Any lump in the breast should be investigated to rule out cancer. Encourage client to see a Physician. In general, encourage all women clients to do regular self-examinations.

References

Danford D. Obstetrics and Gynaecology. 3rd ed. New York: Harper & Row; 1977.

Iglehart JD. The breast. In: Sabiston DC, editor. Textbook of Surgery- the biological basis of modern surgical practice. 14th ed. London: WB Saunders Co; 1991. p. 522-523.

Fibrocystic disease - breast (Mammary dysplasia)

Reproductive system

Development of fibrosis and cyst formation in the breast.

Cause:

It may be caused by the hypersensitivity of the breast tissues to hormones. It may also be due to unresolved proliferation of the breast tissue due to the cyclical hormonal changes. It is believed by some to be a precursor of cancerous changes in the breast.

Notes

It is treated with painkillers. In some clients reduced caffeine intake, low-salt diet and vitamin E are of benefit. In those with severe pain, mastectomy may be done.

For more details see Appendix C: Mastectomy; Painkillers.

Signs and Symptoms:

It is felt as multiple small lumps that are prominent and painful just before menstruation. The lumps may produce heaviness in some while in others it may be very painful.

a Handbook for Massage Therapists

Risk Factors:

It is seen in women of the reproductive age group.

Caution and Recommendations to Therapists:

Any lump/s in the breasts should be investigated and cancer should be ruled out. Encourage client to see a Physician. For clients diagnosed with this condition, heat or cold therapy may be beneficial. Use warm or cold packs wrapped in a towel.

References

Danford D. Obstetrics and Gynaecology. 3rd ed. New York: Harper & Row; 1977.

Iglehart JD. The breast. In: Sabiston DC, editor. Textbook of Surgery- the biological basis of modern surgical practice. 14th ed. WB Saunders Co; 1991. p. 521-522.

Reproductive system	# Fibroid (Leiomyoma; Myoma; Fibromyoma)
	An abnormal growth of the smooth muscles of the uterus.

Cause:

The cause is not known. Estrogen and progesterone levels have been implicated in altering the growth of the tumor.

Signs and Symptoms:

The symptoms and signs will depend on the location of the fibroid ie. whether it is on the surface, in the muscle or under the inner lining of the uterus. Most often it is asymptomatic. The more common symptom is abnormal menstrual bleeding with increased flow, of longer duration (menorrhagia). Swelling in the lower abdomen, interference with passing urine and pelvic pain are some of the other symptoms. Premature labour and recurrent abortions are symptoms that have been associated with leiomyomas.

Risk Factors:

It is common over the age of 35. The incidence is higher in Afro-Americans.

Caution and Recommendations to Therapists:

Do not massage the lower abdominal area. Refer to a Physician if the lower abdominal swelling is prominent. Encourage client to take iron supplements if anemic, due to excessive bleeding.

Notes

Most clients with the condition do not require treatment. Myomas are treated surgically or with nonsurgical measures, according to the size and location of tumor, age of person, pregnancy status and desire for children.

References

Danford D. Obstetrics and Gynaecology. 3rd ed. New York: Harper & Row; 1977

Musculoskeletal, Nervous systems	# Fibromyalgia (Fibromyalgia syndrome; Fibrositis; Fibromyositis)
	A chronic condition that produces musculoskeletal pain.

Cause:

The cause is not known. It has been postulated that it may be due to a disturbance of normal stages of sleep. Psychological disorders, muscle abnormalities and autonomic dysfunction may play a part in this condition. More recently, it has been considered as a disorder of the nervous and endocrine system with chemical

Notes

The treatment is symptomatic and multi-pronged. It is very important for the client to be educated about the disease. As well, family and friends have to be involved in

imbalances that affect how pain is perceived by the body. Abnormalities in neurotransmitters like substance P and serotonin are implicated. Emotional stress, trauma, surgery and disease of the thyroid have been implicated in triggering the symptoms.

Signs and Symptoms:

The symptoms vary from individual to individual and changes in the same individual from day to day. It is characterized by diffuse, ill-defined muscle pain, stiffness, easy fatigability and disturbed sleep. There is generalized ache and stiffness. There may be stiffness of joints and a feeling of swollen joints although there are no visible signs of swelling. The stiffness may be more in the morning. The patient complains of exhaustion and wakes up tired. The symptoms may be precipitated or increased by stress, cold weather and exertion. In some, there may be numbness and tingling in arms and legs. Many experience daily headache. Some exhibit different degrees of memory loss and difficulty in concentrating.

Some individuals have symptoms of irritable bowel syndrome with bouts of constipation, diarrhea, bloating, gas etc. Others may have associated urinary problems with frequency, difficulty and burning while passing urine.

It is diagnosed by the presence of tender sites that are constant in location. The common locations of tender sites are: bilaterally over the suboccipital muscle insertion at the base of the skull, the anterior aspect of the intertransverse process spaces at C5-C7, the midpoint of the upper border of the trapezius, above the scapular spine near the medial border of the scapula, the second costochondral junction, the lateral epicondyle, the upper outer quadrant

Common locations of tender sites

of the buttock, the posterior aspect of the trochanteric prominence, and the medial fat pad of the knee.

According to the American College of Rheumatology, diagnosis is made if there is diffuse muscular pain along with 11 of the 18 tender points described.

Risk Factors:

It is common in women between the ages of 25-45 years of age. It may be associated with rheumatoid arthritis, migraine headache, irritable bowel syndrome or other connective tissue diseases. It may be hereditary.

the treatment program. Massage, acupressure, acupuncture, injection of tender sites with steroids, anti-inflammatory drugs, antidepressants, painkillers, education, rest, physiotherapy, biofeedback and exercise are some of the treatment options.

For more details see Appendix C: Antiinflammatories - steroidal drugs; Antiinflammatories - non steroidal drugs; Antidepressants; Biofeedback; Painkillers.

Caution and Recommendations to Therapists:

A detailed history should be obtained every time the client visits, as the symptoms vary from day to day, and the massage techniques have to be altered accordingly. The frequency and duration of massage should be individualized. Massage may not be beneficial to all clients. It is important to enquire about medications and be informed about the side effects of these medications.

In general, a full body relaxation massage of short duration is indicated. The client may be on painkillers that depress the sensations and inadequate feedback may be given. All strokes should be gentle and rhythmic. Gentle cross fiber friction over entire muscles, stretching and strokes such as effleurage have been shown to be beneficial.. Hot packs can be used in areas that are particularly painful. However, heat and cold may be initiating factors of pain for some clients and has to be avoided in these situations.

In general, massage has been shown to increase relaxation of muscles, decrease fatigue, decrease pain, produce sleep, decrease edema and increase mobility. It has been shown to increase communication, decrease depression and anxiety and produce a general increase in sense of well being. All these effects directly address the symptoms of fibromyalgia.

References

Goldenberg DL. Fibromyalgia syndrome a decade later. What have we learned? Arch Intern Med 1999; 159: 777-785.

Wallace DJ. The fibromyalgia syndrome. Ann Med 1997; 29:9-21.

Wolf F. Fibromyalgia: the clinical syndrome. Rheum Dis Clin North Am 1989; 15: 1-18.

Massage therapy is a unique form of therapy in that it establishes a rapport and strong communication between client and Therapist. This in itself can be a tremendous healing process in these clients who are often depressed by their affliction. Massage Therapists can play a significant role in guiding the client to take charge and fight back. For this, the Therapist has to be well informed about the disorder in order to educate the client and point them to the right resources. See Appendix D for organizations and support groups.

Folliculitis

Integumentary system

A bacterial infection of the hair follicles of the skin.

Cause:

Notes

It is treated with local or oral antibiotics. For more details see Appendix C: Antimicrobial - antibacterial agents.

It is usually caused by the bacteria *staphylococcus aureus*. Other organisms may produce the infection particularly when associated with immersion in contaminated warm water eg. in swimming pools or Jacuzzis.

Signs and Symptoms:

It appears as a small pustule at the base of a hair follicle. There is redness, swelling and pain around the hair follicle. It is more commonly seen in the thighs, lower legs, arms, face and scalp.

Risk Factors:

Any condition that occludes the hair follicles predisposes to the condition. Trauma (eg. hair removal), topical corticosteroids, prolonged antibiotic therapy, excessive sweating and occlusive dressings are all risk factors.

Caution and Recommendations to Therapists:

Since it is very localized, avoid massaging the area with folliculitis. Cover area with a Band-Aid or bandage. Often the folliculitis disappears without treatment. Local application of antibiotic lotions helps. Occasionally, it may spread to other regions - when it will require oral antibiotics. It has to be distinguished from non-infectious conditions such as pustular psoriasis and acne rosacea. Disinfect table, towels and other linen after treating the infected client. Frequently change the water used for heating hot packs etc. to avoid this being a source of bacteria. Refer to Appendix B: Strategies for infection prevention and safe practice.

References

Fitzpatrick TB et al, editors. Dermatology in general medicine. 3rd ed. New York: McGraw-Hill; 1987

Fractures

The interruption to the continuity of bone.

Musculoskeletal system

Cause:

Sudden application of force that is more than what the bone can withstand is the most common cause. Fractures may also be caused by overuse injury (*stress fracture*). *Pathological fractures* occur in bones weakened by tumors or other diseases.

Signs and Symptoms:

Fractures may be *spiral, transverse* or *oblique* according to the type and direction of stress. It is classified as *open/compound* if it is associated with broken skin or *closed* if the skin is intact. It is considered as *comminuted* if the bone is broken to more than one piece, *compression type* if two bones are crushed together or *impacted type* if the bones are wedged together. The rate of healing and chances of complications vary according to the type of fracture.

Inflammation with its' characteristic redness, pain, swelling and loss of function, is seen in the area of fracture. Abnormal movement, grating sound (crepitus) and deformity may accompany it. The bone may be shortened, abnormally rotated or angulated. If the fracture is compound with the skin open to the exterior, bleeding occurs. Soon after the fracture the local area become numb from a few minutes to an hour, and the muscles around the fracture loose their tone.

Symptoms and signs of complications such as compartment syndrome, fat emboli, impaired healing - delayed union, malunion or nonunion may be present. Compartment syndrome is produced when there is a rise in pressure in a confined area of the body that alters blood flow to the region and affects the function of the nerves and muscles in the area. Abnormal sensations like tingling, loss of sensation, severe pain and loss of motor control are some of the symptoms. Fat emboli may present as disorientation or changes in behavior immediately after or up to a week after fracture, if the embolus is lodged in the

Notes

Treatment varies according to the site and type of fracture. Manipulative correction and application of cast or splint, gradual correction by prolonged traction and surgery, are some of the options. Physiological intervention to control the acute inflammatory response - such as application of ice, compression, elevation and relaxation may be used. Care should be taken to avoid and prevent continued trauma and irritation by reducing the load on the part. At the same time, optimal levels of function should be maintained and unnecessary dysfunction should be prevented. Active and passive stretching, exercise and transverse friction massage are other supportive measures used in the long run.

For more details see Appendix C: Plaster cast.

cerebral circulation. If in the pulmonary circulation, difficulty in breathing, rapid heart rate and pain behind the sternum may be present.

If the healing is impaired, the patient may have abnormal mobility even after the normal healing period (4-6 weeks in children, 6-8 weeks in adolescence, 10 to18 weeks in adults). Deformity may be seen in malunion. In nonunion, abnormal mobility, pain on applying pressure, loss of range of motion and atrophy of surrounding muscles are seen. Adhesions and persistent edema are other complications of fractures.

Risk Factors:

Stress fractures are common in occupations that require overuse of one bone. Pathological fractures are common in local areas weakened by infection, cysts or tumors. Generalized diseases like osteoporosis, Paget's disease or tumors that have spread to the bone from other areas predispose to pathological fractures.

Caution and Recommendations to Therapists:

Fractures are treated by reduction, immobilization, preservation and restoration of function (rehabilitation). Massage therapy can play a positive role during the period of immobilization and rehabilitation. The time needed for healing varies in different bones and has to be taken into consideration while treating clients. Healing time depends on the thickness of the bone, blood supply, amount of separation between the bone fragments, part of the bone fractured, age of client, nutrition, degree of immobilization, infection and extent of bone death. In adults, it takes approximately 6 weeks in the upper limb and 12 weeks in the lower limb for consolidation to occur in spiral fractures. It takes 12 weeks in upper limb and 24 weeks in lower limb for transverse fracture to consolidate.

During the immobilization period, the aim of massage is to maintain circulation, joint mobility and muscle power and to reduce edema without slowing or preventing healing. Another role is to watch for complications and report to Physician. The affected limb can be elevated to improve drainage. During the period of immobilization, use hot packs to improve circulation, decrease spasm and reduce pain in the muscles close to the immobilized part. Passively move all joints not fixed by plaster. This helps the venous return and prevents stiffness. However, do not use forced movements. A whole body gentle, relaxation massage helps reduce the general stress level of client. Massaging around the immobilized fracture site helps reduce edema, relieve pain and tension in the muscles. The massage should be gentle and rhythmic. Avoid the fracture site and take care not to disturb the repair process thus leading to delayed or nonunion. Oil should not be used close to the plaster cast as it can soften the cast.

During rehabilitation, the aim is to help client regain mobility of the previously immobilized or restricted joints. Assess the range of motion of joint and compare with the sound joint. The tissue that was under the cast is likely to be fragile and weak. Muscle atrophy will be present too. Avoid testing for range of motion and tone for at least a week after removal of cast. Remember that although union may have occurred in the bone, consolidation/remodelling may not be complete. In some cases this may take from 6 months to a year. Therefore, care must be taken not to put undue pressure over the fracture site. Heat packs can be used to help improve circulation and relieve pain. The part may be immersed in warm water before massage. Use friction strokes around joints and passively move all joints. Active assisted movements can be used after consultation with Physiotherapist or Physician.

One to two treatments a week during the immobilization period, increased to three times a week after removal of cast for two weeks are recommended. This may be followed by massages once a week for as long as required.

References

Mercier LR, editor. Practical orthopedics. 4th ed. New York: Mosby-Year book Inc; 1995.p. 6-27.

Hall C M. Brody LT. Therapeutic exercise moving toward function. Philadelphia: Lippincott Williams & Wilkins; 1999. p. 173-175.

Fungal infections (Mycosis - Systemic pneumocystosis;

Aspergillosis; Mucormycosis; Systemic candidosis)

Respiratory system

It includes infections caused by different fungi.

Cause:

Fungal infections may affect previously healthy individuals or those with lowered immunity. Fungal infections affecting healthy individuals include Histoplasmosis (Ohio Valley disease, Central Mississippi Valley disease, Appalachian Mountain disease, Darling's disease), Blastomycosis (North American blastomycosis, Gilchrist's disease), Cryptococcosis (Torulosis, European blastomycosis), Para coccidioidomycosis (Valley fever, San Joaquin Valley fever). Those fungal infections that typically affect people with lowered immunity are Aspergillosis, Candidiasis to name a few.

Signs and Symptoms:

Symptoms vary according to the disease. Often the symptoms resemble that of tuberculosis with fever, cough, and difficulty in breathing, lethargy, weight loss and fatigue.

Risk Factors:

Immunocompromised individuals with diseases such as AIDS, lymphoma, leukemia, diabetics or malnutrition are at high risk. Healthy individuals in occupations with potential to inhale fungal spores in feces of birds, bats or soil contaminated by feces (near barns, caves, under bridges, farms) are also at risk. Some forms of fungi spread through broken skin from soil, wood, moss and decaying vegetables and are common in gardeners and horticulturists working with bare hands.

Caution and Recommendations to Therapists:

Avoid harboring caged birds for ornamental purposes in clinic area. Keep clinic area well lit - preferably with natural light, and low humidity to inhibit fungal growth. There is risk of contracting fungal infection through inhalation of spores

Notes

The various conditions are treated by using specific antifungal drugs.

For more details see Appendix C: Antimicrobial - antifungal agents.

References

Morello JA, Mizer HE, Wilson ME, Granato PA. Microbiology in patient care. 6th ed. New York: McGraw-Hill; 1998.

from dressings or casts. Do not massage until an infected individual has been treated fully. See Appendix D for organizations and support groups. Also see Appendix B: Strategies for infection prevention and safe practice.

Integumentary system

Furunculitis (Furuncles; Furunculosis; Boil)

A bacterial infection of the skin.

Cause:

It is usually caused by staphylococcus bacteria.

Signs and Symptoms:

It appears as a large pustule in the base of a hair follicle. There is redness, swelling and pus around the hair follicle. The fully formed furuncle "points" and discharges pus. Occasionally, it may spread to other regions - when it will require oral antibiotics.

Risk Factors:

Diabetes mellitus, immunodeficiency, close contact with people who are carriers of the bacteria are all risk factors.

Caution and Recommendations to Therapists:

It is very localized so avoid massaging the area with furunculosis. Cover area with a large Band-Aid or bandage. The lymph nodes draining the area will often be painfully enlarged. Avoid massaging over the lymph nodes. If the Therapist is affected by recurrent folliculitis or impetigo it should be ensured that she/he is not a carrier of such bacteria, by visiting a Physician and getting swabs taken from nose, perineal and axillary areas. Refer to Appendix B: Strategies for infection prevention and safe practice.

Notes

Application of moist heat that promotes drainage is adequate treatment in most cases. Local application of antibiotic lotions may help in the early stages. A furuncle may require surgical incision and drainage, if large. If recurrent, oral antibiotics are used.

For more details see Appendix C: Antimicrobial - antibacterial agents.

References

Morello JA, Mizer HE, Wilson ME, Granato PA. Microbiology in patient care. 6th ed. New York: McGraw-Hill; 1998

Gastrointestinal system

Gall stones (Cholelithiasis)

Stones in the gall bladder.

Cause:

The gallbladder is pear-shaped and located just below the liver. The cystic duct connects it to the common bile duct that in turn opens into the duodenum. The gallbladder can hold 20-50 ml of bile and serves to collect, concentrate and store bile. When food, especially of high fat content, enters the intestines the muscles of the gallbladder contract. The contraction is brought about mainly by secretion of local hormones.

Changes in the composition of bile cause cholesterol and/or bilirubin to precipitate and form stones. Stagnation of bile, and inflammation of the gall bladder that increase the concentration of bile, also promote stone formation.

Notes

This condition is usually treated by surgery where the gall bladder is removed. In selected clients, the gallstones may be dissolved using medicine (eg. bile acid therapy). The stones may be fragmented by using a method known as lithotripsy, where shock waves generated are directed at the stones.

For more details see Appendix C: Cholecystectomy; Lithotripsy.

Signs and Symptoms:

Most people are asymptomatic. Indigestion and colicky pain may be present. The pain is located in the right upper quadrant of the abdomen and may be referred to the back, the right shoulder, right scapula or between the scapula.

Risk Factors:

Gallstones are more common in obese women of the older age group who have had many children and are on contraceptives (Fat, Forty, Fertile, Female). All these factors increase the excretion of cholesterol into bile. The higher incidence of gallstones in Native Americans indicates a genetic predisposition. Diabetes mellitus, by increasing cholesterol excretion predisposes to stone formation in the gall

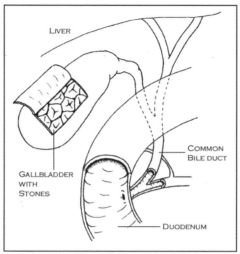

bladder. Conditions that increase the rate of destruction of red blood cells also predispose to bilirubin stones by increasing the excretion of bilirubin in the bile (see Jaundice).

Caution and Recommendations to Therapists:

Encourage client to reduce weight and be active. Avoid massage to the right upper quadrant of the abdomen. Refer to the illustration under Back pain for areas of referred pain due to gall bladder inflammation. See Appendix D for organizations and support groups.

References

Narhwold DL. Chronic cholecystitis and cholelithiasis.In: Sabiston DC, editor. Textbook of Surgery- the biological basis of modern surgical practice. 14th ed. London: WB Saunders Co; 1991. p. 1057-1063.

Ganglion

Musculoskeletal system

A superficial cystic enlargement.

Cause:

Conflicting views exist as to the origin of ganglion. Some believe that it is a separation of small sacs of synovial membrane from the synovial sheaths of tendon or joints. Others claim that it is due to a degenerative process. The sacs are filled with clear viscous fluid. The sac may be attached to a joint capsule or tendon sheath, but no direct communication exists between the joint cavity and the inside of the sac. There is a danger of these sacs getting inflamed.

Signs and Symptoms:

Ganglion presents as a rounded swelling, very small or the size of a walnut,

Notes

In the absence of pain or complications, a ganglion is left untreated. Sometimes it is excised, but it may recur if fragments are left behind. Some use injection of sclerosing agents to treat it. Firm local pressure may disperse the ganglion temporarily. Some treat ganglion temporarily by aspirating its contents with a wide-bore needle. (The term ganglion also refers to a collection of nerve cell bodies eg. dorsal root ganglion.)

For more details see Appendix C: Sclerosing agent.

a Handbook for Massage Therapists

usually over the dorsum of the hand or foot, or on the outer side of the knee. It is usually soft to touch. An ache may be present over the swelling when using the part extensively. Usually it produces no symptoms. Sometimes it may press on local nerves and produce motor and sensory problems.

Risk Factors:

Injury to tendon or joints may predispose to this.

Caution and Recommendations to Therapists:

No special precautions have to be taken, as they are painless. If surgery is done, massage the arm, hand and around the ganglion site postoperatively.

References

Mercier LR, editor. Practical orthopedics. 4th ed. New York: Mosby-Year book Inc; 1995.p. 104.

Cardiovascular system

Gangrene

Death of tissue (necrosis).

Cause:

Gangrene may be classified as *dry, moist/wet* and *gas gangrene*. Dry gangrene is due to reduction of arterial blood flow to the tissue with resultant cell death. Wet gangrene is due to blockage of venous drainage from the tissue. Gas gangrene is due to an infection of tissue by the bacteria *Clostridium*. The incubation period is less than 3 days.

Signs and Symptoms:

In dry gangrene, the tissue becomes dry and shrunken. The skin over the dead tissue is wrinkled. The color of the skin changes to dark brown or black. There is a definite line of demarcation between the dead and healthy tissue where inflammatory reaction occurs. Dry gangrene is more common in the extremities. See Appendix A: page 351.

In the case of wet gangrene, the area is swollen and cold. No pulsation can be felt. The wet, dead tissue may get infected and a foul odor is often present. It is difficult to distinguish the dead and healthy tissue. The gangrene spreads quite rapidly and the person has pain and systemic symptoms like fever.

In gas gangrene, the toxins liberated by the bacteria destroy the tissue. There is a sudden onset of pain in the region of the wound. The gangrene spreads rapidly and severe edema is seen. There is oozing of reddish, frothy fluid from the site. Red blood cells are hemolyzed by the toxin and the person becomes anemic. Hemoglobin liberated as a result of the hemolyses can block the glomeruli of the kidney and result in kidney failure. Hydrogen sulfide gas is liberated as the bacteria metabolises the tissue and the gas forms bubbles in the tissue. The area has a peculiar sweetish smell. If the condition is not treated promptly, the skin becomes brown with blebs filled with dark red fluid.

Risk Factors:

Any condition that affects blood flow to a tissue or blocks venous drainage can

Notes

Amputation if a limb is affected, or surgery to remove the dead tissue is the treatment for gangrene.

Gas gangrene is treated with penicillin or other antibiotics. Amputation may be required if a limb is involved. In some centers, hyperbaric oxygen (oxygen under high pressure) is used, as the clostridium bacteria are anaerobic.

For more details see Appendix C: Amputation; Antimicrobial - antibacterial agents; Hyperbaric oxygen therapy.

lead to gangrene formation. Diabetes mellitus, chronic varicose veins, embolism etc are all predisposing conditions.

Since the Clostridium bacteria is present everywhere, any wound, especially those that result in crushing of tissue if contaminated by dirt is prone to gangrene formation.

Caution and Recommendations to Therapists:

Watch for darkened shrunken tissue in clients with chronic diabetes or chronic varicose veins and refer to Physician. Avoid massaging area of gangrene. Massage the tissue above the lesion with strokes towards the draining lymph nodes and towards the heart to facilitate venous drainage and reduce edema. Refer to the section on Amputation for treating clients who have undergone surgery.

References

Porth CM, editor. Pathophysiology concepts of altered health states. 4th ed. Philadelphia: JB Lippincott Co; 1994. p. 32-33.

Gastritis

Gastrointestinal system

An inflammation of the mucosa of the stomach.

Cause:

Any condition that irritates the gastric mucosa and produces inflammation causes gastritis. Gastritis may be acute or chronic. Stress-induced gastritis has been attributed to reduction of blood flow to the mucosa and entry of the acid secretion into the mucosa. It may also be due to reflux of secretions from the duodenum into the stomach. The destruction of the normal gastric mucosal barrier can cause gastritis. Some form of gastritis is due to the bacillus *H. pylori*, which resides below the mucus gel layer that coats the gastric mucosa. The bacillus secretes proteins that potentiate damage to the gastric mucosa.

Chronic gastritis may be caused by autoimmune reactions or H. pylori infection. The inflammation may be superficial or extend deeper to destroy the glands. Pernicious anemia may be present as intrinsic factor secretion and thereby absorption of vitamin B12 is affected. Eventually, the gastric mucosa atrophies.

Notes

It can be treated by altering the position during sleep with the head higher than the rest of the body. Antacids are given to reduce the acidity of the stomach contents and thus retard the erosion of the esophageal mucosa. Drugs may also be given to increase the pressure of the sphincter. Surgery is resorted to in severe cases.

For more details see Appendix C: Antacids; Antimicrobial - antibacterial agents.

Signs and Symptoms:

The person presents with pain below the sternum (epigastric pain), indigestion, loss of appetite, nausea and vomiting. In chronic cases, there may be intolerance to spicy or fatty food. Blood may be present in the vomitus.

Risk Factors:

Allergy to certain food, ingestion of spicy food, alcohol, smoking, ingestion of anti-inflammatory drugs like aspirin and indomethacin, caffeine and corticosteroid therapy are some of the risk factors. Endotoxins released from bacteria can destroy the mucosa and predispose to gastritis. Acute stress eg. burns, severe infection, surgery are other risk factors.

Caution and Recommendations to Therapists:

Position the client with the leg lower than the head end. A seated massage may

References

McGuigan JE. Peptic ulcer and gastritis. In: Isselbacher KJ et al. Harrison's principles of internal medicine. 13th ed. London: McGraw-Hill Co; 1994. p.1378-1382.

Gastroesophageal reflux

The backflow of the contents of the stomach or duodenum into the esophagus.

Cause:

Dysfunction of the sphincter in the lower part of the esophagus or excessive pressure in the stomach can cause this.

Signs and Symptoms:

The person may have no symptoms. Some individuals may present with a burning sensation behind the sternum that increases on exercising, lying down or bending. The pain is relieved by sitting up or with use of antacids. The pain may be referred to the neck, jaw and arms resembling anginal pain. Rarely, the contents of the stomach may regurgitate into the mouth in the middle of the night, awakening the individual with choking and coughing. Complications such as spasm of the lower end of the esophagus and difficulty in swallowing may result. If the contents regurgitate into the respiratory tract the person may have lung infection.

Risk Factors:

Surgery to the stomach, prolonged nasogastric intubation, alcohol, cigarette smoking, use of drugs that affect the autonomic system, hiatal hernia, positions and conditions that increase the intra-abdominal pressure are all predisposing factors.

Diets high in fat, whole milk, orange juice, chocolate and tomatoes tend to lower the pressure of the lower esophageal sphincter, while protein, carbohydrate and nonfat milk increase the pressure.

Caution and Recommendations to Therapists:

The epigastric (upper abdominal) region may be painful to touch. Avoid the local area. The client may be more comfortable in a seated or half-lying position. See Appendix D for organizations and support groups.

Notes

It is treated by alteration of diet to small frequent meals and avoidance of risk factors. Use of antacids frequently and intake of drugs that may predispose to gastritis, after a meal can reduce incidence. If H. pylori infection is suspected, antibiotics are used. Vitamin B12 has to be administered if pernicious anemia is present.

For more details see Appendix C: Antimicrobial - antibacterial agents; Antacids.

References

Skinner DB. Hiatal hernia and gastroesophageal reflux. In: Sabiston DC, editor. Textbook of Surgery - the biological basis of modern surgical practice. 14th ed. London: WB Saunders Co; 1991. p. 708-715.

(top of page, continued)

be more appropriate. Excessive pressure in the abdomen should be avoided. Encourage client to avoid smoking, alcohol, bedtime snacks and spicy food. See Appendix D for organizations and support groups.

Genu valgum (Knock-knee)

A deformity where the space between the knees is decreased.

Cause:

It may be due to vitamin D deficiency - rickets or osteomalacia, or any condition where there is softening of bone. Laxity of the medial collateral ligament may also cause this condition.

Notes

In infants, bowlegs resolves spontaneously and treatment is not

Signs and Symptoms:

The medial malleoli cannot be brought in contact with each other when the knees are touching. It may be associated with short stature. The gait may be abnormal and there is an increased risk of sprain and fractures.

If the condition is not corrected, osteoarthritis may develop in adulthood as a result of abnormal stress on the knee joints. Pain and swelling of joint may be seen. Recurrent subluxation and dislocation of the patella are other complications that in turn predispose the individual to chondromalacia and joint pain.

Risk Factors:

See Cause.

Caution and Recommendations to Therapists:

Due to the deformity, the posture is affected. As a result, some groups of muscles are shortened while others lengthened. The joint – especially the knee is also stressed. The Therapist has to carefully assess and identify those muscles that are short and tense and those that are elongated and weak. Stimulatory massage is given to the latter while relaxation massage to the former.

required. If the condition is present in children above the age of two, braces may be required.

References

Adams JC, Hamblen DL. Outline of orthopaedics. 11 Ed. New York: Churchill Livingstone; 1990. p. 343-345

Genu varum (Bow leg)

Musculoskeletal system

An outward bowing of the knees.

Cause:

It may be caused by Vitamin D deficiency (osteomalacia or rickets) or other conditions where weakening of bone is present.

Signs and Symptoms:

The knees are separated by more than 1 inch when the medial malleoli of the ankle are in contact with each other. Most infants and toddlers have some form of bowlegs till the age of 2.

If the condition is not corrected, osteoarthritis may develop in adulthood as a result of abnormal stress on the knee joints. Pain and swelling of joint may be seen. The gait may be awkward and there is an increased risk of sprains and fractures.

Risk Factors:

See cause.

Caution and Recommendations to Therapists:

Due to the deformity, the posture is affected. As a result, some groups of muscles are shortened while others lengthened. The joint – especially the knee is also stressed. The Therapist has to carefully assess and identify those muscles that are short and tense and those that are elongated and weak. Stimulatory massage is given to the latter while relaxation massage to the former.

Notes

In infants, bowlegs resolves spontaneously and treatment is not required. If the condition is present in children above the age of two, braces may be required

References

Adams JC, Hamblen DL. Outline of orthopaedics. 11 Ed. New York: Churchill Livingstone; 1990. p. 343-345

a Handbook for Massage Therapists

German measles (Rubella)

A viral disease that produces skin rashes.

Notes

It is important for every female child and adults in the reproductive age group to be immunized against rubella due to the possibility of fetal abnormalities, if infected during the early stages of pregnancy. However, the vaccine should not be given to pregnant women or those who are likely to become pregnant within three months of immunization.

For more details see Appendix C: Immunization.

Cause:

It is caused by the *Rubella virus*. It is transmitted by contact with airborne droplets of the respiratory secretion from an infected individual. The incubation period ranges from 16-18 days. The infected individual may shed the virus through the oropharynx for up to 8 days after the onset of symptoms.

Signs and Symptoms:

The symptoms are very mild. Most often, especially in children, no fever or other systemic illness is seen. Mild skin rash is observed. The rash begins in the head and rapidly spreads down the body in a few days and soon disappears. Some individuals do not develop even a rash. Joint pain and enlargement of the occipital lymph nodes may be seen.

If it affects the fetus in a pregnant woman, it can produce congenital heart abnormalities, mental retardation, cataracts and motor and sensory nervous problems.

Risk Factors:

Exposure to an infected individual increases the risk.

Caution and Recommendations to Therapists:

It is important for all female children and adults in the reproductive age group to be immunized against rubella due to the possibility of fetal abnormalities, if infected during the early stages of pregnancy. Encourage female clients at risk to get vaccinated. Therapists should consider getting vaccinated against this disease. See Appendix D for organizations and support groups. Also see Appendix B: Strategies for infection prevention and safe practice.

References

Morello JA, Mizer HE, Wilson ME, Granato PA. Microbiology in patient care. 6th ed. New York: McGraw-Hill; 1998. p. 388-390

Giardiasis

A protozoal infection that causes diarrhea.

Notes

It is treated with a full course of a suitable antibiotic. It is a very infective condition and carriers and close contacts have to be treated as well.

For more details see Appendix C: Antimicrobial - antibacterial agents.

Cause:

It is caused by a protozoa *Giardia lamblia*. The infection occurs when the person ingests the cysts of the organism. The organisms emerge from the cysts on reaching the small intestine and begin to multiply there. The organism attaches itself to the intestinal mucosa by sucking disks. If the condition in the intestines become adverse, the organism forms cysts. It is these cysts that are found in the feces. The cysts can survive for a long time in cold, fresh water.

The infection spreads by contact. It can also be transmitted by ingestion of contaminated water.

Signs and Symptoms:

The person has diarrhea. Some infected individuals have no signs and symptoms at all.

Risk Factors:

See Cause.

Caution and Recommendations to Therapists:

Do not treat clients with this condition until the full course of antibiotics has been taken. Refer to Appendix B: Strategies for infection prevention and safe practice. See Appendix D for organizations and support groups.

References

Morello JA, Mizer HE, Wilson ME, Granato PA. Microbiology in patient care. 6th ed. New York: McGraw-Hill; 1998. p. 380-381.

Wolfe MS. Giardiasis. Clin microbiol Rev 1992; 5(4): 93-100.

Gingivitis

Gastrointestinal system

An inflammation of the gums.

Cause:

It could be caused by lack of vitamins, diabetes or poor oral hygiene.

Signs and Symptoms:

It presents as redness and painless swelling of tissue around the teeth. The gum bleeds easily. It can affect the underlying ligaments and bone and may be complicated by abscess formation and can eventually lead to loss of teeth. Gingivitis may be associated with plaque formation and calcification of the plaques.

Risk Factors:

See Cause.

Caution and Recommendations to Therapists:

Avoid the area around the mouth and lower part of the face, if painful. Encourage client to go for regular dental checkups.

Notes

Regular brushing of teeth, flossing, antibacterial rinses and removal of impacted food debris can prevent gingivitis. Treatment of gingivitis includes removal of plaques and calculus and elimination of contributing factors.

References

Greenspan JS. Oral manifestations of disease. In: Isselbacher KJ et al, editors. Harrison's principles of internal medicine. 13th ed. London: McGraw-Hill Co; 1994. p. 199.

Glaucoma

Nervous system

A condition where the intraocular pressure is high.

Cause:

The optic nerve is damaged as a result of the increased intraocular pressure. It is of two types. *Open-angle glaucoma* is due to an interference with the drainage of the aqueous fluid. *Angle-closure glaucoma* is due to the iris blocking the passage of fluid.

Signs and Symptoms:

There is progressive loss of vision and ultimately blindness. The disease is

Notes:

Open-angle glaucoma is treated with special eyedrops that result in reduction of intraocular pressure. If this does not control the pressure, surgery may be done to facilitate drainage of intraocular fluid. In acute angle-closure glaucoma, the pressure has to be reduced promptly. Surgery is often curative.

For more details see Appendix C: Eye drops.

usually asymptomatic. In an acute case of angle-closure glaucoma, there is severe pain, nausea and vomiting. The person complains of colored halos around lights and some loss of vision. The pupils are fixed in a mid-dilated position. There is redness of the conjunctiva and edema of the cornea.

Risk Factors:

See Cause. Diabetes and cataract formation are some predisposing factors.

Caution and Recommendations to Therapists:

Encourage client to use the eyedrops regularly as the condition can be controlled. Avoid pressure over the eye. See Appendix D for organizations and support groups.

References

Miller SH. Parsons' diseases of the eye. 18th edition. New York: Churchill Livingstone; 1990. p. 214-221.

Renal system

Glomerulonephritis

An inflammation of the glomeruli of the kidney.

Notes

Treatment is mainly supportive, with maintenance of fluid and electrolyte balance and diet restrictions - reduced water, protein and salt intake.

Glomerulonephritis can progress to nephrotic syndrome and kidney failure.

Cause:

The most common cause is the immune reaction that occurs 10-14 days after a streptococcal infection - impetigo or throat infection. The antigen-antibody complexes formed as a result of the immune system's assault on the bacteria, get entrapped in the capillaries that supply the glomeruli. There is an inflammatory reaction to the complexes in the glomeruli, making the capillary membrane leaky to red cells and proteins.

There is no cause identified for some types of glomerulonephritis.

Signs and Symptoms:

The person usually gives a history of sore throat 1-3 weeks before the onset of symptoms. There is generalized edema and fatigue. The volume of urine excreted is reduced and may be pink (presence of blood) and cloudy (presence of proteins).

Risk Factors:

Untreated streptococcal infections may lead to this condition.

Caution and Recommendations to Therapists:

A very light, soothing massage of short duration is recommended. Do not try to reduce the edema present, as the cause is not inadequate drainage of interstitial fluid. Rather, the edema actually prevents overloading of the heart, which is overly stressed by the accumulation of fluid. Deep pressure especially over the lumbar region has to be avoided. See Appendix D for organizations and support groups.

References

Glassock RJ, Brenner BM. The major glomerulopathies. In: Isselbacher KJ et al, editors. Harrison's principles of internal medicine. 13th ed. London: McGraw-Hill Co; 1994. p. 1295-1308.

Pathology A to Z -

Glossitis

An inflammation of the tongue.

Cause:

The inflammation may be due to streptococcal infection, irritation or injury to the tongue, hypersensitivity or vitamin deficiency.

Signs and Symptoms:

The tongue is red and swollen and may be ulcerated. There is pain on swallowing and chewing. The swelling of the tongue along with the pain can make speech difficult.

Risk Factors:

Irregular biting surface of teeth, ill-fitting dentures, injury to tongue caused during convulsions, spicy food, alcohol, smoking, allergy to toothpaste and vitamin deficiencies are all predisposing factors.

Caution and Recommendations to Therapists:

If the glossitis is due to hypersensitivity, it is possible for the client to be allergic to aromatherapy, or to oils that are used during massage. Obtain a thorough history and avoid use of allergic substances.

Notes

Treatment of underlying cause, good oral hygiene, mouth washes and avoidance of predisposing factors are some of the treatment options used.

References

Greenspan JS. Oral manifestations of disease. In: Isselbacher KJ et al, editors. Harrison's principles of internal medicine. 13th ed. London: McGraw-Hill Co; 1994. p. 205.

Glycogen storage diseases

A group of genetic disorders that affect the enzymatic pathways involved in the metabolism of carbohydrates.

Cause:

Glucose requires a number of enzymes for its conversion to the storage form glycogen. As well, many enzymes are required for the breakdown of glycogen to glucose. In glycogen storage diseases, there is a lack of specific enzymes in the liver or muscle due to genetic defects. The diseases are classified according to the type of enzyme that is affected (eg. *glucose-6-phosphatase deficiency* or *von Gierke disease; debrancher deficiency* or *Cori disease etc*).

Signs and Symptoms:

Hypoglycemia is common. There may be enlargement of the liver. The symptoms vary according to the type of disease. If the disease is a type that affects muscle, symptoms of pain and cramps after exercise are common.

Risk Factors:

See Cause.

Notes

Treatment is mainly by alteration of diet according to the type of disease. Genetic counselling is also required.

For more details see Appendix C: Genetic testing/Counselling.

References

Beaudet AL. Glycogen storage diseases. In: Isselbacher KJ et al, editors. Harrison's principles of internal medicine. 13ᵗʰ ed. London: McGraw-Hill Co; 1994. p. 2099-2105.

Caution and Recommendations to Therapists:

Since hypoglycemia is common, ensure that glucose or some form of carbohydrates is available with the client or in the clinic during the session.

Endocrine system	# Goiter (Simple goiter; Nontoxic goiter)
	An enlargement of the thyroid gland.

Cause:

Notes

The cause of the goiter is identified and treated.

The thyroid gland is located in front of the neck and weighs about 30 grams. It is butterfly-shaped with two lobes on either side of the trachea. The lobes are about 5cm long, 2cm thick and about 3cm wide. A normal thyroid is not visible and is felt as a soft mass in front of the neck above the sternum that moves up on swallowing.

A goitre usually results when the production of thyroid hormone does not meet the metabolic needs. It may be due to lack of adequate iodine in the diet. Such a condition may be seen in communities living in areas with iodine-depleted soil. When the demands are more for the hormone as during pregnancy, adolescence and menopause, the thyroid gland may hypertrophy especially if the iodine needs are not met. Certain foods have a direct effect on thyroxine production. Intake of excess rutabagas, cabbage, soybeans, peanuts, peaches, peas, strawberries, spinach and radishes can reduce thyroxine production.

Signs and Symptoms:

The thyroid enlarges in size slowly and presents as a painless, uniform or nodular swelling in front of the neck. The swelling moves on swallowing. Usually there are no signs of hyper or hypothyroidism - but a goitre may present as either. Due to the compression of the underlying structures, the person may have difficulty in swallowing. Pressure on the neck veins can cause the veins above the swelling to bulge and become prominent.

Risk Factors:

See Cause.

Caution and Recommendations to Therapists:

References

JD Wilson, Foster DW. Editors. Williams' Textbook of Endocrinology. 8ᵗʰ Ed. Philadelphia: WB Saunders Co; 1992.

Encourage client to consult a Physician if a thyroid swelling is noted as the cause has to be found and tumors have to be ruled out. Do not massage over the neck area. The individual may present with no symptoms or have the symptoms of hypo or hyperthyroidism.

Gonorrhea

A sexually transmitted disease caused by bacteria.

Cause:

It is caused by the bacteria *Neisseria gonorrhoeae* that can survive only for a very short duration outside the human body. It is transmitted through intimate physical contact. Infection can also spread from an infected mother to the baby during delivery. The bacteria enter the mucosal membrane producing inflammation. The bacteria can change its form easily and evade local immune reaction. Hence repeated infections are possible in an individual.

Signs and Symptoms:

In men, it presents as inflammation of the urethra 1-8 days after infection. Pain on urination and profuse white discharge is common. The infection may travel upwards and produce inflammation of the epididymis, prostate and other areas.

In women it may present as pain on urination, profuse white discharge, increased and abnormal menstrual bleeding. The infection may spread upwards and cause inflammation of the fallopian tubes and other areas. The resolution of the inflammation by fibrosis can produce narrowing of the tubes and increase the chances of infertility and ectopic pregnancy. There may be lower abdominal pain and pain during intercourse.

Risk Factors:

It is common in the lower socioeconomic group in urban areas. Those with a past history of gonorrhea are at higher risk. The incidence is highest in the sexually active adolescent female.

Caution and Recommendations to Therapists:

Refer client to Physician if they give a history of white discharge and pain on passing urine. Since the infection spreads by intimate physical contact - specifically sexual intercourse, and the bacterium does not live for very long outside the human body, the risk of the Therapist contracting the infection is very low. Refer to Appendix B: Strategies for infection prevention and safe practice. See Appendix D for organizations and support groups.

Notes

The disease is easily treated with antibiotics.

For more details see Appendix C: Antimicrobial - antibacterial agents.

References

Morello JA, Mizer HE, Wilson ME, Granato PA. Microbiology in patient care. 6th ed. New York: McGraw-Hill; 1998. p. 412-416.

Guillain-Barré syndrome (Infectious polyneuritis;

Landry-Guillain-Barré syndrome; Acute idiopathic polyneuritis)

An acute, rapidly progressive disorder that results in muscle weakness and sensory loss.

Cause:

The cause is unknown. But it may be due to the alteration of the body's immunity to attack antigens in peripheral nerves. This seems to follow many forms of viral infections including AIDS and Hepatitis. There is inflammation and swelling around peripheral nerves with destruction of myelin sheath, sensory and motor neurons.

Signs and Symptoms:

There is usually a history of mild fever or respiratory infection preceding the disease. Muscle weakness of legs, followed by weakness of the arms and face are seen. The signs and symptoms appear over a few days. Pain and stiffness may accompany the weakness. There may be loss of sensation. Weakness of the respiratory muscles can result in death.

Autonomic disturbances may also be seen. This presents as postural hypotension, abnormal sweating, flushing of face, bladder and bowel disorders. Typically, the syndrome has three phases - the initial phase lasting for 1-3 weeks when the symptoms are seen, the plateau phase lasting for about 2 weeks when the symptoms do not progress and the recovery phase which may last from months to years. Recovery may not be complete. The debility makes the person prone to infections. Muscle contractures, joint stiffness, deep vein thrombosis (following prolonged immobility) are other complications.

Risk Factors:

Surgery, influenza vaccination, viral illness, Hodgkin's disease and Lupus Erythematosus may precipitate the disease.

Caution and Recommendations to Therapists:

During the active and plateau phase, massage helps improve circulation and reduce pain. Perform passive range of motion exercises within the pain tolerance. Movement of shoulder, thighs and trunk muscles is painful in these individuals. Use tapotement and vibration strokes over the chest to help mucus drainage from the lungs. Since these individuals are in bed they are prone for pressure ulcers. Gently massage areas that are prone for ulcers - these areas are around the sacrum, ankles and heels. Avoid massaging a wide area around the ulcer if an ulcer has already developed. Sensory loss in certain areas of the body will result in the client giving inadequate feedback. Avoid using excessive pressure. Individuals with this disorder are prone to postural hypotension. Support the client well when changing positions. They are also prone to thrombophlebitis (inflammation of veins) especially in the legs. Watch for edema, pain, redness and swelling in the legs. Do not massage the legs if this is present as you may dislodge a thrombus and produce further complications.

If the client has constipation give a stimulatory abdominal massage (always in a clockwise direction). In the recovery phase the aim is to prevent contractures and increase tone of the flaccid muscles. Use stimulatory massage over flaccid muscles. Perform passive range of motion exercises of all joints. Use deep transverse friction around joints to reduce adhesions and stretch tendons. Avoid excessive pressure over areas with sensory loss. If the client is in a wheelchair, spend time massaging muscles that are stressed excessively while maneuvering the wheelchair. See Appendix D for organizations and support groups.

References

Morello JA, Mizer HE, Wilson ME, Granato PA. Microbiology in patient care. 6th ed. New York: McGraw-Hill; 1998. p. 277.

Hay Fever (Allergic rhinitis)

An inflammation of the nose and conjunctiva that occurs seasonally due to allergy.

Cause:

Individuals, who are genetically predisposed, react to certain antigens like pollen, fungal spores, etc. by producing large amounts of immunoglobulins (antibodies). The antigen-antibody reaction is responsible for the symptoms seen.

Signs and Symptoms:

Recurrent sneezing, watery nasal discharge, itching (pruritus), congestion and swelling of the eyes and nose, itching in the throat and headache are the most common symptoms.

Risk Factors:

Hay fever can occur in all age groups, but is more common in children and adolescents. A genetic predisposition is present.

Caution and Recommendations to Therapists:

Individuals with allergic rhinitis may also have other forms of allergy, so a proper and detailed history of allergy should be taken. Keep the clinic area dust free to prevent a fresh episode of rhinitis in these individuals. Proper air conditioning, regular vacuuming, low humidity, avoiding use of dust-collecting items like thick carpets and heavy drapes, minimizing presence or avoidance of flowering plants are some of the simple precautions that can be taken in the clinic to reduce the incidence of allergy in clients. Refer client to local support groups for Allergy. See Appendix D for organizations and support groups.

Notes

The best form of treatment is to avoid exposure to the agent that causes symptoms. The symptoms can be treated with antihistamines. Nose drops may be used to reduce congestion. In some cases, immunotherapy (hyposensitization), where subcutaneous injections of increasing concentration of the allergen are given repeatedly, may be done.

For more details see Appendix C: Nose drops/Nasal decongestants; Antihistamines; Immunotherapy.

References

Li J. Prevention and treatment of rhinitis and common cold by self-massage. Journal of Traditional Chinese Medicine 1992; 12(4): 290-291.

Headache - cluster

Headaches of short duration occurring recurrently for short periods of time.

Cause:

The cause is not known. Cluster headaches are considered to be a vascular type of headache.

Signs and Symptoms:

The headache lasts from 10 minutes to two hours. The pain is confined to the eye and nose of one side. There is watering of the eye and running of the nose associated with the pain. The skin may be reddened on the side of pain. The headache recurs 2-3 times a day for 5-6 weeks. There may be no headaches for weeks to months after the cluster of symptoms.

Notes

Vasoconstrictors or inhalation of pure oxygen is used to treat this type of headache.

For more details see Appendix C: Vasoconstrictors; Oxygen therapy.

References

Polseno CD. The massage therapist's headache lists: everything you need to know. Massage Therapy Journal 1997; 36(1): 53-64.

Wine ZK. Russian medical massage: headache. Massage 1994; 47 (Jan/Feb): 40, 42.

Wine ZK. Russian medical massage: headache. Massage. 1993; 46 (Nov/Dec): 58, 60.

Risk Factors:

It may be induced by stress.

Caution and Recommendations to Therapists:

It is usually not treated as it lasts only for a short while. During an attack the same techniques as for tension headache may be used (see Headache -Tension). See Appendix D for organizations and support groups.

Headache - migraine

Nervous system

A throbbing pain in the head that is often confined to one side associated with or without an aura and provoked by stimuli.

Cause:

The cause is unknown. Recent evidence indicates that the headache is brought on by the leakiness of the blood vessels of the brain due to polypeptides called neurokinin that dilate blood vessels. Abnormal metabolism and decrease of serotonin (5 hydroxytryptamine) in the brain have also been implicated. Migraine has been associated with dilatation and constriction of arteries inside and outside the cranium.

Notes

Analgesic drugs such as aspirin, ibuprofen etc. are beneficial. Many drugs specific for migraine are available and one or more may be used. If the frequency of attacks is more, drugs that have the capacity to stabilize migraine may be taken daily.

For more details see Appendix C: Painkillers; Craniosacral therapy; Imagery.

Signs and Symptoms:

Initially, the pain is usually confined to one side of the head. Later it spreads to other areas. The headache is typically preceded by flashing lights, dark spots, double vision and hallucinations. These auras are due to the reduced blood flow to specific areas of the brain. Nausea, vomiting, hypersensitivity to light, sound and smell are other typical symptoms. Migraine can also occur without auras.

Risk Factors:

Different factors precipitate an attack in susceptible individuals. Red wine, cheese, canned food, hot dog, salami, bacon - food containing preservatives, bean pods, chocolate, avocados, bananas, citrus fruits, yogurt, sour cream, fresh bread, coffee cake, doughnuts, nuts, peanut butter, fermented, pickled and marinated foods are some of the food types that may precipitate an attack. In some, changes in weather and pressure can cause a headache. In women, the hormonal changes during the menstrual cycle can also trigger an attack. In the younger age group both males and females are equally affected. In adults, women are attacked more than men. There may be a family history of migraine headache.

References

Launso L, Brendstrup E, Arnberg S. An exploratory study of reflexological treatment for headache. Alternative therapies May 1999; 5 (3): 57-65.

Di Concetto G, Sotte L. Treatment of headache by acupuncture and Chines herbal therapy – conclusive data concerning 1000 clients. J Tradit Chin Med 1991; 11(3): 174-176.

Caution and Recommendations to Therapists:

During the headache, a whole body relaxation massage is most helpful. Use same techniques as for tension headache when massaging over the neck, scalp and face. Do not apply heat over the area as it causes changes in the arteries that may increase the pain. During the headache apply cold compresses or gel packs to the face, scalp, eyes, wrist and feet. Use deep moist heat at the end of treatment.

The treatment regimen followed is once a week for one month followed by once every other week for a total of eight weeks. Thirty-minute sessions have been found to be adequate. Other recommended treatment schedules are a total of 10-12 sessions lasting about 15 minutes each scheduled every other day.

Consider keeping brochures of local migraine associations in the clinic. Encourage client to make dietary and life-style changes. Advice client to do aerobic exercises regularly. This promotes circulation. Teach clients to massage the scalp and neck muscles.

Many alternative forms of therapy exist and have been found to be beneficial. Craniosacral therapy is one form of treatment. Deep breathing exercises and imagery have been found to be effective by some.

Recent research indicates that reflexology and acupuncture can have a positive effect on these clients. These interventions have been shown to reduce the number of episodes experienced, relieve pain, reduce medication consumption, improve mood state and reduce sleeplessness. See Appendix D for organizations and support groups.

Tavola T, Gala C, Conte G. Traditional Chinese acupuncture in tension-type headache: a controlled study. Pain 1992;48(3):325-329.

Vincent CA. A controlled trial of the treatment of migraine by acupuncture. Clin J Pain 1989;5(4):305-312.

Wine ZK. Russian medical massage: headache. Massage 1994; 47 (Jan/Feb): 40, 42.

Wine ZK. Russian medical massage: headache. Massage. 1993; 46 (Nov/Dec): 58, 60.

Carlsson J, Augustinsson LE, Blomstrand C et al. Health status in clients with tension headache treated with acupuncture or physiotherapy. Headache 1990; 30(9): 593-599.

Polseno CD. The massage therapist's headache lists: everything you need to know. Massage Therapy Journal 1997; 36(1): 53-64.

King R. Tension headache and neck pain relieved by seated myofascial techniques. Massage Therapy Journal 1997; 36(1): 43-50.

Headache - others

Includes headaches that are not tension or migraine.

Nervous, Musculoskeletal, Cardiovascular systems

Cause:

Headaches can be caused by infection of the meninges - meningitis, tumors that increase the intracranial tension, disorders of the cranium, neck, eyes, ears, nose, sinuses, teeth, mouth or other facial/cranial structures. Pressure, reduced blood supply or inflammation of the main sensory nerve - the trigeminal nerve can also cause severe pain (see Trigeminal neuralgia). Headaches may also be caused by withdrawal syndrome associated with alcohol or substance abuse. Sometimes, the pain may be referred from the temporomandibular joint or problems with the cervical spine.

Signs and Symptoms:

Headaches due to meningitis, or other intracranial problems are often associated with motor or sensory problems. Neck stiffness and pain on flexing the hip with the knee extended, accompany it. The stretching of the inflamed meninges when performing this maneuver produces the pain. Those caused by tumors are typically associated with nausea and forceful vomiting. The patient will also give a history of recent onset of headache.

Risk Factors:

See Cause.

Notes

The cause is treated.

References

Polseno CD. The massage therapist's headache lists: everything you need to know. Massage Therapy Journal 1997; 36(1): 53-64.

Wine ZK. Russian medical massage. headache. Massage 1994; 47 (Jan/Feb): 40, 42.

Wine ZK. Russian medical massage: headache. Massage 1993; 46 (Nov/Dec): 58, 60.

Caution and Recommendations to Therapists:

It is very important to take a careful and detailed history when dealing with headache. Refer to Physician if the history indicates any of the above lesions. Massage is indicated only for tension or migraine headaches. See Appendix D for organizations and support groups.

Musculoskeletal, Nervous systems

Headache - tension (Fibrositic headache)

A symptom of pain in the head, face and/or neck regions due to muscle contraction and psychological causes.

Cause:

This is the most common type of headache. Contraction/spasm of the neck and scalp muscles caused by stress of any kind produce this type of headache. The pain is produced by the pressure of the contracted muscle on the nerves and blood vessels in the area. The resultant reduced blood flow increases the accumulation of waste products like lactic acid in the region and perpetuation of the pain.

Notes

A good history has to be taken to identify the precipitating cause of the headache. Imagery and biofeedback are other techniques employed to combat headache.

For more details see Appendix C: Imagery; Biofeedback.

Signs and Symptoms:

The patient complains of a dull, persistent ache and a feeling of tightness around the head, temple, forehead and occiput. The pain is typically more in the evenings. There is no loss of sensation, muscle weakness, or aura associated with this type. Headache that starts suddenly in a person who has not experienced such headache before is not tension headache.

Risk Factors:

Noise, bright lights, crowds, mental strain, menstruation, alcohol intake, fasting and fatigue can precipitate an attack. Any occupation which requires the head to be held in a fixed position such as typing, jewellery repair or microscope work can increase the risk of contracting this type of headache. Prolonged exposure to cold, sleeping with the head held in a strained position also predisposes to this condition.

Caution and Recommendations to Therapists:

Encourage client to sleep in a warm room and tie a scarf around the neck if venturing out in the cold. Massage can help only temporarily, but identifying and avoiding precipitating factors alone can produce long-term effects. Ask client to actively contract the shoulder and neck muscles and then relax it as much as possible. This helps the client to consciously relax muscles that are being involuntarily tensed. Position the client in a seated position with the head resting on a pillow in front, supported by elevated arms. This helps to relax the shoulder and neck muscles. The aim is to relax the muscles in spasm and thereby relieve the pressure on the nerves and blood vessels. The aim is also to promote venous and lymphatic drainage from the area. Moist heat application over the tense muscles during the treatment has been found to be beneficial. Use effleurage, friction and vibration strokes in the shoulder and neck region. Effleurage should be long and continuous beginning from the occiput to the shoulder joint and from below, over the scapula to the neck - ie. in the direction of the muscle fibres of the trapezius.

Friction is done on either side of the spinous process of the cervical vertebrae. Start friction in areas that are less tense and then slowly progress to that under spasm. Use the pads of your fingers and start with lighter strokes and then proceed to deeper strokes. Make the strokes continuous ie. do friction from one area to the adjacent area without loosing contact with the skin. Alternate the friction strokes with effleurage from time to time. Do not neglect to massage the neck muscles - scalene and sternocleidomastoid, which are in front of the neck. More time should be spent over the origin and the insertion of these muscles, which will be closer to the clavicle and sternum and the mastoid process (the protrusion just behind the ear) respectively. The massage should also focus on the trapezius, erector spinae, levator scapulae and rhomboids muscles that are usually tense.

Use vibration over the trigger point areas for five to ten seconds, repeating the vibration after eight to ten seconds while maintaining contact with the skin during the break. Repeat the procedure three to four times. Passively move the head and neck in all directions. Gentle traction of the head also helps. Initially, spend half the duration of massage using effleurage with the rest of the time divided equally for vibration and friction strokes. Increase the duration spent on friction in subsequent sessions up to three fourth of the time. Gentle scalp and face massage has also been found to be very beneficial. Spend time over the temporalis (the fan shaped muscle located above the ears), masseters and frontalis (located in the forehead region) using fingertip kneading strokes.

Four to five sessions for the first week followed by less frequent sessions for a total of twelve treatment sessions have been found to be beneficial. The duration of each session should be short not lasting for more than 15 minutes. Other treatment schedules practised are two times a week for two weeks followed by once a week for one month. Individualize the treatment according to the clients' feedback. There may be a need to charge the client on a treatment schedule basis rather than individual sessions. The client may be on painkillers and therefore give inadequate feedback. Adjust pressures accordingly.

Recent research indicates that reflexology and acupuncture can have a positive effect on these clients. These interventions have been shown to reduce the number of episodes experienced, relieve pain, reduce medication consumption, improve mood state and reduce sleeplessness. See Appendix D for organizations and support groups.

References

Launso L, Brendstrup E, Arnberg S. An exploratory study of reflexological treatment for headache. Alternative therapies May 1999; 5 (3): 57-65.

Di Concetto G, Sotte L. Treatment of headache by acupuncture and Chines herbal therapy – conclusive data concerning 1000 clients. J Tradit Chin Med 1991; 11(3): 174-176.

Tavola T, Gala C, Conte G. traditional Chinese acupuncture in tension-type headache: a controlled study. Pain 1992; 48(3): 325-329.

Vincent CA. A controlled trial of the treatment of migraine by acupuncture. Clin J Pain 1989; 5(4): 305-312.

Carlsson J, Augustinsson LE, Blomstrand C et al. Health status in clients with tension headache treated with acupuncture or physiotherapy. Headache 1990; 30(9): 593-599.

Keller E, Bzdek UM. Effects of Therapeutic Touch on tension headache pain. Nursing Research 1986; 2(35): 101-105.

Wine ZK. Russian medical massage: headache. Massage 1994; 47 (Jan/Feb): 40, 42.

Wine ZK. Russian medical massage: headache. Massage 1993; 46 (Nov/Dec): 58, 60.

Heart attack (Myocardial infarction)

Death of myocardial tissue due to insufficient blood flow in the coronary arteries.

Notes

The prognosis is related to whether the electrical activity of the heart has been affected and/or there is heart failure. Heart failure depends on the extent of tissue death. The aim of the treatment is to prevent death due to arrhythmias and reduce the extent of tissue death. Arrhythmia can be managed if trained individuals and the right equipment are at hand. Usually, time is wasted by the client delaying seek for help. This can be avoided by proper client education. By continuous monitoring of the functioning of the heart in coronary care units, the mortality rates have been reduced markedly.

Administration of intravenous drugs (to remove/reduce occlusion by thrombosis) within the first hour of symptoms has been shown to markedly reduce mortality. Drugs to reduce the pain, reduce spasm of arteries, reduce coagulation of blood (eg. aspirin) and oxygen inhalation are other forms of treatment. The client has to avoid activities that increase the work of the heart until healing of the infarct has occurred ie. 6-8 weeks.

For more details see Appendix C: Painkillers; Anticoagulants; Vasoconstrictors; Oxygen therapy.

References

Pasternak RC, Braunwald E. Acute myocardial infarction. In: Isselbacher KJ et al, editors. Harrison's principles of internal medicine. 13th ed. London: McGraw-Hill Co; 1994. p. 1066-1077.

Cause:

Insufficient coronary blood flow due to thrombosis, vasospasm or increased oxygen demand by the myocardium causes this condition.

Signs and Symptoms:

The person presents with an abrupt onset of suffocating, squeezing or crushing pain below the sternum, or radiating to the left arm, jaw or neck. The pain is not relieved by rest or drugs for angina. It may be associated with nausea and vomiting or indigestion. Palpitations, restlessness and anxiety may accompany the pain. The skin may be pale and moist. Complications include sudden death, shock, rupture of the heart, thromboemboli, ventricular aneurysms and pericarditis.

Risk Factors:

Atherosclerosis, cigarette smoking, hypertension, among others predispose to myocardial infarction. (See Risk factors for Atherosclerosis and Angina.)

Caution and Recommendations to Therapists:

Avoid using stimulatory or painful techniques in clients with atherosclerosis, angina or previous myocardial infarction. A whole body, gentle relaxation massage alleviates stress, a common precipitator of heart attack.

If a client has an anginal attack, severe chest pain, sweating or difficulty in breathing on the table, bring him/her up to a sitting or standing position as this reduces the load on the heart and call for help. Ensure that a contact address and the telephone number of the treating Physician has been recorded for clients with a history of myocardial infarction. See Appendix D for organizations and support groups.

Heart failure (Cardiac failure)

A syndrome where the heart is unable to cope with the demands made by the body.

Notes

The underlying pathology has to be identified for proper treatment. Diuretics and low salt intake are some of the other supportive measures used.

For more details see Appendix C: Diuretics.

Cause:

Heart failure may be due to many conditions. The dysfunction may be due to damage to the heart muscle as in coronary artery disease and myocardial infarction. It may be due to mechanical disturbances as in stenosis (narrowing) of the opening between the ventricle and atrium. Rapid beating of the heart as in atrial fibrillation can lead to inefficiency in pumping the blood from the heart. Heart failure can also occur when the organ is overloaded by increased pressure in the blood vessels (hypertension, aortic stenosis) or leaky valves.

With time, to compensate for the reduced blood that is pumped, the heart increases in size by dilation and/or hypertrophy. Another compensatory mechanism is the increase in heart rate due to increased sympathetic activity.

Signs and Symptoms:

The signs and symptoms produced by heart failure depend on whether the right, the left or both sides of the heart fail. If the right ventricle is affected, there is a tendency for the blood to dam up in the venous circulation. This results in edema of the legs, sacral region and enlargement of the liver and spleen. Fluid may collect in the abdomen (ascites).

In left heart failure, pressure tends to build up in the pulmonary circulation causing pulmonary edema and difficulty in and noisy breathing.

The inadequate blood flow to the brain and kidney can produce other symptoms.

Risk Factors:

See Cause.

Caution and Recommendations to Therapists:

It is important to find out the cause of edema in any edematous client. If cardiac edema is suspected, refer to a Physician. Techniques to reduce edema are not beneficial, and in fact may be detrimental in a client in cardiac failure. For those under medications, massage should be done only after clearance from a Physician. Relaxation massage of short duration, with the client seated may be beneficial. See Appendix D for organizations and support groups.

References

Braunwald E. Heart failure. In: Isselbacher KJ et al. editors. Harrison's principles of internal medicine. 13ᵗʰ ed. London: McGraw-Hill Co; 1994. p. 998-1011.

Helminthic infection - Abdominal Angiostrongyliasis

Gastrointestinal system

An infection produced by the worm Angiostrongylus costaricensis.

Cause:

The infection is caused by the ingestion of contaminated vegetation. The worm is normally found in rodents. Slugs and snails are intermediate hosts. The slime from the slugs and snails containing the larvae may be left on fruits and vegetables. If the contaminated fruits and vegetables are ingested by humans, infection is produced. The larvae enter the intestinal wall and develop into adult worms in the blood vessels. The eggs and worms trigger immune reactions in the body that are responsible for the symptoms.

Signs and Symptoms:

The immune reaction in the gut causes abdominal pain, tenderness, fever and vomiting. The inflammatory reaction may present as a swelling in the right iliac fossa.

Notes

Antihelminthic drugs are not very effective. If the symptoms are severe, surgery may have to be done to remove the thickened region of the intestines.

For more details see Appendix C: Antihelminthics.

Risk Factors:

It is more common in Latin America and Africa.

Caution and Recommendations to Therapists:

These infections are not spread by contact as in massage. Treatment has to be planned according to the presenting symptoms. Avoid abdominal massage. Refer to Appendix B: Strategies for infection prevention and safe practice for some useful guidelines. Also see Appendix D for organizations and support groups.

References

Morello JA, Mizer HE, Wilson ME, Granato PA. Microbiology in patient care. 6ᵗʰ ed. New York: McGraw-Hill; 1998.

Helminthic infection - Anisakiasis

Gastrointestinal system

An infection caused by ingestion of the larvae of worms that are found in the tissue of fishes.

Cause:

The larvae are found in the tissue of a variety of fishes. The worm has a complex life cycle that involves marine organisms. When uncooked fish is eaten, the larvae enter the walls of the stomach and intestines.

Notes

The infection can be prevented by proper cooking of fish. The worm can be visualized and removed using endoscopy.

Signs and Symptoms:

There is severe abdominal pain, nausea and vomiting within hours of ingestion.

Risk Factors:

Eating raw fish (eg. sushi, pickled herring etc).

Caution and Recommendations to Therapists:

Avoid massage when acute symptoms are present. These infections are not spread by contact as in massage. Refer to Appendix B: Strategies for infection prevention and safe practice for some useful guidelines. Also see Appendix D for organizations and support groups.

References

Morello JA, Mizer HE, Wilson ME, Granato PA. Microbiology in patient care. 6ᵗʰ ed. New York: McGraw-Hill; 1998.

Helminthic infection - Ascariasis

Gastrointestinal system

(Roundworm infection)

An infection by worms that reside in the intestines.

Cause:

The infection is due to the worm *Ascaris lumbricoides*. It is one of the largest worms that infect humans and can grow to a length of 40 cms. The eggs produced by the female worms are excreted in the feces. Each female can produce about 200 000 eggs per day! They mature in the soil and become infective after many weeks. The eggs are highly resistant and can remain viable

Notes

It is treated with antihelminthic drugs.

For more details see Appendix C: Antihelminthic agents.

Pathology A to Z -

for years. When the eggs are ingested (fecal-oral contamination), the larvae emerge in the intestine, penetrate the mucosa and enter the circulation. In the lungs, the larvae migrate into the alveoli, ascend up the bronchi and enter the gut once again, where they become adult worms in 2-3 months. The migrating larvae and the adult worms in the intestines produce the signs and symptoms.

Signs and Symptoms:

When the larvae enter the lungs (about 9-12 days after ingestion of eggs), they tend to produce dry cough. It may be associated with mild fever. The eosinophil count is increased during this period. When the number of adult worms in the intestines are few, there are no intestinal symptoms. But if they are numerous, they can produce abdominal pain and symptoms of intestinal obstruction, especially in children. Occasionally, the worm may migrate into the bile duct producing symptoms of bile duct obstruction or move up the esophagus resulting in cough and expulsion of the worm through the mouth.

Risk Factors:

It is more common where there are no proper sanitary facilities and in places where human manure is used as fertilizer. Improper washing of vegetables grown in contaminated soil is a potential risk. Children are more at risk as they tend to play in soil.

Caution and Recommendations to Therapists:

These infections are not spread by contact as in massage. Refer to Appendix B: Strategies for infection prevention and safe practice for some useful guidelines. Also see Appendix D for organizations and support groups.

References:

Morello JA, Mizer HE, Wilson ME, Granato PA. Microbiology in patient care. 6th ed. New York: McGraw-Hill; 1998.

Beutel WD, Allison JG. Ascariasis. Consultant 1983; 23(7): 213,216-217,220-222.

Helminthic infection - Capillariasis

Gastrointestinal system

An infection produced by the worm Capillaria philippinensis.

Cause:

The infection is caused when infected raw fish is eaten. The larvae present in the fish enter the body and mature into adult worms in the intestines where they produce an inflammatory reaction.

Notes

It is treated with antihelminthic drugs. For more details see Appendix C: Antihelminthic agents.

Signs and Symptoms:

It presents as a slow onset of diarrhoea and abdominal pain. The villi get destroyed as a result of the inflammatory reaction. If it is not treated, it can eventually result in malabsorption syndrome and malnutrition.

Risk Factors:

It is more common in the Philippines and Thailand.

Caution and Recommendations to Therapists:

These infections are not spread by contact as in massage. Refer to Appendix B:

References

Ash LR, Orihel TC. Atlas of human Parasitology. 3d ed. Chicago: ASCP Press; 1990.

Strategies for infection prevention and safe practice for some useful guidelines. Also see Appendix D for organizations and support groups.

Helminthic infection - Dracunculiasis

Gastrointestinal system

(Guinea worm infection)

An infection caused by the worm Dracunculus medinensis.

Cause:

Notes

The worm can be extracted from the skin by winding a few centimeters of the worm at a time, on a stick.

The infection is produced when water contaminated by the larvae is ingested. The larvae enter the stomach and intestines where they mature. The worm is long, ranging from 300 cm to 1 m. The female worm migrates to the skin. A blister forms in the region where the worm is located. The blister later bursts and ulcerates, releasing numerous larvae.

Signs and Symptoms:

Usually there are no symptoms until the worm reaches the skin and forms blisters. At this time, there may be associated fever, wheezing and swelling.

Risk Factors:

It is more common in the Middle East, India, Pakistan and Africa.

References

Ranque P, Hopkins D: Current status of the global campaign to eradicate dracunculiasis (guinea worm disease) Ann Parasitol Hum Comp 1991; 66(suppl 1):37.

Caution and Recommendations to Therapists:

These infections are not spread by contact as in massage. Refer to Appendix B: Strategies for infection prevention and safe practice for some useful guidelines. Also see Appendix D for organizations and support groups.

Helminthic infection - Enterobiasis

Gastrointestinal system

(Pinworm infection)

An infection caused by the worm Enterobius vermicularis.

Cause:

Notes

It is treated with antihelminthic drugs. Family members may have to be treated as well. For more details see Appendix C: Antihelminthic agents.

The infection is caused by the worm *Enterobius vermicularis* that lives in the lumen of the gut. At night, the female worm moves to the skin around the anus and lays thousands of eggs. When the person scratches the perianal region, the eggs get lodged in the hand or under the nails and if proper precautions are not taken, eventually get transported to the mouth and are ingested to begin the cycle again.

Signs and Symptoms:

The most common symptom is itching in the perianal region, especially at night. If the infection is severe, abdominal pain and weight loss may be seen.

Risk Factors:

Since the eggs are easily transmitted by contact, it is common among family members.

Caution and Recommendations to Therapists:

Eggs from the perianal region can be dislodged and can infect another individual if they are caught under the nail and inadvertantly ingested. It is important to ensure that these clients have their underclothes on during the session. Take special precautions to wash hands thoroughly with soap and disinfect the linen. In general, it is very important for the Therapist to adhere to hygeinic techniques. Refer to Appendix B: Strategies for infection prevention and safe practice for some useful guidelines. Also see Appendix D for organizations and support groups.

References

Ash LR, Orihel TC. Atlas of human Parasitology, 3d ed. Chicago: ASCP Press; 1990.

Morello JA, Mizer HE, Wilson ME, Granato PA. Microbiology in patient care. 6th ed. New York: McGraw-Hill; 1998

Helminthic infection - Filariasis (Elephantiasis)

Lymphatic system

A disease of the lymphatic system caused by the filarial worm.

Cause:

The organisms causing this type of filariasis are *Wuchereria bancrofti*, *Brugia malayi* and *Brugia timori*. The adult worms produce microfilariae that circulate in the blood. The microfilariae enter the body of the mosquito when it bites infected humans. It develops into larvae in the mosquito. The larvae are injected into the bloodstream of humans when the mosquito bites. They then migrate to the lymphatics and become adult worms.

Symptoms are produced by obstruction to lymphatic flow by the long, threadlike filarial worms. Further problem results from inflammatory damage to the lymphatics due to the immune response of the body to the adult worms that live in afferent lymphatic vessels and the lymph node.

Notes

It is treated medically with drugs. Some of the symptoms may be treated by elevation of the affected limb, use of elastic stockings and massage. If the swelling is extensive and disfiguring, surgery is done. Use of insect repellent, mosquito nets, spraying of mosquito breeding areas are some preventive measures that can be taken.

Signs and Symptoms:

It presents as a slow onset of swelling and heaviness of a limb, scrotum or labia accompanied by high fever with chills. The swelling persists even after treatment, and lasts for years. Legs may appear as large as an elephants' - thus its name. Prolonged accumulation of protein and fluid in the interstitial fluid compartment (area between the cells) causes thickening of skin in the region. The local lymph nodes may be enlarged. Inflammation of the lymphatic vessels (lymphangitis) may be seen radiating from the lymph nodes.

If the genital region is involved, scrotal pain, tenderness and swelling result.

Risk Factors:

It is more common in those living in tropical countries where this condition is endemic.

Caution and Recommendations to Therapists:

These infections are not spread by contact as in massage. Massage may be beneficial to help drain the toxins from the edmatous area and to reduce fibrosis and adhesion. Keep the affected limb elevated for soemtime before the massage. Avoid areas that are fissured and ulcerated. Refer to Appendix B: Strategies for infection prevention and safe practice for some useful guidelines. Also see Appendix D for organizations and support groups.

References

WHO expert committee on Lymphatic filariasis: Fifth report. Technical report series No. 821, Geneva: WHO; 1993.

Helminthic infection - Hookworm

Gastrointestinal system

(Hookworm infection)

An infection by the intestinal worm - hookworm.

Cause:

The infection is produced by one of two species *Ancylostoma duodenale* or *Necator americanus*. The worms are about 1 cms long with blood-sucking devices that help them attach to the mucosa of the small intestine. The adult worms produce eggs that are expelled in the feces. In the soil, the eggs hatch and larvae are released. The larvae mature and become infective. They enter the human body by penetrating the skin. They then enter the circulation and reach the lungs from where they migrate up the bronchi to enter the pharynx. They are swallowed and reach the intestines where they mature into adult worms capable of producing eggs. It takes about 6-8 weeks for the cycle ie. from entering the body to producing eggs in the intestines. The worms can survive for many years inside the human body.

Signs and Symptoms:

Usually, there are no symptoms. There may be inflammation and itching of the skin, at the site of penetration of the larva. Inflammation may be present along the course the larva took while migrating under the skin. Dry cough may be produced when the larva migrates through the lungs. In individuals whose intake of iron is inadequate, iron deficiency anemia may be produced. Symptoms due to the anemia such as weakness, shortness of breath result. There may be associated hypoproteinemia.

Risk Factors:

Poor sanitary facilities and contamination of soil with feces are risks. Walking barefoot in contaminated soil can increase the risk of infection.

Caution and Recommendations to Therapists:

These infections are not spread by contact as in massage. Refer to Appendix B: Strategies for infection prevention and safe practice for some useful guidelines. Also see Appendix D for organizations and support groups.

Notes

Many safe and effective antihelminthic drugs are available for treatment. Iron deficiency and hypoproteinemia, if present, have to be treated concurrently.

References

Schad GA, Warren KS, editors. Hookworm Disease: Current status and new directions. London: Taylor and Francis; 1990.

Helminthic infection - Larva migrans

An infection produced by the migration of larvae of worms through tissues.

Cause:

The larvae are those of worms that are normally parasites of other species. So they do not develop into adult worms in the human body. The more common type of larva migrans is *toxocariasis* - due to the larva of *Toxocara canis* - a worm that infects dogs. The eggs are found in the feces of infected dogs that contaminate the soil. Humans acquire the disease by the ingestion of eggs. It is more common in children who tend to play with soil.

A cutaneous form of larva migrans is due to the larvae of animal hookworms (dogs and cats) that burrow under the skin. The larvae hatch from eggs found in the feces of infected animals and enter the human body when the skin comes in contact with infected soil.

Signs and Symptoms:

The larvae hatch from the eggs that have been ingested and penetrate the intestinal mucosa from where they are carried by blood to all parts of the body. They produce an immune reaction in the tissue. Fever, loss of appetite, lethargy, weight loss, cough, wheezing and rashes are common symptoms. There may be enlargement of the spleen and liver. Seizures may be seen if the brain is involved. Sometimes, the larva migrates into the eye and produces various forms of inflammatory reactions there.

The cutaneous form of larva migrans produces reddish lesions along the tortuous course that the larva takes under the skin. The area is very itchy and vesicles may be formed. With time, the larva dies and the lesions resolve.

Risk Factors:

See Cause.

Caution and Recommendations to Therapists:

These infections are not spread by contact as in massage. Refer to Appendix B: Strategies for infection prevention and safe practice for some useful guidelines. Also see Appendix D for organizations and support groups.

Notes

In those with severe symptoms, glucocorticoids may be given. Antihelminthic drugs are not effective. Deworming dogs and laws against littering public parks and playground with dog excreta are some preventive measures.

For more details see Appendix C: Antihelminthic agents; Antiinflammatories - steroidal drugs.

References

Ash LR, Orihel TC. Atlas of human Parasitology, 3d ed. Chicago: ASCP Press; 1990.

Helminthic infection - Loiasis

(African eye worm infection)

An infection produced by the worm Loa loa.

Cause:

The worm lives in the subcutaneous tissue of infected humans. The microfilariae

It is treated with antifilarial drugs. Protective garments to prevent insect bites are helpful.

are found in the blood between 12 noon and 2 PM. The microfilariae enter the body of insects (deerflies) when they bite humans. The infection spreads when the insect bites another human.

Signs and Symptoms:

It may be asymptomatic in people living in endemic areas. If the adult worm migrates to the eye, there is an inflammatory reaction produced there. Redness and swelling (*Calabar swelling*) due to allergic reaction of the body to the adult worms, may be seen in the limbs. Other symptoms may be produced, depending on where the worm migrates.

Risk Factors:

It is more common in the rain forests of West and Central Africa.

References

Klion AD et al. Loiasis in endemic and non-endemic populations: Immunologically mediated differences in clinical presentation. J Infect Dis 1991:163;1318.

Caution and Recommendations to Therapists:

These infections are not spread by contact as in massage. Refer to Appendix B: Strategies for infection prevention and safe practice for some useful guidelines. Also see Appendix D for organizations and support groups.

Helminthic infection - Onchocerciasis

Integumentary system

(River blindness)

An infection produced by the worm Onchocerca volvulus.

Cause:

Notes

The aim is to prevent irreversible changes. Nodules may be removed surgically. Special drugs (eg ivermectin) are available for treating this condition.

Measures to reduce the breeding of blackflies by spraying insecticides and use of protective garments to prevent bites are some forms of preventing the infection.

The infection is produced when the larvae are deposited on the skin of humans by infected blackfly. The larvae develop into adult worms under the skin. The female worms release infective microfilariae that disseminate throughout the body. The microfilariae produce inflammatory reactions in the body.

Signs and Symptoms:

In the skin, itching is produced over the area where the worm lies. The inflammatory reaction results in wrinkling of the skin, loss of elastic tissue and changes in pigmentation. The fibrous reaction produced around the adult worm results in the formation of nodules under the skin. Often, the larvae enter the eye and produce inflammatory reactions there. There may be impairment of vision and in severe cases atrophy of the eye and blindness. Lymph nodes draining the area where the adult worm is located may be enlarged. Other symptoms may be produced depending on the location affected.

Risk Factors:

It is more common in Africa and Latin America. Since the blackfly breeds near rivers and streams, the disease is more common in regions close to water.

Caution and Recommendations to Therapists:

These infections are not spread by contact as in massage. Ensure that your clinic is 'insect proofed' if practicing in an area where this condition is present. Refer to Appendix B: Strategies for infection prevention and safe practice for some useful guidelines. Also see Appendix D for organizations and support groups.

References

WHO expert committee on Onchocerciasis: Third report. Technical Report Series No 752, Geneva: WHO; 1987.

Helminthic infection - Schistosomiasis
Gastrointestinal system

An infection produced by trematodes (flukes).

Cause:

The condition is due to flukes (*Schistosoma mansoni, Schistosoma haematobium, Schistosoma japonicum* etc) that infect humans and live in organs such as the intestines, lungs, bladder, ureter, bile duct, liver etc. The site of infection varies with the species.

Humans are infected when they come in contact with water that contains the infective stage (*cercariae*) of the parasite. In humans, the adult worms lay eggs that eventually get excreted via urine or feces as ova. In water, this free swimming ciliated stage of the parasites (*mircadium*) seek out snails and penetrate the soft tissue. The mircadium form cercariae, the stage that can infect humans by penetrating intact skin. From the skin, the cercariae migrate to various organs where they mature into adult worms and the cycle repeats.

Signs and Symptoms:

The signs and symptoms are variable. In visitors to endemic areas, fever (*Katayama fever*), headache, weakness, loss of weight, abdominal pain, diarrhea etc. may be seen due to the immune response evoked. The symptoms produced are due to the inflammatory and immune reaction of the body to the eggs deposited in various organs. One of the complications of Schistosomiasis is fibrosis of the liver leading to portal hypertension. Other manifestations include, chronic cystitis (inflammation in the urinary bladder), ureteritis, dermatitis etc.

Risk Factors:

Exposure to cercariae found in infected water increases the risk. Schistosomiasis is more common in parts of South America, Africa, Middle East, China and Philippines.

Caution and Recommendations to Therapists:

These infections are not spread by contact as in massage. Refer to Appendix B: Strategies for infection prevention and safe practice for some useful guidelines. Also see Appendix D for organizations and support groups.

Notes

The condition is treated with specific drugs.

Measures to prevent contamination of ponds, lakes etc. by urine and feces can reduce the incidence. The intermediary host - snails can be destroyed by using Molluscicides.

References

Rollinson O, Simpson AJG, editors: The biology of schistosomes. From Genes to Latrines. New York: Academic; 1987.

Helminthic infection - Strongyloidiasis

An infection produced by the worm Strongyloides stercoralis.

Cause:

Notes

Even if asymptomatic, this infection is treated with antihelminthic drugs.

For more details see Appendix C: Antihelminthic agents.

This worm is unusual as it can reproduce in the intestine and life cycles can repeat there. In addition, cycles can continue in the soil without the presence of hosts. The adult worm is about 2 mm in size. It lays eggs in the intestinal walls. The eggs produce larvae that are excreted in the feces. Alternately, the larvae can mature in the colon or in the skin around the anus and enter the circulation. If the larvae is excreted in the feces, they can mature in the soil and enter the human body by penetrating the skin. From the skin they enter the circulation, reach the lungs, enter the alveoli, ascend up the bronchi to be eventually swallowed. When they reach the gut, the larvae mature into adult worms and the cycle repeats.

Signs and Symptoms:

Usually there are no symptoms. Itching and inflammation may be present at the site of penetration of skin. The route taken by the larvae as it migrates under the skin may also produce irritation and may be seen as a tortuous, inflamed, itchy area. Some cough may be produced as the larvae pass through the lungs. In the intestines, the presence of the adult worms may cause burning pain in the epigastrium (similar to peptic ulcer pain). Abdominal discomfort, nausea, diarrhea, mild gastrointestinal bleeding, malabsorption and weight loss may be produced. In those who are immunocompromised, the larvae may migrate all over the body and produce severe symptoms. The infection can be fatal in these individuals.

Risk Factors:

References

Ash LR, Orihel TC. Atlas of human Parasitology. 3d ed. Chicago: ASCP Press; 1990.

Morello JA, Mizer HE, Wilson ME, Granato PA. Microbiology in patient care. 6th ed. New York: McGraw-Hill; 1998.

See Cause.

Caution and Recommendations to Therapists:

These infections are not spread by contact as in massage. Refer to Appendix B: Strategies for infection prevention and safe practice for some useful guidelines. Also see Appendix D for organizations and support groups.

Helminthic infection - Taeniasis

(Tapeworm infection)

An infection due to segmented worms (tapeworms) that live in the intestines.

Cause:

The infection is produced by many species of tapeworms. In some types, the human is the definitive host where the adult worm lives in the gastrointestinal tract. In other types, humans are intermediary hosts and the larval stage of the parasite is found in the tissues.

Notes

Effective antihelminthic drugs are available for treatment. Surgery may be required to treat cysticercosis.

For more details see Appendix C: Antihelminthic agents.

The worm attaches to the intestinal mucosa by cup-like structures located on the head. Behind the head, segments begin to form that may extend upto many meters. Each segment matures and forms eggs that are excreted in the feces. When the eggs are ingested by an intermediate host (eg. vegetation contaminated by the eggs), it develops into larvae that penetrate the intestinal mucosa and migrate to tissues where they form cysts. When the tissue containing the cysts are ingested by the definitive host (eg. humans), they form adult worms in the intestines and the cycle repeats.

Taeniasis saginata (beef tapeworm) is due to ingestion of raw or undercooked (infected) beef. *Taeniasis solium* and *cysticercosis* is caused by the pork tapeworm and is due to the ingestion of infected, undercooked pork. There are many other forms of tapeworms that have dogs, cats and fish etc. as intermediary hosts and accidentally infect humans causing symptoms. For example, *echinococcosis* is an infection caused by the larval stage of a tapeworm that affects dogs. When humans ingest the eggs, the larvae migrate to organs like the liver or lungs where they form large fluid-filled cysts (*hydatid cysts*) that produce symptoms due to the size or when they rupture.

Signs and Symptoms:

Passage of tapeworm segments in the feces may alert individuals to infection. Sometimes, it may present as abdominal pain, nausea, loss of appetite, weakness and weight loss. In some forms of tapeworm infection (eg. pork tapeworm), eggs may be ingested (fecal contamination) and the larval form may enter the body from the intestine and produce inflammatory reactions where they lodge. This type of infection - *cysticercosis*, may produce seizures, headache, nausea and vomiting etc. if the brain is involved.

Risk Factors:

Eating properly cooked meat and living in areas with proper sanitary facilities are some preventive measures.

Caution and Recommendations to Therapists:

These infections are not spread by contact as in massage. Refer to Appendix B: Strategies for infection prevention and safe practice for some useful guidelines. Also see Appendix D for organizations and support groups.

References

Ash LR, Orihel TC. Atlas of human Parasitology. 3d ed. Chicago: ASCP Press; 1990.

Morello JA, Mizer HE, Wilson ME, Granato PA. Microbiology in patient care. 6th ed. New York: McGraw-Hill; 1998.

Helminthic infection - Trichinosis

Gastrointestinal system

An infection caused by the worm Trichinella spiralis.

Cause:

The condition develops after ingestion of infected pork or other meat (dog

Prevention is best. Antihelminthic drugs are effective only against the worm in the gut and not those in the muscle. In many lightly infected individuals, recovery may be produced with bed rest, painkillers and steroids.

For more details see Appendix C: Antihelminthic agents; Painkillers; Antiinflammatories - steroidal drugs.

meat; horse meat; bear, wild boar and walrus meat). The worms form cysts in the tissue of carnivorous/omnivorous animals. When the infected meat is ingested, the acid and pepsin in the stomach digest the walls of the cysts and the larvae are liberated. The larvae enter the walls of the small intestine and mature into adult worms. After a week, the female worms release larvae that reach skeletal muscles via the bloodstream. The larvae form cysts in the muscle.

Signs and Symptoms:

The signs and symptoms vary according to the phase of infection. In the first week, diarrhea, abdominal pain, constipation, nausea and vomiting are some of the symptoms seen when the worm invades the small intestines. When the larva migrates to the muscle, fever, facial edema, rash, headache, cough, difficulty in breathing and difficulty in swallowing may be present. When the worm enters the muscle, about 2-3 weeks after the infection, muscle pain, edema and weakness may develop.

Risk Factors:

See Cause.

Caution and Recommendations to Therapists:

These infections are not spread by contact as in massage. Refer to Appendix B: Strategies for infection prevention and safe practice for some useful guidelines. Also see Appendix D for organizations and support groups.

References

Beaver PC et al. Clinical Parasitology. 9th ed. Philadelphia: Lea & Febiger; 1984.

Morello JA, Mizer HE, Wilson ME, Granato PA. Microbiology in patient care. 6th ed. New York: McGraw-Hill; 1998.

Gastrointestinal system

Helminthic infection - Trichuriasis

(Whipworm infection)

An infection produced by the worm Trichuris trichiura.

Cause:

Notes

It is treated with antihelminthic drugs. For more details see Appendix C: Antihelminthic agents.

The worm Trichuris trichiura is shaped like a whip - with a broader posterior and a thinner anterior portion. The adult worms that grow to 3-5 cms in length, live in the cecum and colon, attached to the mucosa. The adult worms lay eggs that are excreted in the feces. If the eggs are ingested, the larvae hatch in the small intestines and later migrate and mature in the large intestines. It takes about 3 months for the cycle to be completed.

Signs and Symptoms:

Usually, there are no symptoms. If the number of worms in the intestine is large, there may be abdominal pain, loss of appetite and weight and blood and mucus in stools.

Risk Factors:

Poor sanitary facilities and contamination of soil with feces increases the risk.

Caution and Recommendations to Therapists:

These infections are not spread by contact as in massage. Refer to Appendix B: Strategies for infection prevention and safe practice for some useful guidelines. Also see Appendix D for organizations and support groups.

References

Beaver PC et al. Clinical Parasitology. 9th ed. Philadelphia: Lea & Febiger; 1984.

Morello JA, Mizer HE, Wilson ME, Granato PA. Microbiology in patient care. 6th ed. New York: McGraw-Hill; 1998.

Hemangiomas

A type of benign vascular tumors.

Cardiovascular, Integumentary systems

Cause:

They are due to abnormal growth of vascular tissue. Unlike malignancies, these tumors are confined to specific areas and do not spread to other organs and tissues.

Signs and Symptoms:

They often occur in the skin and subcutaneous tissue. They may be seen in deeper tissues too including the brain, liver etc. Their appearance differs according to the size, location and microscopic pattern. *Capillary hemangiomas* are made up of capillary vessels or capillary-like structures. *Cavernous hemangiomas* are made up of dilated vessels filled with blood. Intramuscular hemangiomas present as soft tissue tumors that may have the appearance of capillary or cavernous hemangiomas. Apart from these types, there are many other types of hemangiomas. See Appendix A: Figure 26.

If superficial, they appear as a red patch on the skin. Deeper tumors tend to appear blue. There may be a tendency to bleed. Disseminated intravascular coagulation has been associated with large lesions.

Risk Factors:

Hemangiomas are one of the common tumors of infancy. They are more common in the head and neck region.

Caution and Recommendations to Therapists:

Do not massage directly over very large lesions as thrombosis, if present may be dislodged. Excessive pressure over hemangiomas may cause bleeding under the skin.

Notes

Most often, hemangiomas involute by themselves and no treatment is required. Treatment depends on the location and size. Small superficial lesions are often excised while large lesions are monitored, as widespread excision may not be acceptable to the individual aesthetically.

References

Sabiston DC, editor. Textbook of Surgery 14th ed. Philadelphia: WB Saunders Company; 1991. p. 1394.

Morelli JG. Disorders of vascular tissue. In: Sams WM, Lynch PJ, editors. Principles and practice of Dermatology. 2nd ed. New York: Churchill Livingstone; 1996. p. 275.

Hemophilia

Hereditary bleeding disorders due to deficiency of a specific clotting factor in the blood.

Cardiovascular system

Cause:

Hemophilia A, one of the types, is caused by a lack of Factor VIII, one of the clotting factors. Lack of factor IX is said to be responsible for *Hemophilia B*.

a Handbook for Massage Therapists

Drugs like aspirin that affect coagulation should be avoided. Factor VIII/IX concentrates prepared from the plasma of many donors is given to hemophiliac clients. Since these individuals require frequent transfusions, there is a risk of Human Immunodeficiency Virus infection, hepatitis etc. through blood products. Complications of hemophilia such as bleeding into joint cavities, internal bleeding have to be treated promptly.

For more details see Appendix C: Blood transfusion.

The clotting mechanism is complex and requires the activation of many inactive factors present in the blood. Absence of any of these factors can result in dysfunction of the clotting mechanism. Hemophilia is inherited from the mother - ie. the gene responsible for the deficiency is present in the X chromosome. Since it is recessive, it does not present in the daughter if the other X chromosome is normal. However, the daughter can be a carrier of the gene and transmit it to her son. As there is only one X chromosome in males, presence of the gene results in presentation of the disease in the form of bleeding.

Signs and Symptoms:

Depending on the degree of deficiency, the person presents with mild, moderate or severe forms of abnormal bleeding. In the mild form, prolonged bleeding may be seen only after major trauma. In the severe form the person may bleed spontaneously. Large hematomas may form in the muscle or under the skin with the mildest of trauma. Bleeding into the joints can lead to severe pain, swelling and joint stiffness that is permanent. Internal bleeding can lead to shock and death.

Risk Factors:

A family history of the disease increases the risk.

Caution and Recommendations to Therapists:

Suspect a bleeding disorder in a client with large hematomas. Elevation of the limb and cold compresses may be of benefit to slow the bleeding process. Massage is contraindicated in those with severe forms of hemophilia. In the milder forms, very superficial, light strokes may not produce harm to the client. In any event, it is advisable to consult the Physician before any form of massage is undertaken. Refer client to a local support group. Encourage daughters born into families with a history of hemophilia to have genetic counseling. Refer to Appendix D for resources.

References

Kasper CK, Dietrich SL. Comprehensive management of haemophilia. Clin Haematol 1985; 14: 489.

Gastrointestinal, Cardiovascular systems

Hemorrhoids (Piles)

A condition with abnormal dilatation of veins in the rectum.

Cause:

It is caused by increased pressure in the venous network of the rectum.

Signs and Symptoms:

Hemorrhoids usually present with no symptoms or as passage of fresh blood during defecation. If the hemorrhoids are chronic, they may be seen or felt as soft swellings in the anus. Itching around the anus is often present. If the hemorrhoid gets obstructed, a sharp pain may be experienced in the anal area. Chronic bleeding through the anus can result in anemia in the patient.

Notes:

It is treated with painkillers. Measures to reduce the pressure include regulation of bowel habits, alteration of diet to include raw vegetables, fruits and whole grain cereal. The pain can be reduced by local anaesthetic creams and sitting in a warm water bath. Injection of sclerosing agents and surgery are strategies used for severe cases.

For more details see Appendix C: Painkillers; Anaesthetics; Sclerosing agents.

Risk Factors:

Occupations that involve prolonged standing or sitting; chronic constipation or diarrhea where straining occurs; chronic cough that recurrently increases the intra-abdominal pressure; any condition that results in damming up of blood in the veins such as cirrhosis of the liver and heart failure are all predisposing factors. Conditions that weaken the pelvic floor - old age, rectal surgery, pregnancy and episiotomy (an incision that is made in the pelvic floor to widen the outlet for the baby during labor) also increase the risk of hemorrhoids.

Caution and Recommendations to Therapists:

Encourage client to alter diet and avoid prolonged standing, sitting and straining. Obtain a good history to determine the cause of hemorrhoids. Massage is not contraindicated, but avoid excessive pressure in the abdominal area. See Appendix D for organizations and support groups.

References

Sabiston DC, editor. Textbook of Surgery 14th ed. Philadelphia: WB Saunders Company; 1991. p. 962-965.

Hepatitis

Gastrointestinal system

An inflammation of the liver.

Cause:

There are many factors that can cause this condition, a few of which are infectious. Alcohol, drugs and toxins can cause inflammation of the liver. Malaria, infectious mononucleosis, typhoid, amebiasis are infectious causes of hepatitis. More commonly, hepatitis is due to infection by the hepatitis virus. The hepatitis virus exists as many strains. *Hepatitis A, B, B associated delta, C* and *E viruses* are some of the well-known strains. The mode of transmission and incubation period varies from strain to strain.

Hepatitis A infection, also known as *infectious hepatitis* or *short incubation hepatitis* is highly contagious and is transmitted by the fecal-oral route. It is transmitted by ingestion of contaminated food, water or milk. It is often spread by eating shellfish from infected water. In homosexuals it can spread by oral-anal contact. It is rarely transmitted through intravenous blood or plasma as the virus is present in the blood during symptoms - a period when the patient is unlikely to donate. The incubation period is 15-45 days. In the infected person the virus can be seen in the feces even two weeks before the onset of symptoms and persists in the feces for many weeks after symptoms begin.

Hepatitis B infection also known as *serum hepatitis* is more serious than Hepatitis A. It lasts longer and can lead to cirrhosis, cancer of the liver and a carrier state (carrier state is the state of a person when the virus continues to be excreted even though no symptoms are seen). It has a long incubation period of 1.5 to 2 months. The symptoms may last from weeks to months. The virus is usually transmitted through infected blood, serum or plasma. However, it can spread by oral or sexual contact, as it is present in most body secretions. Infants can contract it from infected mothers. Infected individuals can be carriers

Notes

Immunoglobulin (antibodies) against Hepatitis A can be given to people in close contact with an infected person, or to those travelling to areas (India, Africa, Asia or Central America) where hepatitis A is endemic. The immunity is short lived and booster doses are required.

Vaccines are available for Hepatitis B in the form of Hepatitis B immunoglobulin (antibodies). This provides protection for 3-6 months. Another form of Hepatitis B vaccine provides long-term immunity. The latter is recommended for people in occupations at high risk.

Hepatitis is treated symptomatically, with bedrest, regulation of fat intake and avoidance of alcohol and drugs that are toxic to the liver.

For more details see Appendix C: Immunization.

for months and years ie. they are capable of transmitting the disease during this period.

Hepatitis C is known as *non-A, non-B hepatitis* and can cause acute or chronic hepatitis. This can also lead to a carrier state and liver cancer. It is transmitted through blood transfusions or exposure to blood products.

Hepatitis D virus infection or B associated delta virus affects individuals who are infected by the B virus. It makes the symptoms associated with Hepatitis B infection more severe. Carrier states are also seen. It is prevented by taking measures against Hepatitis B infection.

Hepatitis E is transmitted by the fecal-oral route and the symptoms are short-lived, similar to that of Hepatitis A.

Signs and Symptoms:

The symptoms are a result of the direct liver cell injury by the virus as well as the immune response of the body to the infection. The symptoms vary from no symptoms to severe jaundice, liver failure and death. In the early stages, the person experiences muscle and joint pain, easy fatigability, loss of appetite, nausea, vomiting, diarrhea or constipation. Dull pain in the right upper abdomen may be present. Slowly this leads to jaundice, liver and spleen enlargement. The acute illness usually lasts for 2-3 weeks. The recovery of the person depends on the type of hepatitis. A person with Hepatitis A recovers in about 9 weeks while an individual with Hepatitis B and C takes about 16 weeks.

Risk Factors:

The incidence is higher in intravenous drug abusers, those requiring blood products (people with bleeding disorders), homosexuals and heterosexuals. Healthcare workers exposed to blood products or high risk individuals, infants born to infected mothers, AIDS victims, hemodialysis patients and individuals on immunosuppressants are all at risk.

Caution and Recommendations to Therapists:

Always contact Physician about the infectivity of an individual with history of hepatitis. Hepatitis as a side effect of drugs or alcohol intake is not infective. Hepatitis A, B, C, D and E are all infective with potential for the person to be in a carrier state. It is advisable to massage individuals with history of this condition with the underclothes on. Take special precautions to wash hands thoroughly with soap and disinfect the linen. Avoid massage to abdomen (especially the right upper quadrant) if there is a history of chronic Hepatitis (hepatitis lasting for more than 6 months). It is advisable for all Therapists to be vaccinated against hepatitis B. Three doses are given at 0, 1 and 6 months. Refer to Appendix B: Strategies for infection prevention and safe practice for some useful guidelines. Also see Appendix D for organizations and support groups.

References

Hollinger FB et al, editors. Viral Hepatitis and Liver Disease. Baltimore: Williams & Wilkins; 1991.

Morello JA, Mizer HE, Wilson ME, Granato PA. Microbiology in patient care. 6th ed. New York: McGraw-Hill; 1998. p372-373.

Hernia - femoral

A protrusion of an organ lying inside the abdominal cavity, through an abnormal opening around the femoral artery as it goes into the leg in the groin area.

Musculoskeletal, Gastrointestinal systems

Cause:

Weakness of the muscles and fascia of the abdomen along with increased intraabdominal pressure results in the intestines, omentum or bladder to protrude through this potential weak spot called the femoral canal.

Signs and Symptoms:

It presents as a swelling that is soft and reducible located just below the crease in the upper part of the thigh. Rarely, it can cause severe pain with nausea and vomiting, if a part of the intestines get obstructed.

Risk Factors:

Straining, lifting weights or chronic persistent cough can predispose to this.

Caution and Recommendations to Therapists:

Advice the client to consult a Physician if a painless reducible or irreducible swelling is seen. Do not massage over the hernia or try to reduce the swelling as obstruction or perforation can be produced in the bowel. Encourage client to reduce weight and get treated for cough, if present. Advice the client to avoid lifting and straining. A normal relaxation massage to other parts of the body is beneficial. If a client has just had surgery, avoid the area until the wound has healed completely. After complete healing, friction massage over the scar may help reduce adhesions.

Notes

Hernia is treated with a truss to support and reduce the swelling if in an elderly individual or in those who cannot have surgery. Surgically, steel mesh, wires or fascia can be used to reinforce the weakened area and/or to close the opening after the contents are pushed into the abdomen.

References

Sabiston DC, editor. Textbook of Surgery 14th ed. Philadelphia: WB Saunders Company; 1991. p. 1143-1144.

Hernia - hiatal (Hiatus hernia)

An abnormal opening in the diaphragm that allows a portion of the stomach to enter the thoracic cavity.

Gastrointestinal, Musculoskeletal systems

Cause:

It is commonly caused by weakening of the diaphragmatic muscle. Other conditions that increase the intra-abdominal pressure also cause this.

Signs and Symptoms:

Usually it does not produce any symptoms. If it is associated with esophageal reflux, there is burning pain below the sternum especially a few hours after a meal. If part of the stomach is caught in the opening such that the blood flow is compromised, there is severe pain and the person may go into shock.

Risk Factors:

It is more common in the older age group. The incidence is higher in women.

Notes

It is managed conservatively by avoiding activities that increase the intraabdominal pressure. Drugs may be given to improve the pressure of the esophageal sphincter. Diet is also modified by encouraging the individual to eat small quantities at a time, but increasing the frequency. Antacids are given to reduce the acidity. Surgery is another treatment option.

For more details see Appendix C: Antacids.

Kyphoscoliosis, trauma, obesity, pregnancy, extreme physical exertion, tight clothing that tend to constrict the abdomen, chronic cough and straining predispose to this condition.

Caution and Recommendations to Therapists:
Massage should be given in a seated or half-lying position if the individual is uncomfortable supine or prone.

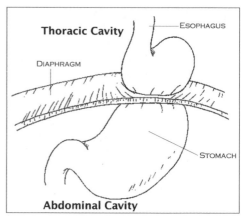

References

Sabiston DC, editor. Textbook of Surgery 14ᵗʰ ed. Philadelphia: WB Saunders Company; 1991. p. 704-708.

Musculoskeletal, Gastrointestinal systems

Hernia - incisional

Protrusion of an organ lying inside the abdominal cavity, through an incision site of a previous surgery.

Cause:

This occurs usually if the incision site on the abdominal wall is weak.

Signs and Symptoms:

It presents as a painless, reducible or irreducible swelling in and around the incisional site. Movements of the intestines can be seen if the swelling is produced by intestines. The swelling becomes more prominent on coughing or straining and may reduce on lying down. Severe pain, nausea and vomiting is produced if the intestines are obstructed or twisted and emergency surgery is required.

Risk Factors:

Infection of the incision site or delayed wound healing increases the risk. Straining, lifting weights or chronic persistent cough before proper healing of the wound can also predispose to this.

Caution and Recommendations to Therapists:

Advice the client to consult a Physician if a painless reducible or irreducible swelling is seen. Do not massage over the hernia or try to reduce the swelling as obstruction or perforation can be produced in the bowel. Encourage client to reduce weight and get treated for cough if present. Advice the client to avoid lifting and straining. A normal relaxation massage to other parts of the body is beneficial. If a client has just had surgery, avoid the area until the wound has

Notes

Hernia is treated with a truss to support and reduce the swelling if in an elderly individual or in those who cannot have surgery. Surgically, steel mesh, wires or fascia can be used to reinforce the weakened area and/or to close the opening after the contents are pushed into the abdomen.

References

Sabiston DC, editor. Textbook of Surgery 14ᵗʰ ed. Philadelphia: WB Saunders Company; 1991. p. 303.

healed completely. After complete healing, very gentle friction massage over the scar may help reduce adhesions

Hernia - inguinal

The protrusion of an organ lying inside the abdominal cavity, through an abnormal opening in the inguinal (upper part of the groin) region.

Cause:

Weakness of the muscles and fascia of the abdomen along with increased intraabdominal pressure results in the intestines, omentum or bladder to protrude through this potential weak spot. In males, the testis descends from the abdomen into the scrotum through the inguinal canal during the seventh month of gestation. If this inguinal canal does not close properly, the organs from the abdomen can be forced into the canal to appear as a swelling in the groin area. Inguinal hernias can also occur in females as the round ligament (a ligament that supports the uterus) passes through this canal.

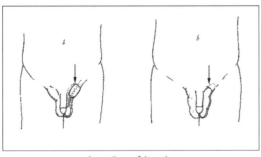

Location of hernia

Notes

Hernia is treated with a truss to support and reduce the swelling if in an elderly individual or in those who cannot have surgery. Surgically, steel mesh, wires or fascia can be used to reinforce the weakened area and/or to close the opening after the contents are pushed into the abdomen.

Signs and Symptoms:

It usually presents as a painless swelling that becomes more prominent on straining. Sometimes if the intestine has herniated, peristalsis (movement of the intestines) can be seen. Most hernias are reducible and can be pushed back manually or reduce on lying down. If adhesions are present between the organ and the surrounding tissue, the hernia cannot be reduced. If the protruding part of the intestines become blocked or twisted, there is severe pain over the area along with nausea and vomiting. In such cases, emergency surgery has to be performed.

Risk Factors:

Weakness of the abdominal wall with aging, obesity and pregnancy predispose to this condition. Occupations that involve heavy lifting and straining increase the intraabdominal pressure. Chronic constipation, chronic cough are other predisposing factors. Birth malformations and nonclosure of the inguinal canal can also be risk factors.

Caution and Recommendations to Therapists:

Advice the client to consult a Physician if a painless reducible or irreducible swelling is seen. Do not massage over the hernia or try to reduce the swelling as

References

Sabiston DC, editor: Textbook of Surgery 14th ed. Philadelphia: WB Saunders Company; 1991. p. 1139-1140.

a Handbook for Massage Therapists

obstruction or perforation can be produced in the bowel. Encourage client to reduce weight and get treated for cough if present. Advice the client to avoid lifting and straining. A normal relaxation massage to other parts of the body is beneficial. If a client has just had surgery, avoid the area until the wound has healed completely. After complete healing, friction massage over the scar may help reduce adhesions.

Hernia - umbilical

Musculoskeletal, Gastrointestinal systems

Protrusion of an organ lying inside the abdominal cavity, through an abnormal opening around the umbilicus (belly button/navel).

Cause:

Notes

Hernia is treated with a truss to support and reduce the swelling if in an elderly individual or in those who cannot have surgery. Surgically, steel mesh, wires or fascia can be used to reinforce the weakened area and/or to close the opening after the contents are pushed into the abdomen.

Weakness of the muscles and fascia of the abdomen along with increased intraabdominal pressure results in the intestines, omentum or bladder to protrude through this potential weak spot.

Signs and Symptoms:

It presents as a painless, reducible or irreducible swelling around the umbilicus. Movements of the intestines can be seen if the swelling is produced by intestines. The swelling becomes more prominent on coughing or straining and may reduce on lying down. Severe, pain, nausea and vomiting is produced if the intestines are obstructed or twisted and emergency surgery is required.

Risk Factors:

In the newborn, weak or abnormal muscle structures around the umbilical cord can result in an umbilical hernia that disappears before the age of five. Obese individuals or those who have had multiple pregnancies are prone. This hernia is also seen in those in occupations that involve lifting and straining or in those with chronic constipation or cough.

Caution and Recommendations to Therapists:

Advice the client to consult a Physician if a painless reducible or irreducible swelling is seen. Do not massage over the hernia or try to reduce the swelling as obstruction or perforation can be produced in the bowel. Encourage client to reduce weight and get treated for cough if present. Advice the client to avoid lifting and straining. A normal relaxation massage to other parts of the body is beneficial. If a client has just had surgery, avoid the area until the wound has healed completely. After complete healing, friction massage over the scar may help reduce adhesions.

References

Sabiston DC, editor. Textbook of Surgery 14th ed. Philadelphia: WB Saunders Company; 1991. p 1145-1146.

Herniated disc (Disc prolapse; Ruptured disc; Herniated nucleus pulposus; Slipped disc)

Musculoskeletal, Nervous systems

Abnormal protrusion of parts of the intervertebral disc with pressure on spinal nerves/spinal cord.

Cause:

Degenerative changes in the intervertebral disc can cause protrusion of the soft, inner nucleus pulposus through the outer, fibrous annulus pulposus. Depending on the direction of the protrusion, the spinal nerve root or spinal cord is compressed. Sometimes, the degenerative changes can result in the disc loosing height with formation of bony spurs that press on adjacent structures.

Signs and Symptoms:

Disc prolapse is more common in the lumbar and cervical regions. In most patients, herniated disc occurs in the L5-S1 or L4-L5 regions. In the neck, it is most frequent in the C6-C7 level.

Typically, a person with lumbar herniation presents with intermittent low back pain. The pain is made worse on moving the back, sitting or standing for a long period of time, lifting heavy objects or coughing and straining. Bed rest relieves the pain. Tingling, numbness and weakness of

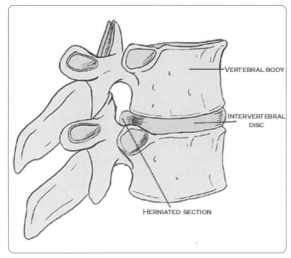

VERTEBRAL BODY

INTERVERTEBRAL DISC

HERNIATED SECTION

specific groups of muscles (depending on the nerve affected) are other symptoms. There may be spasm of muscles on either side of the spine, lumbar scoliosis and tenderness over the lumbar spines.

A person with cervical herniation may experience pain in the neck that may radiate to the upper arm. The pain is increased on moving the neck, coughing or straining and reduced by bed rest. As in lumbar herniation, tingling, numbness and weakness of muscles may be present.

If the herniation is towards the midline, the spinal cord is compressed (cervical region) and motor and sensory function is affected at and below the level of compression (see

Notes

Initially, bed rest on a firm mattress is beneficial. Painkillers and muscle relaxants may be given along with antiinflammatory drugs. Local application of heat, traction and support (eg. lumbosacral corsets) are helpful. Later the patient is encouraged to do back exercises to strengthen the back muscles and increase support to the spine.

If the symptoms are severe or if there is evidence of spinal cord compression, surgery may be required to decrease the compression. Simpler procedures such as injection of chymopapain, an enzyme that reduces the size of the protrusion or removal of the prolapsed disc using a small incision in the skin (percutaneous lumbar discectomy) may be resorted to. Laminectomy is a major procedure where the posterior arch (vertebral lamina) is removed to reduce compression.

For more details see Appendix C: Painkillers; Antiinflammatories - steroidal drugs

Spinal cord injury). Sexual function and voluntary control of bowel and bladder may be affected.

Risk Factors:

Trauma (eg.Whiplash injury) and degenerative diseases of the spine (eg. Ankylosing spondylitis) predispose to this problem.

Caution and Recommendations to Therapists:

If a person with acute low back pain complains of tingling, numbness or weakness of muscles or if the pain radiates or increases on coughing or straining, do not massage, but advice the client to seek medical help. Work in conjunction with the Physiotherapist on those under treatment for this condition. Identify the muscles that have gone into spasm. Some muscles would be under strain because of compensations made to the posture. Hot packs are beneficial and help to reduce spasm and pain. Encourage the client to do regular exercises to strengthen the back.

References

Sabiston DC, editor. Textbook of Surgery 14th ed. Philadelphia: WB Saunders Company; 1991. p. 1262-1267.

Integumentary system

Herpes simplex (Cold sore; Fever blister)

A viral infection of the skin and mucous membrane.

Notes

Antiviral chemotherapy is used to treat the infection.

It is infectious in an active state so contact should be avoided. Herpes can be spread from one part of the body to another by direct contact. Once infected, a high incidence of recurrence is seen.

For more details see Appendix C: Antimicrobial - antiviral agents.

Cause:

It is caused by *Herpes simplex virus type I* and *II*. Infections of the genitalia are caused by type I and II while those above the waist are caused by type I. It is spread by direct, intimate contact, oral sex and kissing, when the virus is inoculated into the small cracks in the skin or mucous membrane. The virus may produce symptoms straightaway (primary herpes) or migrate to the ganglia of sensory nerve where it may lie dormant and later get reactivated (secondary herpes). The incubation period for primary herpes is 5-14 days.

Signs and Symptoms:

In the primary type the patient presents with high fever, sore throat and vesicles all over the mucous membrane. In the general form, pain, itching, vaginal discharge and painful enlargement of the lymph node may be present. The virus may be shed from the lesions up to 12 days after the symptoms are seen. The virus persists in the ganglia and is reactivated in some people. This is secondary herpes. The patient complains of burning and itching sensations in the affected area. Soon the area reddens with formation of vesicles that progress to pustules, ulcer and crusts. There may be accompanying pain. The lesion disappears in 10-14 days. It commonly affects the face, mouth or lips.

Risk Factors:

Previous infection by herpes virus is a risk factor. There is a recurrence of infection precipitated by stress, exposure to sunlight, menstruation or injury.

Caution and Recommendations to Therapists:

It is infectious in an active state so avoid massage. Herpes can be spread from one part of the body to another by direct contact and is an occupational hazard for Therapists. Therapists who have this condition should avoid contact with clients, when in an active state. Massage may be given during the intermittent phases when there is no visible lesion. Refer to Appendix B: Strategies for infection prevention and safe practice for some useful guidelines. Also see Appendix D for organizations and support groups.

References

Corey L. Herpes simplex viruses. In: Isselbacher KJ et al, editors. Harrison's principles of internal medicine. 13th ed. New York: McGraw-Hill Inc; 1994. p. 782-787.

Morello JA, Mizer HE, Wilson ME, Granato PA. Microbiology in patient care. 6th ed. New York: McGraw-Hill; 1998. p.104-105,436-437.

Herpes zoster (Shingles)

Integumentary, Nervous systems

A viral infection of spinal or cranial nerves, affecting a dermatome segment of the skin.

Cause:

It is caused by the herpes virus that causes chickenpox. The virus, which may lie latent in the dorsal root ganglion of a nerve for years in a person who has been exposed to chicken pox, is reactivated and travels along the dermatome causing an inflammatory reaction.

Notes

Antiviral chemotherapy may be used to speed up healing.

For more details see Appendix C: Antimicrobial - antiviral agents; Painkillers.

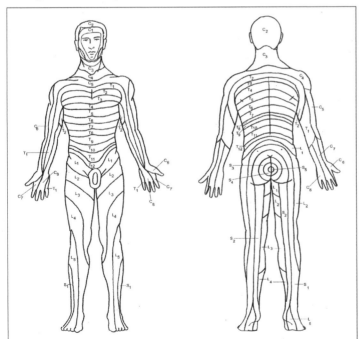

Distribution of dermatomes on the skin

Signs and Symptoms:

Vesicles with reddened bases erupt unilaterally, confined to a single or adjacent group of dermatomes, over a period of 3-4 days. It may be preceded by fever, itching, pain and tenderness in the area. The vesicles dry and form crusts over a period of 2-3weeks. If the branch of the trigeminal nerve supplying the eye is involved it may result in blindness. Older patients may experience prolonged pain in the area even in the absence of vesicles. The severity varies from person to person. Pain may vary from mild to excruciating and may be permanent pain. See Appendix A: page 351.

Risk Factors:

Immunocompromised individuals, the elderly and those highly stressed are more prone.

Caution and Recommendations to Therapists:

It is contagious when the vesicles erupt. Contact with the virus results in chicken pox in a person who has never been exposed to it. Avoid massage during the acute phase. Massage may be given during the intermittent phases when there is no visible lesion, and is beneficial to the client. No specific precautions need be taken when there are no vesicles. Often, elderly clients may be on painkillers if experiencing neuralgia. Always enquire about the use of painkillers before massage. Excessive pressure during massage can damage skin and tissue in clients with reduced sensitivity to pain sensations. Refer to Appendix B: Strategies for infection prevention and safe practice for some useful guidelines. Also see Appendix D for organizations and support groups.

References

Weller TH: Varicella and herpes zoster: Changing concepts of the natural history, control and importance of a not-so-benign virus. N Engl J Med 309: 1362, 1983.

Whitley RJ. Varicella-zoster virus infections. In: Isselbacher KJ et al, editors. Harrison's principles of internal medicine. 13th ed. New York: McGraw-Hill Inc; p. 787-789.

Morello JA, Mizer HE, Wilson ME, Granato PA. Microbiology in patient care. 6th ed. New York: McGraw-Hill; 1998. p. 291-292.

Lymphatic system

Hodgkin's disease (Lymphoma - Hodgkin's)

A malignant disorder of the lymphatic structures.

Notes

Special criteria exist for staging the disease and the treatment varies according to the stage. Radiation and/or chemotherapy may be used.

For more details see Appendix C: Radiation therapy; Cancer chemotherapy.

References

Kaplan HS. Hodgkin's disease. 2nd ed. Cambridge: Harvard University; 1990.

Ferrell-Torry AT, Glick OJ. The use of therapeutic massage as a nursing intervention to modify anxiety and the perception of cancer pain. Cancer Nursing 1993; 16(2):93-101.

McNamara P. Massage for people with cancer. London: 1993. Wandsworth Cancer Support Center; 1993.

Cause:

The cause is not known. It is suspected that it starts as an inflammatory reaction to an infectious agent in an individual whose immunity is lowered or deficient.

Signs and Symptoms:

It presents as a painless, progressive enlargement of a single or group of lymph nodes with a potential to spread to other areas. Fever, night sweats, unexplained weight loss, fatigue, itching and anemia are some of the symptoms. In advanced stages, due to the effect of the abnormal lymphocytes of the immune system, the immunity is lowered and the patient becomes more susceptible to infections.

Risk Factors:

It is more common in young adults between 15 and 35 years of age. There is a higher incidence in males. There is a higher risk in people with immunodeficiencies and autoimmune diseases.

Caution and Recommendations to Therapists:

The disease is not contagious. However, massage is contraindicated as Hodgkin's disease is a form of cancer and massage can help spread it. Consult Physician if the client is under treatment. Both the disease and its treatment reduce the activity of the immune system and there is danger of exposure to mild infections having serious consequences. See Appendix D for organizations and support groups.

Chamness A. Massage therapy and persons living with cancer. Massage Therapy Journal 32(3): 53-65.

MacDonald G. Massage for cancer patients: a review of nursing research. Massage Therapy Journal 34(3): 53-56

Homocystinurias

Musculoskeletal, Nervous systems

A group of genetic disorders that affects the metabolism of the sulfur-containing amino acid homocystine.

Cause:

It is due to the absence or defect of genes that code for certain enzymes involved in the metabolism of homocysteine.

Homocystine interferes with the normal cross-linkages of collagen.

Signs and Symptoms:

The presence of altered collagen in the lenses of the eye result in dislocation of the lens. Osteoporosis is produced due to collagen abnormalities in the bone. There is a tendency to form thrombosis as the metabolism of the connective tissue in the walls of blood vessels is affected. In some forms of the disease, the central nervous system is affected and may present as mental retardation.

Risk Factors:

It is a genetic disorder.

Caution and Recommendations to Therapists:

Get clearance from a Physician, as osteoporosis and thrombus formation is common.

Notes

Infants diagnosed with the disorder can be treated with special diets. Genetic counselling is important.

For more details see Appendix C: Genetic testing / Counselling.

References

Rosenburg LE. Inherited disorders of amino acid metabolism and storage. In: Isselbacher KJ et al, editors. Harrison's principles of internal medicine. 13th ed. New York: McGraw-Hill Inc; 1994. p 2122-2123.

Huntington's disease (Huntington's chorea;

Hereditary chorea; Chronic progressive chorea; Adult chorea)

Nervous system

A degenerative disease of the cerebral cortex and basal ganglia.

Cause:

The cause is unknown but this type of chorea (Greek: *chorea*- to dance) is transmitted genetically. Both sexes can inherit it. There is a 50% chance of a child getting it from a parent who has the disease. If the child does not inherit

Notes

This disease often requires institutionalization of the person. It progresses to death within 15 years of onset. Treatment is only supportive.

it there is no chance of it being transmitted down the generation. It may be due to destruction of neurons that produce the neurotransmitter GABA (gamma amino butyric acid) that inhibits activity in the basal ganglia.

Signs and Symptoms:

The symptoms start slowly with loss of motor control. It then progresses to rapid, involuntary, purposeless movements. The movements are often graceful hence the name chorea. The movement is initially confined to one side of the face, tongue or arm and then progresses to other areas. The disease then progresses to personality changes like carelessness, moodiness, inappropriate behavior, loss of memory and lack of concentration.

Risk Factors:

It usually affects people between the ages of 25-55. There is a family history of the disease.

Caution and Recommendations to Therapists:

Consult treating Physician. Special training may be required by a Therapist who wishes to deal with clients with such problems.

References

Harper P. Huntington's disease. Philadelphia: Saunders; 1992.

Reproductive system	# Hydrocele
	Accumulation of fluid in the sac surrounding the testis.

Cause:

When the fetal testis descends from the abdominal cavity into the scrotum, part of the peritoneal cavity is drawn into the scrotum. Later this extension known as the *processus vaginalis* is occluded. Hydrocele is fluid accumulation in some parts of the processus vaginalis. In the congenital type of hydrocele, there is a communication between the peritoneal cavity and the processus vaginalis resulting in fluid around the testis. Inflammation of the testis and epididymis can also produce hydrocele in some.

Signs and Symptoms:

There is a painless enlargement of the scrotum. It is asymptomatic.

Risk Factors:

See Cause.

Caution and Recommendations to Therapists:

Massage is not harmful in these clients.

Notes

Surgery may be done to reduce the hydrocele.

References

Sabiston DC, editor. Textbook of Surgery 14th ed. Philadelphia: WB Saunders Company; 1991.

Hydrocephalus

An excessive accumulation of cerebrospinal fluid (CSF) within the ventricles of the brain.

Cause:

Any condition that results in obstruction to the flow of CSF from the ventricles of the brain into the venous sinuses or reduces absorption or results in overproduction of CSF can cause hydrocephalus. This usually occurs in children, but can be seen in adults too. The increased pressure on the brain tissue results in atrophy and resultant mental retardation, motor function abnormalities and loss of vision.

It is treated with surgery that shunts the excess fluid from the ventricles of the brain to the atrium of the heart or into the abdominal cavity.

For more details see Appendix C: Shunts.

Signs and Symptoms:

In infants the head appears abnormally large. This is due to the increased pressure separating the unfused sutures of the bones of the skull. The skin is thin and shiny and the neck muscles are weak. If the pressure is very high it can depress the orbits of the eye and the eyes look small and sunken. Motor dysfunction - spasticity of

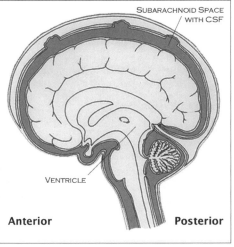

SUBARACHNOID SPACE WITH CSF

VENTRICLE

Anterior   Posterior

Sagittal section of the brain

the lower legs may also occur. In adults, there may be slowing of the intellect, irritability, reduced consciousness, headache, forceful vomiting, seizures, incoordination and difficulty in maintaining balance. Since the sutures are fused in adults, there is no increase in the size of the head.

Risk Factors:

Obstruction to flow can occur as a complication of meningitis, syphilis, brain tumor or aneurysm of cerebral arteries. Congenital defects in the formation of ventricles can also predispose to this. Tumor of cells that produce the CSF can increase the formation of CSF and predispose to hydrocephalus.

Caution and Recommendations to Therapists:

In infants with hydrocephalus, rhythmic stroking and holding has a positive effect emotionally. The gentle, repetitive and rhythmic strokes also help reduce the spasticity of the muscles. Rhythmic movements that are slow and relaxed with the hand broad and flat are very effective. The skin over the head and face are very fragile and break down easily. Use very gentle strokes. While changing position reduce the strain on the neck by moving the head, neck and shoulders

a Handbook for Massage Therapists

References

Adams JC, Hamblen DL. Outline of orthopaedics. 11 ed. New York: Churchill Livingstone; 1990.

simultaneously as the body. In adults, the aim is to reduce the spasticity and prevent contractures. Passively move all joints. Gently stretch the spastic muscles. Do not use force. Start with 15-minute sessions and then proceed to a longer duration. If treating after surgery, avoid area of incision.

Hyperaldosteronism (Conn's syndrome)

Endocrine system

A condition where there is increased secretion of the steroidal hormone aldosterone from the adrenal cortex.

Notes

This endocrine disorder is managed by surgery or by administration of drugs that retain potassium and at the same time increase water and sodium excretion by the kidneys. Dietary salt intake is also restricted.

Aldosterone along with antidiuretic hormone of the posterior pituitary gland regulates the level of sodium and water. It reduces the excretion of water and sodium, and increases the excretion of potassium from the body, by having a direct effect on the tubules of the kidney.

For more details see Appendix C: Diuretics.

Cause:

It is usually caused by growth of an aldosterone-secreting tumor in the adrenal cortex. In some cases the cause is unknown. Other conditions that reduce the volume of fluid or sodium in the blood vessels can also produce increased secretion of aldosterone.

Signs and Symptoms:

The symptoms are due to excess sodium and water retained in the body and decreased potassium. The expanded volume of fluid overloads the heart and can lead to hypertension and cardiac failure. Decreased potassium makes the muscles and nerves hyperirritable. There is muscle weakness, fatigue and headache. The sensations are reduced. Diabetes mellitus is common in these individuals as the low potassium level interferes with the secretion of insulin.

Risk Factors:

See Cause.

Caution and Recommendations to Therapists:

Massage is not contraindicated. Take a detailed history. The massage techniques have to be altered on an individual basis according to presenting symptoms.

References

JD Wilson, Foster DW, editors. Williams' textbook of Endocrinology. Philadelphia: Saunders; 1992.

Hyperparathyroidism

Endocrine system

A condition where there is overactivity of the parathyroid gland with secretion of excess parathormone.

Notes

The treatment aims to reduce calcium levels in the blood. Surgery may be resorted to if a tumor is suspected.

Cause:

It is usually caused by a tumor in the parathyroid gland. Increased secretion also occurs when there is a deficiency of vitamin D or renal failure.

Parathormone is one of the important regulators of calcium and phosphate metabolism and maintains the normal levels of calcium in the blood. Parathormone causes calcium to be absorbed into the blood from the bone and gut and reduces its excretion by the kidney. It is secreted by the 4 parathyroid glands that are located on the posterior aspect of the thyroid gland.

Calcium is one of the important elements required by the body. Some of the more important functions of calcium are for muscle contraction, transmission of impulses through nerves and for blood clotting.

Signs and Symptoms:

The high levels of calcium in the blood promote stone formation in the kidneys. The rapid absorption of calcium from the bone causes thinning of bones and tendency to fracture. Bone pain, and low back pain are common symptoms. Severe abdominal pain and formation of peptic ulcers are other associated problems. The muscle atrophies and is weak. Psychological problems such as depression and personality disturbances are also seen.

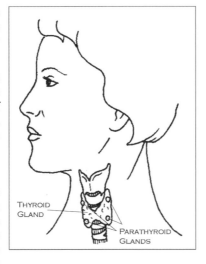

THYROID GLAND

PARATHYROID GLANDS

Risk Factors:

See Cause.

Caution and Recommendations to Therapists:

The thinning of bones makes the client very vulnerable to fractures. Techniques using very light strokes are the only type of massage that should be employed till the underlying condition is treated. Encourage client to drink large volumes of water.

References

JD Wilson, Foster DW, editors. Williams' textbook of Endocrinology. Philadelphia: Saunders; 1992.

Hyperpituitarism (Acromegaly; Gigantism)

A condition where there is an increased production of human growth hormone by the anterior pituitary gland.

Endocrine system

Cause:

It is caused by a tumor in the anterior pituitary. The cause of the tumor is not known.

Signs and Symptoms:

If the overproduction occurs before puberty, there is abnormal lengthening of the bones resulting in an unusual height of the person (*gigantism*).

Notes

Treatment is surgical with removal of the tumor. After surgery, the person may require replacement of various hormones produced by the endocrine glands whose secretions are controlled by the pituitary.

a Handbook for Massage Therapists

189

For more details see Appendix C:
Hormone therapy/replacement.

Overproduction after puberty when the epiphysial plates of the bone have been fused results in thickening of bones, overgrowth of cartilage and connective tissue. Typically, there is protrusion of the jaw (*acromegaly*) with coarsening of the facial features - thick ears and nose. The enlarging tumor in the skull produces pressure symptoms such as headache and vomiting. The proximity of the enlarging pituitary gland to the optic nerve causes deterioration of sight. The effects of overproduction of growth hormone include osteoporosis, hypertension and diabetes mellitus. The high levels of cholesterol in the blood, due to the excess hormone causes atherosclerosis - thickening of the arterial wall and narrowing of lumen. Psychological disturbances may also occur.

Risk Factors:

Rarely, there may be a family history of overproduction.

Caution and Recommendations to Therapists:

Massage is not contraindicated and may be beneficial to alleviate the stress produced by the sudden body change. Headaches due to this condition cannot be relieved by massage. Suspect increased intracranial pressure when a client with no history of headache suddenly develops one associated with vomiting. Encourage client to see a Physician if typical signs and symptoms are seen. Emphasize the importance of following the Physicians' orders regarding hormone replacement therapy after surgery.

References

JD Wilson, Foster DW, editors. Williams' textbook of Endocrinology. Philadelphia: Saunders; 1992.

Hypertension (High blood pressure)

Cardiovascular, Renal, Endocrine systems

A condition where the systolic blood pressure is 140 mmHg or higher and the diastolic pressure is 90 mm Hg or higher consistently. (The age, sex and race are other factors that have to be considered.)

Cause:

In *primary, idiopathic* or *essential hypertension*, the more common type, there is no evidence of other diseases. In *secondary hypertension*, kidney disorders may be associated. Secondary hypertension may be due to acute brain lesions that raise the intracranial pressure. Alterations in endocrine function and hormone levels as in increased activity of adrenal cortex and medulla can cause hypertension. Vascular disorders like arteriosclerosis or coarctation of the aorta are other causes of high blood pressure. A person is said to have *malignant hypertension* if the complications are rapidly progressive.

In adults, a diastolic pressure below 85 mmHg is considered to be normal; 85-89 mmHg as high normal; 90 to 104 mmHg as mild hypertension; 105-114 mmHg as moderate hypertension; 115 mmHg or more as severe hypertension.

A diastolic pressure below 90 mmHg and a systolic pressure below 140 mmHg is considered to be normal; 140-159 mmHg as borderline isolated systolic hypertension; 160 mmHg or higher as isolated systolic hypertension.

Notes

General measures for treating hypertension include relief of stress; dietary management; regular aerobic exercise; weight reduction and control of other risk factors. Restriction of sodium intake; increase of calcium and potassium intake; caloric restrictions in obese individuals; reduction of intake of cholesterol and saturated fats are part of the dietary management.

Drugs such as diuretics (to reduce blood volume and sodium levels); antiadrenergic drugs (to reduce sympathetic nervous system activity); vasodilators; angiotensin-converting enzyme inhibitors (to inhibit the potent vasoconstrictor angiotensin) and calcium channel blockers (to produce vasodilation) are used alone or in combination.

Pathology A to Z -

Signs and Symptoms:

Essential or primary hypertension is asymptomatic and diagnosis is made by chance. Early morning headache located in the back of the head or neck may be a symptom. Other complaints may be related to the complications in other systems. Complications include heart failure, atherosclerosis, aneurysms, angina, retinal changes and stroke.

Risk Factors:

Hypertension is more common in African-Americans. Family history, advancing age, high salt intake, obesity, excess alcohol consumption, stress and use of oral contraceptives are other risk factors.

Hypertension is seen in 10% of all pregnancies.

Caution and Recommendations to Therapists:

Obtain a detailed history and rule out complications due to hypertension. If complications exist, clearance from the treating Physician may be required.

Massage helps reduce blood pressure by relaxing the client and lowering stress. The sympathetic nervous system is also inhibited by massage. Sometimes, massage can reduce the blood pressure so much that the client can experience giddiness on getting off the massage table - postural hypotension. Clients on anti- hypertensives are also more prone to postural hypotension. The Therapist should make sure that these clients get up slowly from the table, sit for some time before getting off. This enables the regulatory mechanisms of blood pressure to come into play effectively against gravity, which tends to pool the blood towards the leg. Get brochures from your local Hypertension Society and have it handy for your clients to read. Encourage clients to get their blood pressure and cholesterol levels checked regularly. Refer to Appendix D for resources.

For more details see Appendix C: Antihypertensives; Diuretics; Vasodilators.

References

Williams GH. Hypertensive vascular disease. In: . In: Isselbacher KJ et al, editors. Harrison's principles of internal medicine. 13th ed. New York: McGraw-Hill Inc; 1994. p. 1116-1131.

Hyperthyroidism (Thyrotoxicosis; Grave's disease;

Basedow's disease; Parry's disease)

Endocrine system

A condition resulting from overproduction of thyroid hormones.

Cause:

Grave's disease, a form of hyperthyroidism, is caused by the production of antibodies that resemble the thyroid stimulating hormone (TSH) of the pituitary. The thyroid stimulating hormone stimulates the thyroid gland to produce thyroxin. There is a tendency of members of a family to have this disease.

Hyperthyroidism may also be caused by tumors of the thyroid gland, excessive secretion of TSH, secretion of thyroid hormones by tumours in the ovary etc.

Notes

Hyperthyroidism is treated with drugs that block the formation of hormones, radioactive iodine and/or surgery.

For more details see Appendix C: Antithyroid drugs.

Signs and Symptoms:

Symptoms are exaggerations of the normal function of the thyroid hormones and resemble hyperactivity of the sympathetic system.

The thyroid gland secretes thyroxine (T4) and triiodothyronine (T3), which require iodine for formation. These hormones are necessary for normal growth and development. They increase the metabolic activity of most tissues.

Classically, the thyroid gland is enlarged (*goiter*) and appears as a swelling in front of the neck. Thyroxine excess makes the person irritable and nervous. In spite of increased appetite and intake of food, there is loss of weight. Hyperactivity of the gut causes diarrhea. Sweating, intolerance to heat, tremors, rapid heart rate are some of the typical symptoms. The accumulation of fluid and connective tissue behind the eyeball causes the eyes to bulge out (*exophthalmus*) in most people with hyperthyroidism. The blood vessels to the skin are dilated to dissipate the excess heat produced by the rapid metabolism and the skin appears red and flushed. There is atrophy, weakness and fatigue of muscles. The menstrual cycle is irregular in females.

Risk Factors:

See Cause. Grave's disease is more common in women between the ages of 20 and 40 years.

Caution and Recommendations to Therapists:

Massage can help reduce stress in these individuals. The clients' intolerance to heat has to be taken into account. If under proper medications, the metabolism can be brought to near normal. Encourage client to take medications regularly.

References

JD Wilson, Foster DW, editors. Williams' textbook of Endocrinology. Philadelphia: Saunders; 1992.

Gastrointestinal system

Hypervitaminoses – Vitamin A and D

Excessive accumulation of Vitamin A/D in the body.

Cause:

It usually results from excessive intake of supplement vitamins.

Signs and Symptoms:

Excess intake of vitamin A can cause irritability, loss of hair, headache, itching, loss of appetite, bone pain, fragility of bone, peeling and dryness of skin. The skin may appear yellow or orange. In Vitamin D excess, the person has nausea, vomiting, loss of appetite, loss of weight, headache, excessive urination and thirst.

Risk Factors:

See Cause.

Caution and Recommendations to Therapists:

Encourage clients to take a well balanced diet, in which case vitamin supplements are unwarranted. Educate clients about the existence of such a condition as hypervitaminosis.

Notes

The symptoms are relieved by discontinuation of intake of excessive vitamins.

References

Combs GF. The vitamins. San Diego: Academic; 1992.

Hypoadrenalism (Adrenal hypofunction; Adrenal insufficiency; Addison's disease)

A condition where there is a decreased secretion of hormones from the adrenal cortex ie. lower blood levels of corticosteroid, aldosterone and androgen.

Endocrine system

Cause:

Usually, it is due to destruction of the adrenal cortex by an autoimmune reaction. Antibodies produced by the body fail to recognize the tissue of the adrenal cortex as self and destroy it. Rarely, infections or lack of blood supply to the adrenals can cause this. Since the adrenal cortical secretion is regulated by the adrenocorticotrophic hormone (ACTH) secreted by the anterior pituitary, lack of ACTH can result in this condition.

In individuals being treated with corticosteroids on a long-term basis for other diseases, abrupt stoppage of the therapy can cause this. This is because of the atrophy of the adrenal glands and suppression of ACTH by the externally administered steroids.

Signs and Symptoms:

Typically, it produces weakness, fatigue, loss of weight and gastrointestinal symptoms like vomiting, diarrhea and loss of appetite. There is excessive pigmentation of the skin and the person looks tanned with darkening of the elbows, creases of the palms and foot and previous scars. This is because of the excess ACTH and melanocyte stimulating hormone (secreted by the pituitary) in order to stimulate the adrenals to start functioning adequately. The person is prone to postural hypotension and the pulse is weak and irregular. Apart from a tendency to have postural hypotension, these individuals can go into an adrenal crisis where there is severe weakness, fatigue, nausea, vomiting, low blood pressure and dehydration. The patient may finally collapse. It can lead to kidney failure, coma and death.

The person is intolerant to stress, even if mild. There is a craving for salty food (loss of sodium and water due to lack of aldosterone). The decrease in androgen presents as changes in menstruation and lack of sex drive.

Risk Factors:

See Cause.

Caution and Recommendations to Therapists:

Do not massage without clearance from a Physician. Apart from a tendency to have postural hypotension, these individuals can go into an adrenal crisis where there is severe weakness, fatigue, nausea, vomiting, low blood pressure, and dehydration and finally collapse. It can lead to kidney failure, coma and death. Also, the individuals are unable to withstand any form of stress.

Notes

Hypoadrenalism is treated by lifelong hormonal replacement.

For more details see Appendix C: Hormone therapy/replacement.

References

JD Wilson, Foster DW, editors. Williams' textbook of Endocrinology. Philadelphia: Saunders; 1992.

Hypoglycemia

A reduction of blood glucose levels below the normal range.

Notes

The best treatment is immediate administration of glucose orally or intravenously. The cause of the hypoglycemia has to be identified and treated. People who are prone should avoid fasting.

Cause:

Any condition that interferes with the metabolism of glucose can lead to hypoglycemia. Glucose is derived from lactate/pyruvate, amino acids and glycerol. Many adaptive mechanisms exist to maintain glucose levels. The hormone insulin is responsible for reducing glucose levels in the blood if it is elevated. When levels increase, glucose is mobilised to utilization and storage sites and is converted to glycogen, proteins and triglycerides. If levels drop below normal, the hormones glucagon, epinephrine, growth hormone and cortisol come into play to bring the levels back to normal. Norepinephrine is released by the sympathetic nervous system.

Hypoglycemia can develop if there is underproduction of glucose as in deficiencies of hormones, defects in enzymes required for its production, reduced availability of glucose (severe malnutrition), disease of the liver or due to certain drugs (alcohol, salicylates etc.). It may also be due to overutilization of glucose as may occur when there is increased insulin secretion or injection of insulin, defective dosage of antidiabetic drugs etc.

Signs and Symptoms:

The symptoms are due to the secretion of epinephrine and the effect of hypoglycemia in the central nervous system. The secretion of epinephrine results in rapid heart rate, sweating, anxiety, hunger and tremors. Dizziness, headache, confusion, loss of consciousness, convulsions are all due to the effect on the nervous system.

Risk Factors:

See Cause.

Caution and Recommendations to Therapists:

References

JD Wilson, Foster DW, editors. Williams' textbook of Endocrinology.Philadelphia: Saunders; 1992.

It is important to identify those clients who are prone to spells of hypoglycemia and ensure that glucose or other forms of carbohydrates are available with the client or in the clinic during the session. Ensure that the address of a treating Physician and a contact address is recorded in your clinic.

Hypoparathyroidism

A decreased secretion of parathormone from the parathyroid glands.

Notes

This condition is treated with calcium and vitamin D supplements.

Cause:

Hypoparathyroidism may be caused by accidental removal or injury to the parathyroid gland during thyroid surgery or radiation therapy to thyroid. Rarely, antibodies formed by the body (autoimmunity) may depress the function.

Signs and Symptoms:

There are no symptoms in mild forms. The symptoms are related to the role of calcium in the body. The muscles become hyperirritable and go into spasm. There is tingling in the fingertips and feet. The skin is scaly and dry, with brittle fingernails. The teeth tend to stain and decay easily. The rhythm of the heart becomes irregular and rapid.

Risk Factors:

See Cause.

References

JD Wilson, Foster DW, editors. Williams' textbook of Endocrinology. Philadelphia: Saunders; 1992.

Caution and Recommendations to Therapists:

Encourage client to take calcium rich diets. Use massage oil liberally as the skin tends to be scaly and dry.

Hypopituitarism (Panhypopituitarism; Dwarfism)

A condition where there is decreased secretion of hormones by the pituitary with resultant hyposecretion from other endocrine glands regulated by it (panhypopituitarism).

Endocrine system

Cause:

The most common cause is a tumor. Rarely, the blood supply to the pituitary is compromised in women who have extensive hemorrhage soon after delivery. Brain surgery and exposure to radiation are other rare causes. Lack of regulatory hormones from the hypothalamus (which controls the secretions by the pituitary) can also be responsible for this condition.

Notes

The cause of the condition has to be identified and addressed. In the case of pituitary tumour surgery may be required. Lifelong hormonal replacement may be necessary.

For more details see Appendix C: Hormone therapy / replacement.

Signs and Symptoms:

This is related to the inadequate levels of various hormones secreted by the pituitary. The anterior pituitary secretes *adrenocorticotrophic hormone* (*ACTH*) - affects the adrenal cortex secretion; *thyroid stimulating hormone* (*TSH*) - affects thyroid gland secretion; *follicle stimulating hormone* (*FSH*) and *luteinizing hormone* (*LH*) - affects hormonal secretion from the ovaries and testis; *growth hormone* (*GH*) - affects overall growth; and *prolactin* - affects milk production in lactating women.

The posterior pituitary secretes *Antidiuretic hormone* (*ADH*), also known as *Vasopressin* - affects the concentration of body fluids by regulating the excretion of water by the kidney. It also causes the blood vessels to constrict thus increasing blood pressure. *Oxytocin* is another hormone secreted by the posterior pituitary. This stimulates the contraction of the uterus during labor and is also responsible for the expulsion of milk while breast-feeding.

The symptoms develop slowly resulting in dwarfism in children. In males, the external genitalia are underdeveloped with a small penis. In females, the menstrual cycles are absent. In both sexes, there is no or underdevelopment of pubic and axillary hair. If the onset is in adulthood, infertility, cessation of menstrual cycle and impotence are seen due to the hyposecretion from the ovaries and testis. The decreased thyroid secretion presents as lethargy, intolerance to cold, dry and thickened skin, and menstrual disturbances - all signs of hypothyroidism. The lowered levels of hormones from the adrenal cortex cause hypoglycemia, loss of appetite, hypotension and abdominal pain.

Other symptoms of increased intracranial pressure are produced if it is caused by a growing tumor. Sudden onset of headache associated with vomiting and loss of sight are some of the symptoms.

Risk Factors:

See Cause.

Caution and Recommendations to Therapists:

A detailed history should be obtained in order to identify the extent of the hormonal insufficiency. Encourage client to take the replacement hormones without fail. While massaging, ensure that the client is well covered (intolerance to cold may be present). Use oil liberally during massage as the skin is likely to be dry (hypothyroid symptoms). Make sure that the client changes position slowly and sits on the table for a while before getting off after massage (they may have postural hypotension). Range of motion exercises are very useful, as arthritis is common. Due to the fluctuating levels of glucose these clients are prone for hypo or hyperglycemia. Keep glucose/sugar handy. Ensure that the address of a treating Physician and a contact address is recorded in your clinic.

References

JD Wilson, Foster DW, editors. Williams' textbook of Endocrinology. Philadelphia: Saunders; 1992.

Cardiovascular system

Hypotension

A term given to blood pressure that is lower than normal.

Cause:

Notes

The cause of the hypotension should be treated. Salt intake may be increased. In some cases, drugs that mimic the effects of the sympathetic nervous system may be given. Drugs given for other disorders that may cause hypotension have to be avoided.

For more details see Appendix C: Sympathomimetic drugs.

Orthostatic or *postural hypotension* is the abnormal drop in pressure when a person assumes an upright posture from a supine position. A drop of 20mmHg systolic pressure or 10mmHg diastolic pressure is considered abnormal.

The body has baroreceptors (receptors that detect changes in the stretch of blood vessels) located between the heart and brain that reflexly increase blood flow to the brain whenever the blood pressure drops in the arteries supplying the brain.

In addition, antidiuretic hormone from the posterior pituitary helps maintain the blood volume and pressure by reducing the loss of fluid in the urine. In hypotension, the regulatory mechanisms are affected in various ways.

The most common cause of hypotension is a reduction in the blood volume due to

Pathology A to Z -

fluid loss or depletion. Hypotension can also be seen in conditions where the sympathetic nervous system activity is not adequate.

Signs and Symptoms:

The person feels dizzy or faints on getting up from a lying position or on changing posture.

Risk Factors:

Prolonged vomiting, diarrhoea, or blood loss predisposes to hypotension. Hypertensive patients on antihypertensive drugs, those on diuretics (drugs that increase the formation of urine) and those with diabetes are also prone to hypotension. Prolonged bed rest and the aging process are risk factors as they reduce the sympathetic activity and sensitivity of the baroreceptors. Disorders of the autonomic nervous system - viz. the sympathetic and parasympathetic system also predispose to hypotension.

Caution and Recommendations to Therapists:

Since massage tends to lower the blood pressure, clients with severe orthostatic hypotension - those who give a history of fainting on getting up quickly from a lying position, should be massaged in a seated posture. In general, caution all clients to get up slowly from a lying posture, preferably, sit on the table for a while and move the legs to help venous return, before getting off the table.

References

Isselbacher KJ et al, editors. Harrison's principles of internal medicine. 13th ed. New York: McGraw-Hill Inc; 1994.

Hypothermia

A reduction in the core temperature of the body to 35°C (95°F) or lower.

Nervous system

Cause:

It is usually due to accidental, prolonged exposure to cold especially in the winter months. In some patients, hypothermia may be secondary to congestive heart failure, diabetes mellitus, drug overdose, hypoglycemia etc. Here, it is due to the failure of the thermoregulatory mechanisms.

Signs and Symptoms:

The person appears pale and cold. The muscles are stiff. Respiration is shallow and slow. The heart rate is very slow and there is associated reduction of blood pressure. There may be generalized edema. If the temperature is very low, the person becomes unconscious. Hypoglycemia and acidosis are associated complications.

Risk Factors:

It is more common in the elderly. Alcohol consumption speeds up the process of hypothermia as alcohol increases heat loss by vasodilation and inhibiting shivering.

Notes

Hypothermia is a medical emergency. The aim is to warm the person, maintain airways, maintain blood volume and prevent arrhythmias. Broad-spectrum antibiotics may be needed, as systemic infection is common in these individuals. Use of humidified warm air, peritoneal dialysis with warmed fluid, irrigation of the stomach with warm fluid are some measures that may be used to speed up the elevation of core temperature.

For more details see Appendix C: Antimicrobial - antibacterial agents; Dialysis - peritoneal dialysis.

References

Jolly et al. Accidental hypothermia. Emerg
Med Clin North Am 1992: 10:311.

Caution and Recommendations to Therapists:

It is highly unlikely for a Massage Therapist to come across a client with this condition.

Endocrine system

Hypothyroidism (Myxedema; Cretinism)

A deficiency of thyroid hormone secretion.

Cause:

In infants, it is caused by underdevelopment of the thyroid gland. Rarely, there may be an absence of one of the enzymes required for the synthesis of thyroxine. If the mother is on antithyroid drugs for hyperthyroidism during pregnancy, it may result in hypothyroidism in the infant. In adults, hyposecretion may be a result of inflammation, infection, production of antibodies against the hormone (autoimmunity), exposure to radiation, or thyroid surgery for other reasons. Lack of adequate iodine in the diet can also result in hypothyroidism.

Signs and Symptoms:

The symptoms resemble hypoactivity of the sympathetic nervous system ie. metabolism is slowed down. In children it results in mental retardation if left undiagnosed and untreated within the first few months after birth. The baby is inactive and sleeps excessively. Growth is slow and dwarfism results.

In adults, the person is lethargic, overweight, with intolerance to cold. The skin is dry and scaly with the hair coarse and brittle. The face, hands and legs are puffy. The heart rate is slow. Thickening of the vocal cords produces a deepening and hoarseness of voice in women. One of the complications of hypothyroidism is coma. This may be precipitated by stress.

Risk Factors:

It is more common in women.

Caution and Recommendations to Therapists:

References

JD Wilson, Foster DW, editors. Williams'
textbook of Endocrinology. Philadelphia:
Saunders; 1992.

Ensure that the client is properly covered, as they are intolerant to cold. Use oil liberally as the skin is coarse and dry. They are prone to osteoporosis, so excessive pressure should not be used. Abdominal massage helps relieve constipation that these individuals are prone to. Massage helps alleviate the depression, a psychological effect of the disease. Encourage client to take medications regularly. Medications are required to be taken throughout life.

Hypoxia

A decrease in the availability of oxygen to the tissues.

Cause:

Hypoxia may be due to many factors. *Hypoxic hypoxia* is due to reduced oxygen levels in the artery. This could result from less oxygen in the environment (high altitude) or disease of the respiratory system where the oxygen is not delivered to the pulmonary capillaries. *Anemic hypoxia* is due to reduced availability of hemoglobin to carry the oxygen, even if it is made available. There may be reduced hemoglobin or the hemoglobin may not be available (carbon monoxide poisoning). In *stagnant* or *ischemic hypoxia* blood flow to the tissue is reduced so that inadequate oxygen is available. In *histotoxic hypoxia*, the oxygen supplied to the tissue is adequate, but the tissue cells are unable to utilize it (eg. cyanide poisoning).

Signs and Symptoms:

If the hypoxia is generalized, the brain is the first organ to be affected. Hypoxia lasting for more that 20 seconds result in loss of consciousness. If it is less severe, impaired judgement, drowsiness, excitement, disorientation and headache may be seen. Nausea, vomiting, rapid heart rate and increase in blood pressure are other symptoms. Death usually occurs from respiratory failure.

Prolonged hypoxia is compensated by increase in hemoglobin levels by stimulation of the bone marrow by the hormone erythropoietin.

Risk Factors:

See Cause.

Caution and Recommendations to Therapists:

It is important to identify the cause. Massage may be useful in improving circulation in local, stagnant or ischemic hypoxia.

Notes

The cause has to be identified promptly and treated. Administration of oxygen-rich gas mixtures is helpful in some forms of hypoxic hypoxia.

For more details see Appendix C: Oxygen therapy.

References:

Ganong WF. Review of medical physiology. 15th ed. California; Appleton & Lange; 1991. p. 634-635.

Ichthyosis (Disorders of cornification)

A group of disorders characterized by formation of visible scales over the body.

Cause:

The condition is due to defective formation and maintenance of the stratum corneum of the epidermis. The stratum corneum prevents water from entering and leaving the body via the skin. It also serves as a physical barrier that prevents physical damage. As many as 24 types of Ichthyosis have been identified.

Notes

Genetic counselling should be given to parents. In young children, the primary concern is to maintain temperature, electrolyte balance and prevent infection. In the older age group, the aim is to keep the skin moisturized, reduce scale formation and prevent inflammation and infection. Application of lubricants in the form of oil or cream and use of steroid creams to reduce inflammation are some forms of treatment.

For more details see Appendix C: Genetic testing/Counselling; Antiinflammatories - steroidal drugs.

Signs and Symptoms:

The distribution of the lesions varies with the type of ichthyosis. Typically, the skin is dry and invisible scales are formed on the surface of the skin. The scales may be shed in clumps in some cases. In some types, fluid-filled lesions (bullae) may be formed.

Risk Factors:

In most cases it is genetic. Sometimes ichthyosis is acquired and associated with intake of certain drugs, some types of cancers or certain chronic disorders (eg. AIDS, hypothyroidism).

Caution and Recommendations to Therapists:

It is not an infectious condition. Massage may be helpful in improving the condition of the skin and reducing its dryness. Avoid inflamed areas. Local application of steroids tends to make the skin susceptible to infection. Use aseptic techniques. Refer to the section on Strategies for infection prevention and safe practice (Appendix B).

References

Williams MLK, Lynch PJ. Generelized disorders of cornification: The ichthyoses. In: Sams WM, Lynch PJ, editors. Principles and practice of Dermatology. 2nd ed. New York: Churchill Livingstone; 1996. p. 383-389.

Integumentary system	# Impetigo

A bacterial infection of the epidermis of the skin.

Cause:

It is caused by *staphylococci* or a type of *streptococci (group A beta-hemolytic) bacteria*.

Signs and Symptoms:

The infection may start in an apparently normal skin or superinfect a scratch or insect bite. It starts as a rounded, raised, fluid-filled cavity in a reddened area. Soon a pustule is seen. The pustule discharges a honey-colored or yellowish fluid that dries and forms a crust. New lesions appear rapidly in surrounding areas (appendix A: page 352).

If impetigo is left untreated, complications affecting the kidney - glomerulonephritis can occur. It may also spread to the dermis to form ecthyma.

Risk Factors:

It is more common in children, but adults can be infected too. It is often seen secondary to scabies in regions with hot, humid climates.

Caution and Recommendations to Therapists:

The infection can spread by contact - especially in individuals with lowered immunity. Massage is contraindicated locally if the lesion is confined to a very small area. Make sure that the infected area is covered with a bandage and does not come in contact with you or the linen. If the lesions are extensive do

Notes

It is treated with topical or oral antibiotics according to the severity.

For more details see Appendix C: Antimicrobial - antibacterial agents.

References

Hirschmann JV. Bacterial infections of the skin. In: Sams WM, Lynch PJ, editors. Principles and practice of Dermatology. 2nd ed. New York: Churchill Livingstone; 1996. p. 79-81.

not massage. Since the infection can be treated and responds well to antibiotics advise client to seek medical help. Impetigo has to be distinguished from eczema (not contagious) which typically appears as multiple patches in skin flexures. Refer to Appendix B: Strategies for infection prevention and safe practice for some useful guidelines. Also see Appendix D for organizations and support groups.

Impotence

Failure to achieve erection of penis, ejaculation or both.

Reproductive, Endocrine, Nervous systems

Cause:

The process of erection and ejaculation is complex and involves many regions. Sexual desire, which in turn is regulated by androgen-related psychic factors, intact parasympathetic, sympathetic, sensory and motor nerves, spinal cord and brain are all important. Erection is produced by vasodilation of the arteries and sinusoidal spaces in the penis and ejaculation by rhythmic contraction of the epididymis, vas deferens, seminal vesicle and contraction of the internal sphincter of the bladder. Therefore any condition that affects any of these structures and processes can lead to impotence.

Some common causes are: drugs such as antihypertensives, antidepressants, antipsychotics, alcohol, heroin, tobacco, neurologic diseases such as spinal cord injury, loss of sensory input, diabetic neuropathy, vascular diseases in the region, psychic factors, endocrine causes etc.

Signs and Symptoms:

Inability to achieve erection and/or ejaculation.

Risk Factors:

See Cause.

Caution and Recommendations to Therapists:

Massage helps to reduce anxiety and depression that is common in these individuals and generally increase the sense of well being.

Notes

It is important to identify the cause of the problem and distinguish psychological causes from organic. Treatment varies with the cause. A variety of substances that alter blood flow to the penis are available. Some are in the form of injections that are injected into the penis. Many types of commercially available mechanical devices such as those that utilize a vacuum to produce erection, occlusive devices that prevent venous return from the penis are used by many. Psychotherapy is often beneficial.

References

Mcconnell JD, Wilson JD. Impotence. In: Isselbacher KJ et al, editors. Harrison's principles of internal medicine. 13th ed. New York: McGraw-Hill Inc; 1994. p. 263-265.

Korenman SG. Sexual dysfunction. In: JD Wilson, Foster DW, editors. Williams' textbook of Endocrinology. Philadelphia: Saunders; 1992. p. 1033-1048.

Incontinence

Inability to retain urine in the urinary bladder.

Renal, Nervous systems

Cause:

Urination or micturition is related to the normal functioning of the smooth muscles of the bladder; its innervation by parasympathetic nerves arising from the sacral region of the spinal cord (S2,3,4); sensory nerves from the bladder that sense distention, pain and temperature; sympathetic nerves (arising from

Notes

The cause has to be identified and treated.

a Handbook for Massage Therapists

201

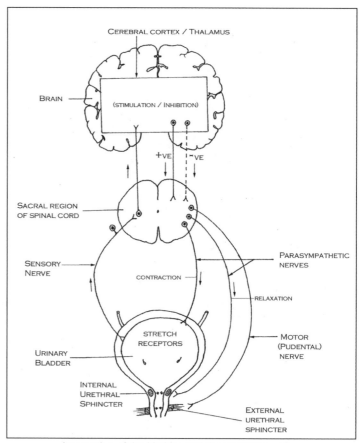

Innervation of the bladder and the micturition reflex

T11-L2) that innervate the internal sphincter of the bladder; motor nerves to the pelvic muscles and external sphincter of the bladder and intact communication between the brain and the sacral region of the spinal cord (voluntary control of micturition).

Any condition that affects the structures involved or nervous communications can produce incontinence. Incontinence is common in the elderly where the bladder becomes prone to uncontrollable contractions due to damage to the nerve pathways that inhibit automatic emptying of the bladder when it is distended. In postmenopausal women, *stress incontinence* is common as the female urethra atrophies and the women are unable to resist escape of some urine while intraabdominal pressure is increased. In men, stress incontinence may follow prostatic surgery. Sometimes, congenital abnormalities (eg. abnormal ureteral openings) may cause *mechanical incontinence.*

Overflow or *paradoxical incontinence* may arise due to large volume of urine being retained in the bladder due to obstruction at the bladder neck or neurologic damage.

Pathology A to Z -

In some cases, incontinence may be psychogenic.

Signs and Symptoms:

The person is unable to retain urine in the bladder.

Risk Factors:

See Cause.

Caution and Recommendations to Therapists:

It is important to understand the cause of the incontinence. Suitable precautions have to be taken to avoid accidents. Massage can be given to the client with catheters in place. Excessive pressure over the abdomen has to be avoided. The Therapist should be sensitive to the clients' condition and strive to put the client at ease. Approximately 80% of people with incontinence can be helped with noninvasive techniques such as basic bladder training, biofeedback, electrical stimulation and pelvic floor strengthening exercises as used by Physiotherapist, Occupational Therapist, and Nurses among others. Encourage client to seek help from such health practitioners.

References

Turner-Warwick R, Whiteside CG, editors. Symposium on Clinical Urodynamics: The Urologic Clinics of North Am. Philadelphia: Saunders; 1979. Vol. 6.

Indigestion (Dyspepsia)

Gastrointestinal system

A term used to describe a variety of symptoms related to the upper part of the gastrointestinal tract.

Cause:

It is important to find out the patients' definition of indigestion. To some it is actual abdominal pain or pressure. To others it may be heartburn or a feeling that digestion has not occurred properly or that they are intolerant to specific types of food. Abdominal distention, repetitive belching, bloating and flatulence are other definitions given by patients. The location of pain, duration, its relation to food intake and type of food ingested should be identified.

Notes

In most cases, no clear explanations can be given for the indigestion. The cause is treated, if identified.

Pain originating from the viscera is due to distention or pressure in the hollow organ. The location of pain may be related to the organ affected. For example, pain originating from the esophagus or stomach is located behind the sternum. Pain in the epigastric region may be due to the stomach, duodenum, bile duct or pancreas. Pain from the gall bladder and bile duct may be referred to the tip of the scapula or the right upper quadrant of the abdomen. Pain from the pancreas may be referred to the back or to the left upper quadrant. Pain related to the small intestines is usually felt around the umbilicus. Pain from the appendix, colon or organs in the pelvis is felt below the umbilicus.

History of the duration of the pain may give clues as to its origin. For example, pain from the biliary tract or gastritis tends to be intermittent. Pain tends to be increased on lying down or at night if a person has reflux esophagitis. Pain related to the esophagus or stomach tends to come on soon after eating. Pain that comes on several hours after eating may be due to obstruction of the stomach outlet. Pain due to duodenal ulcers is often reduced on ingestion of food.

Heartburn is usually due to reflux of acid or bile into the esophagus or abnormal distention of the esophagus or irritation of the esophagus. In some people specific types of food tend to be related to indigestion. For example, acidic food may aggravate the symptoms in a person with peptic ulcer. In some, indigestion may result after intake of food that is not easily digested by them eg. fatty food in people with biliary disease. In others, due to that absence of specific enzymes, certain types of food are not digested easily eg. deficiency of lactase and ingestion of milk. A person may be allergic to certain types of food and may present with indigestion along with other allergic reactions.

In many, indigestion may be described as repetitive belching. In most cases, it is due to air being swallowed. Another source of gas in the intestines is due to the fermentation of food by intestinal bacteria. Food that results in a large quantity of residue reaching the large intestine serve as substrate for the bacteria to ferment eg. legumes, beans, grains.

Certain drugs can cause indigestion. Indigestion may be associated with other systemic diseases in some cases.

Signs and Symptoms:

It is important to obtain a proper history (see Cause).

Risk Factors:

See Cause.

Caution and Recommendations to Therapists:

References

Friedman LS, Isselbacher KJ. Anorexia, nausea, vomiting, and indigestion. In: Isselbacher KJ et al, editors. Harrison's principles of internal medicine. 13th ed. New York: McGraw-Hill Inc; 1994. pp. 210-213.

Abdominal massage may be helpful in reducing abdominal distention, bloating and other such uncomfortable symptoms. Those with heartburn may prefer massage in a seated or half-lying position. Encourage clients with chronic symptoms of indigestion to seek medical help.

Respiratory system

Infectious mononucleosis (Kissing disease)

An acute viral infection primarily affecting the upper respiratory tract.

Notes

It is treated with aspirin and other forms of supportive treatment as it resists prevention and antimicrobial treatment. Contact sport should be avoided for 6-8 weeks, as splenic rupture is an infrequent complication.

For more details see Appendix C: Antimicrobial - antiviral agents; Antiinflammatories - non steroidal drugs.

Cause:

It is caused by the *Epstein-Barr virus*. The virus is spread through salivary secretions. It may also spread by blood transfusion. It is highly contagious and individuals are contagious even before the symptoms develop and continue to be infectious through the symptomatic phase, as well as for an indefinite period after the symptoms subside. The incubation period ranges from 10-50 days.

Signs and Symptoms:

Typically it presents with fever (higher in the evening), sore throat and enlargement of cervical lymph nodes. As the name suggests there is an increase in monocytes and lymphocytes in the blood. There may be enlargement of the spleen and liver. A rash may accompany it. Jaundice may also be present. Complications though rare, may occur and include splenic rupture, meningitis, encephalitis, anemia and thrombocytopenia (platelet deficiency). The symptoms subside in 6-10 days. However, in some individuals it may persist for weeks.

Risk Factors:

It is more common in young adults and children. There is a higher incidence of infectious mononucleosis in the United States, Canada and Europe.

Caution and Recommendations to Therapists:

Since it is difficult to prevent and treat the disease due to its' long incubation period and persistence even after symptoms subside, avoid massaging individuals who have been diagnosed with infectious mononucleosis at least until the symptoms subside (which may be a few weeks to months). Be careful while massaging the abdomen in individuals who have just recovered from the disorder as the splenic enlargement may persist. Excessive pressure in the left upper quadrant of the abdomen may result in splenic rupture. Gentle massage with the use of heating pads help relieve persisting body ache. Refer to Appendix B: Strategies for infection prevention and safe practice for some useful guidelines. Also see Appendix D for organizations and support groups.

References

Morello JA, Mizer HE, Wilson ME, Granato PA. Microbiology in patient care. 6th ed. New York: McGraw-Hill; 1998 p. 294.

Inflammatory Bowel Disease (IBD) - Crohn's disease (Regional enteritis; Granulomatous colitis)

Gastrointestinal system

A chronic inflammatory disease of the gastrointestinal tract affecting all layers of the intestinal wall.

Cause:

The exact cause is not known. Immune disorders and allergies have been implicated. The blockage of lymphatic flow in the gut leads to edema, inflammation, ulceration, healing by fibrosis, infection and abscess formation. The wall eventually thickens and has the appearance of a hose. The most common region to be affected is the ileum (last part of the small intestine). However, any region from the mouth to the anus can be affected.

Signs and Symptoms:

Initially, the symptoms are vague with mild pain in the abdomen. The symptoms vary according to the location affected and can range from fever and nausea to flatulence and diarrhoea. There may be blood in the stools. In chronic cases, the person has diarrhea, pain in the lower right quadrant of the abdomen, loss of

Notes

The patients have to be encouraged to keep a close watch on the kind of diet that triggers or worsens symptoms. Frequent small meals are helpful. Increase in the intake of water to two to three liters per day is beneficial.

The treatment for this condition is symptomatic. The aim is to reduce inflammation and replace nutritional losses. The malabsorption is compensated with intravenous supplements. Steroids and drugs that suppress immunity are also given along with anti-inflammatory drugs. Surgery is done to reduce symptoms in severe cases. Here, portions of the affected gut is cut and joined with normal bowel. In severe cases, the ileum is opened on to the surface of the abdominal wall (*ileostomy*).

Inflammatory Bowel Diseases may be associated with arthritis and muscle pain.

For more details see Appendix C: Antiinflammatories - steroidal drugs; Antiinflammatories - non steroidal drugs; Ileostomy.

References

Glickman RM. Inflammatory bowel disease (Ulcerative colitis and Crohn's disease). In: Isselbacher KJ et al, editors. Harrison's principles of internal medicine. 13th ed. New York: McGraw-Hill Inc; 1994. p.1403-1417.

weight, and fatty, foul-smelling stools. Other signs of malabsorption are also there (see Malabsorption syndrome). The symptoms may be altered by complications of stricture formation. Fistulas (abnormal communications between two structures) between the intestine and other areas like bladder or the surface of the skin may form. Formation of abscess is common. The disease progresses with remissions and exacerbations.

Risk Factors:

It is more common between the ages of 20-40. There is a genetic predisposition with higher incidence in those with a family history. Stress can make the symptoms worse. Crohn's affects men and women equally.

Caution and Recommendations to Therapists:

The aim of the massage is to reduce stress and relax the client. Avoid massage over the abdominal area during a flare-up of the condition. In general, deep or vigorous treatment of the abdomen and back should be avoided. Since these clients may be on corticosteroids and drugs that suppress immunity, they are prone to infection. Do not treat if you have even a mild infection. The malnutrition due to malabsorption makes their skin bruise easily. Do not use excessive pressure. The skin is dry due to poor nutrition as well as dehydration. The oil used for massage may be helpful. Clients with this condition are also prone to osteoporosis, reiterating that only light pressure should be used. Encourage them to keep a close watch on the kind of diet that triggers or worsens symptoms. Frequent small meals are helpful. Advice client to increase the intake of water to two to three liters per day. Encourage clients to join local support groups. See Appendix D for organizations and support groups.

Gastrointestinal system	# Inflammatory Bowel Disease (IBD) - Ulcerative colitis

A chronic inflammatory disease of the gastrointestinal tract primarily affecting the superficial (mucosal) layer of the large intestines.

Notes

Treatment is similar to that of Inflammatory Bowel Disease - Crohn's disease. There is a higher incidence of cancer in people with ulcerative colitis.

The patients have to be encouraged to keep a close watch on the kind of diet that triggers or worsens symptoms. Frequent small meals are helpful. Increase in the intake of water to two to three liters per day is beneficial.

The treatment for this condition is symptomatic. The aim is to reduce inflammation and replace nutritional losses. The malabsorption is compensated with intravenous

Cause:

The cause is not known. It is believed to be caused by an abnormal immune response in the gastrointestinal tract. The inflammation of the mucosa of the colon and rectum results in ulceration of the mucosa and thickening of the gut.

Signs and Symptoms:

The symptoms are seen as remissions and exacerbations and can be of varying severity. Diarrhoea, blood and mucus in stools, abdominal pain, and fever are some of the symptoms seen. Signs of malabsorption and malnutrition like weight loss and fatigue are often seen. The person may have arthritis.

Pathology A to Z -

Risk Factors:

It is more common in women between the second and third decade of life with a higher incidence in Caucasians.

Caution and Recommendations to Therapists:

The aim of the massage is to reduce stress and relax the client. Avoid massage over the abdominal area during a flare-up of the condition. In general, deep or vigorous treatment of the abdomen and back should be avoided. Since these clients may be on corticosteroids and drugs that suppress immunity, they are prone to infection. Do not treat if you have even a mild infection. The malnutrition due to malabsorption makes their skin bruise easily. Do not use excessive pressure. The skin is dry due to poor nutrition as well as dehydration. The oil used for massage may be helpful. Clients with this condition are also prone to osteoporosis, reiterating that only light pressure should be used. Encourage them to keep a close watch on the kind of diet that triggers or worsens symptoms. Frequent small meals are helpful. Advice client to increase the intake of water to two to three liters per day. Encourage clients to join local support groups. See Appendix D for organizations and support groups.

supplements. Steroids and drugs that suppress immunity are also given along with anti-inflammatory drugs.

Surgery is done to reduce symptoms in severe cases. Here, portions of the affected gut is cut and joined with normal bowel. In severe cases, the ileum is opened on to the surface of the abdominal wall (*ileostomy*).

Inflammatory Bowel Diseases may be associated with arthritis and muscle pain.

For more details see Appendix C: Antiinflammatories - steroidal drugs; Antiinflammatories - non steroidal drugs; Ileostomy.

References

Glickman RM. Inflammatory bowel disease (Ulcerative colitis and Crohn's disease). In: Isselbacher KJ et al, editors. Harrison's principles of internal medicine. 13th ed. New York: McGraw-Hill Inc; 1994. p.1403-1417.

Influenza (Grippe; Flu)

Respiratory system

A highly contagious respiratory tract infection.

Cause:

It is a viral infection produced by different strains of three different types of *Myxovirus influenzae*. It is transmitted by inhalation of the droplets expelled into the air as infected individuals cough or sneeze. It may also spread by sharing glasses with an infected person. The virus enters the system through the respiratory epithelium and produces an inflammatory response.

Signs and Symptoms:

It takes 1-2 days after infection for symptoms to be produced. There is a sudden onset of fever with chills, headache, dry cough, body ache, laryngitis, congestion and watery discharge from nose and eyes. There may be enlargement of the cervical lymph nodes. Fatigue and general weakness may persist for weeks even though the acute symptoms subside in a few days. Complications like pneumonia, worsening of obstructive pulmonary disease (if present) may occur. Rarely, it may lead to pericarditis and nervous system complications like encephalitis.

Risk Factors:

It is more common in the colder months. The symptoms are more severe in young children, the elderly, immunocompromised individuals and those with other chronic diseases.

Notes

In uncomplicated cases, it is treated symptomatically.

Susceptible individuals can be vaccinated to prevent infection. Influenza vaccine is reformulated every year according to the type of virus that is likely to affect the society. Side effects of vaccination are usually restricted to local irritation and fever for a short duration.

For more details see Appendix C: Immunization.

References

Kaplan MM, Webster RG. Epidemiology of Influenza. Sci Am 1977; 237(6): 88-92.

Caution and Recommendations to Therapists:

Be informed about outbreaks of influenza in your area. It may be wise to have annual inoculations of flu vaccines (not advisable if pregnant) at the start of the flu season ie. in late autumn. Do not massage clients with influenza until they have fully recovered. Therapists with influenza should not massage clients until all symptoms have disappeared. Proper disposal of tissues, hand washing, covering mouth while sneezing or coughing are simple techniques that can prevent spread of disease. Refer to Appendix B: Strategies for infection prevention and safe practice for some useful guidelines. Also see Appendix D for organizations and support groups.

Intestinal obstruction

Gastrointestinal system

The impairment of movement of the contents of the intestine in the direction of the rectum and anus.

Cause:

Notes

The cause of the obstruction has to be identified and treated. Intussusception, volvulus, strangulation of herniated gut and other acute obstructions require emergency surgery, as they can be fatal.

The obstruction could be due to mechanical reasons or due to inadequate activity of the autonomic nervous system. Mechanically, the lumen of the intestine can be obstructed by hernias, growths, strictures (common in Ulcerative Colitis), foreign bodies like gall stones, worms, fruit pits and adhesions between organs (can occur after abdominal surgery). Rarely, the gut can telescope onto itself (*intussusception*) or twist (*volvulus*) causing obstruction.

Paralysis and loss of all movements of the bowel usually occurs after abdominal surgery (*paralytic ileus*). However, paralytic ileus is temporary and disappears after 2-3 days. It can also occur after back injuries and spinal cord injuries or thrombosis in the vessels that supply the gut.

Signs and Symptoms:

There is abdominal distention due to accumulation of fluids and gases. Constipation, colicky abdominal pain and vomiting are also present. The obstruction perpetuates the growth of bacteria. The toxins produced by bacteria and death of tissue are absorbed into the blood resulting in further complications. The loss of fluid leads to symptoms of dehydration - reduced urine formation, dry and loose skin texture and intense thirst. There is weakness, excessive sweating and anxiety.

Risk Factors:

It can be a complication of hernia or abdominal surgery.

References

Silen W. Acute intestinal obstruction. In: Isselbacher KJ et al, editors. Harrison's principles of internal medicine. 13th ed. New York: McGraw-Hill Inc; 1994. p. 1431-1433.

Caution and Recommendations to Therapists:

Do not massage if intestinal obstruction is suspected. Refer to a Physician immediately.

Irritable bowel syndrome (IBS)

A collection of symptoms due to hypermotility and increased sensitivity of the intestines.

Cause:

It is due to abnormal motility of the intestines. In those with diarrhea there is faster movement of feces along the ascending and transverse colon. In those with constipation, there is a delay in movement. There is increased visceral perception to stimuli in these patients. As a result, reflex intestinal contraction is increased. It is believed that the altered perception may be due to the input from the central nervous system and stress may be a trigger of symptoms.

Signs and Symptoms:

Typically, there is a history of intermittent constipation, diarrhoea or both over months or years. The diarrhea is more frequent in the morning and patients may have no symptoms the rest of the day. Some patients may complain of lower abdominal pain and a bloated feeling that is relieved by defecation or passage of gas. Back pain, heartburn, weakness, and palpitations are other symptoms that may be present.

Risk Factors:

There is a higher incidence of depression, hysteria and other psychological disturbances in patients with IBS. It is more common in women and young and middle-aged adults are affected more.

Caution and Recommendations to Therapists:

Since stress tends to aggravate the symptoms, massage, by alleviating stress can be beneficial to these individuals. Depending on the client, abdominal massage may have to be varied – with stimulatory massage for those with constipation and perhaps avoidance of the abdomen in those whose primary symptoms include diarrhea. If the symptoms are severe, clearance from the Physician is advisable. See Appendix D for organizations and support groups.

Notes

The condition is chronic and no cure is available. The patient has to be encouraged to identify triggers such as stress that exacerbate the symptoms. Those with constipation may respond to dietary changes that increase the bulk and fibre content. Drugs that alter the motility of the colon may be given.

For more details see Appendix C: Laxatives; Antidiarrhoeal drugs.

References

Lamont JT, Isselbacher KJ. Diseases of the small and large intestine. In: Isselbacher KJ et al, editors. Harrison's principles of internal medicine. 13th ed. New York: McGraw-Hill Inc; 1994. p. 1421-1422.

Jaundice (Icterus)

The yellow discoloration of the skin due to abnormally high levels of the pigment bilirubin in the blood.

Cause:

Bilirubin is a breakdown product of hemoglobin of the red blood cells. It is metabolized in the liver and secreted in the bile along with bile salts. Therefore, any condition that increases the breakdown of red blood cells, and/or affects its metabolism in the liver, or retards its excretion in the bile can result in abnormal increase of bilirubin in the blood. Thus jaundice (French: *jaune* - yellow) can be

Notes

Those with severe prehepatic jaundice may require frequent blood transfusions. Supportive treatment is given for hepatic jaundice. Posthepatic jaundice is usually treated surgically.

Neonatal jaundice may be treated with exposure of the infant to strong white or blue light. The light facilitates conversion of bilirubin to a more soluble form that is rapidly excreted. Exchange transfusion may be needed in some cases.

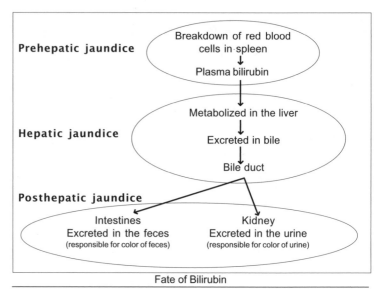

Prehepatic jaundice

Breakdown of red blood cells in spleen
↓
Plasma bilirubin

Hepatic jaundice

Metabolized in the liver
↓
Excreted in bile
↓
Bile duct

Posthepatic jaundice

Intestines
Excreted in the feces
(responsible for color of feces)

Kidney
Excreted in the urine
(responsible for color of urine)

Fate of Bilirubin

classified as *prehepatic*, *hepatic* or *posthepatic* according to the cause.

Signs and Symptoms:

Bilirubin has an affinity for elastic tissue and usually presents as a yellow discoloration of the white of the eye. Mucous membrane of the mouth also appears yellow. In prehepatic jaundice, there will be associated anemia. History of hepatitis along with other signs of hepatitis will be present in the hepatic type (see Hepatitis). There may be severe itching of the skin especially in the posthepatic type of jaundice. In addition, in the latter, due to the obstruction to the flow of bile, digestion of fat is affected and feces is foul-smelling and clay-colored. The urine is dark in color as a result of increased excretion of bilirubin in the urine.

Risk Factors:

Transfusion of incompatible blood, hereditary disorders of the red blood cells like sickle cell anemia, thalassemia and spherocytosis predispose to prehepatic jaundice. Jaundice in the newborn (neonatal jaundice) is usually due to the inability of the immature liver to cope up with the breakdown of red cells. However, other causes such as Rh incompatibility have to be ruled out if severe jaundice is noticed at birth. In the newborn, bilirubin can cross the blood-brain barrier, get deposited in the brain and produce irreversible nervous system complications (*erythroblastosis foetalis*).

Hepatic jaundice is the most common type and is due to viral hepatitis. This type can also be caused by liver failure due to toxic agents, drugs, cirrhosis or cancer. Rarely, hereditary absence of liver enzymes required for the metabolism of bilirubin can predispose an individual to jaundice.

Bile duct abnormalities, gallstones or tumors obstructing the flow of bile can predispose to posthepatic jaundice.

Caution and Recommendations to Therapists:

The cause of the jaundice should dictate the treatment plan. Prehepatic jaundice is not contagious and can be treated on an individual basis. A soothing massage of short duration is indicated. Avoid massage to the upper abdomen as both the spleen and the liver are likely to be enlarged in these individuals. The massage should be gentle and soothing. Undue pressure should not be used as the individual may have a bleeding disorder and bruise and bleed easily. The cause of hepatic jaundice should be obtained. If due to Viral Hepatitis, the precautions given under hepatitis should be followed. If the jaundice is posthepatic, the massage oil may reduce the intense itching experienced by these individuals. Abdominal massage should be avoided.

References

Premkumar K. The Massage Connection – Anatomy, Physiology and Pathology. Calgary: VanPub Books; 1998. p. F2-F3.

Ganong WF. Review of medical physiology. 15th ed. California; Appleton & Lange; 1991. p. 467-468.

Kyphosis

Musculoskeletal system

A deformity of the spine that produces a rounded back.

Cause:

Kyphosis is classified as *primary, functional* or *first degree* if the deformity is of muscular origin and can be corrected; *secondary, structural* or *second degree* if due to connective tissue change and *tertiary* or *third degree* if due to bony changes.

There are numerous causes. In children and adolescents it is due to bad posture. It may be also be brought about by arthritis, lung problems like emphysema, paralysis or weakness of back muscles. Tuberculosis of the spinal column, compression fracture of the vertebral body, ankylosing spondylitis, tumour of the spinal column and osteoporosis are other causes.

Notes

Treatment is geared towards the specific cause of the problem.

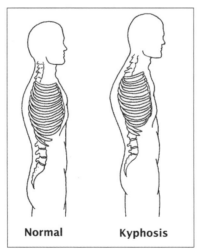

Normal   **Kyphosis**

Signs and Symptoms:

The back is rounded and the chest flattened. There may be difficulty in breathing due to the shortening of the pectoral muscles that interferes with thoracic movement. The rhomboids, trapezius and the longitudinal muscles of the back are stretched and weakened. The scapula is pulled forward and the person has a forward head posture.

a Handbook for Massage Therapists   211

Risk Factors:

Occupations that require a hunched posture can predispose to kyphosis. Also see Cause.

Caution and Recommendations to Therapists:

Work in close conjunction with the Physiotherapist and Physician. A proper assessment is required to identify the extent of spasm, range of motion, trigger points and adhesions. In kyphosis, the neck extensors, hip flexors, lumbar spinal extensors, shoulder adductors, pectoralis minor and the intercostals are shortened but strong. The neck flexors, upper back spinal extensors, external oblique, hamstrings, middle and lower trapezius are elongated and weak. This is due to the compensation made to posture such as forward head, cervical lordosis, abducted scapulae, lumbar lordosis, anterior pelvic tilt, hip joint flexion, knee joint hyperextension and ankle plantar flexion.

The client should be encouraged and taught to stretch the shortened muscles and strengthen the weak and elongated muscles. The trapezius, rhomboids, latissimus dorsi, erector spinae, pectoralis minor and major are some of the large muscles that have to be tested for strength and length.

The aim is to produce general relaxation, reduce pain by increasing circulation in the tense muscles, and stretch shortened muscles and fascia. Position the client in as comfortable posture as possible with supporting pillows. Heat packs may help reduce pain and spasm. Start with the client supine and use techniques to stretch the shortened pectorals. Massage the tense neck and pectoral muscles addressing trigger points if present. In the prone position, use techniques to stimulate the rhomboids and trapezius. The rotator cuff muscles, gluteal and back muscles should also be massaged thoroughly. Deep diaphragmatic breathing helps mobilize the thoracic cavity.

Avoid mobilizing techniques if the kyphosis is due to changes in bone or connective tissue.

References

Hall CM, Brody LT. Therapeutic exercise moving toward function. Philadelphia: Lipppincott Williams & Wilkins; 1999. p. 570-572.

Mercier LR. editor. Practical orthopedics. 4th ed. New York: Mosby-Year book Inc; 1995. p. 155-157.

Respiratory system

Laryngitis

An inflammation of the vocal cords.

Cause:

It is usually caused by viral or bacterial infection. Excessive use of the voice can also produce this condition.

Signs and Symptoms:

It presents with hoarseness or complete loss of voice, cough and pain on swallowing.

Notes

It is treated with voice rest, painkillers and humidification of air breathed. If it is due to bacterial infection, antibiotics are given. If there is excessive edema, there is a potential for obstruction of the airways and more serious measures such as administration of glucocorticoids, oxygen and intubation are needed.

Pathology A to Z -

Risk Factors:

It is more common in occupations like teaching, public speaking or singing. Loud cheering, constant dust, smoke or fume inhalation, smoking and alcoholism are other predisposing conditions.

Caution and Recommendations to Therapists:

If the laryngitis is due to viral or bacterial infection it spreads by inhalation of droplets from the infected person. Do not massage clients with laryngitis of infective origin. Encourage rest to the voice. Increase humidification of air, reduce air conditioning (which tends to dehumidify) while treating clients with laryngitis of noninfective origin. Refer to Appendix B: Strategies for infection prevention and safe practice for some useful guidelines. Also see Appendix D for organizations and support groups.

For more details see Appendix C: Painkillers; Antimicrobial - antibacterial agents; Antiinflammatories - steroidal drugs; Oxygen therapy; Intubation.

References

Maran AGD, editor. Logan Turner's diseases of the nose, throat and ear. 10th ed. London: Wright; 1988. p. 160-162.

Lead poisoning (Plumbism)

Abnormally high levels of lead in blood.

Nervous system

Cause:

Lead is used in paints as coloring agents and stabilizers. It may also be a contaminant of tap water. Organic lead salts are added to gasoline and many other consumer products. Lead in the form of inorganic salts is absorbed through the lungs (if particles very small) or gut. Organic lead salts can be absorbed through the skin. After absorption, lead is found in association with the red blood cells or taken up by bone. It may also be found in the kidneys and brain.

Lead is toxic to enzymes and interferes with transport of calcium, formation of neurotransmitters and in high concentration it can affect intracellular proteins and cause cell death.

Notes

It is important to identify and remove the source of exposure. Chelating agents are used to remove lead from the body. For more details see Appendix C: Chelating agents.

Signs and Symptoms:

In adults it presents as abdominal pain, anemia, kidney disease, headache, loss of memory and unsteady gait. The peripheral nerve function is affected as it causes demyelination of neurons. The effect on the central nervous system is more severe in children and is related to the age and duration of exposure. Some of the symptoms seen in children are lethargy, loss of appetite, ataxia, slurred speech and in severe cases convulsions and coma. Mental retardation may also occur.

Risk Factors:

See Cause.

Caution and Recommendations to Therapists:

Special tests are required to estimate the lead content in the body. Spend some time to investigate if there is any possible source of lead that could be contaminating the environment in the vicinity. Rarely, a client may present

References

Graef JW. Heavy metal poisoning. In: Isselbacher KJ et al, editors. Harrison's principles of internal medicine. 13th ed. New York: McGraw-Hill Inc; 1994. p. 2463-2464.

with the residual effects of lead poisoning. The sensory and motor deficit has to be assessed and treatment plan altered accordingly.

Integumentary system

Lentigo

A lentigo is a well-circumscribed macule on the skin that is present at birth or appears in childhood.

Cause:

It is due to excessive numbers of melanocytes and melanin pigment in the area. There are many types of lentigines. One of the common types is the solar (senile) lentigines (liver spots) that is seen in most elderly and occurs in response to exposure to the sun.

Signs and Symptoms:

The darker, brown-black macules are usually less than 1 cm and found in any part of the body. They do not darken on exposure to the sun (unlike freckles).

Risk Factors:

See Cause. Some types of lentigines are associated with gastrointestinal polyps.

Caution and Recommendations to Therapists:

Lentigo does not produce any symptoms and is of no consequence to the Therapist. However, if a hyperpigmented patch is of recent onset or appears to be increasing in size in a client who frequents the clinic, advice the client to seek medical help.

Notes

It is treated with laser therapy, cryotherapy or by special bleaching agents.

For more details see Appendix C: Laser therapy; Cryotherapy.

References

Fitzpatrick TB et al, editors. Dermatology in general medicine. 3rd ed. New York: McGraw-Hill; 1987.

Integumentary, Nervous systems

Leprosy (Hansen's disease)

A chronic infection that affects the skin and peripheral nerves.

Cause:

It is caused by the organism *Mycobacterium leprae*. The incubation period is 2-6 years. It is probably transmitted by droplet infection and enters the body through the mucosa of the upper respiratory tract or skin. The reaction seen in an individual is based on his/her immunity. There are many types of clinical presentations - the *indeterminate* or *early leprosy*, *tuberculoid* (good prognosis, normal immunity), the *lepromatous* (poor prognosis, poor immunity) and *borderline*.

Notes

It is treated with drugs and Dapsone is the treatment of choice. More than one drug is given depending on the type of leprosy. Analgesics, antipyretics, antibiotics and anti-inflammatory drugs may be needed if there are severe reactions. In addition to drugs, physical therapy, surgery and occupational therapy may be needed depending on the type of lesions and complications. Nerve and tendon transplants and

Signs and Symptoms:

In early or indeterminate leprosy, one or more hypopigmented patches are seen on the skin. The patches may be anesthetic. Usually, they are found while screening close contacts of patients already diagnosed with leprosy.

In tuberculoid leprosy, hypopigmented patches are seen on the skin. These patches are well demarcated and anesthetic. The lesions slowly enlarge with elevation of the margins and atrophy and depression of the central regions. The peripheral nerves are enlarged and can be palpated as a thickened cord. Muscle atrophy may be seen when the nerves are involved, often resulting in contractures of the hand and foot. Due to the loss of sensation in areas, ulcers can be produced especially after injury.

In the type lepromatous leprosy, shiny, brown or red, symmetric macules, plaques and nodules may be seen on the skin. The lesions are not anesthetic. Usually, cooler areas of the body like the nose, ears, wrists, elbow, buttocks and knees are affected. Subsequent collapse of the nasal bridges may occur. The skin may become thickened - especially of the face, giving the characteristic leonine appearance. Lymph nodes may be enlarged.

Borderline leprosy presents in a variety of ways. Sometimes, there is an exacerbation of the immune response (erythema nodosum leprosum) and many systems are affected (arthritis; nephritis; enlargement of the liver and spleen etc). The lesions become tender and inflamed associated with fever and lymphadenopathy.

Leprosy is complicated by the development of contractures. Trauma and secondary infection can lead to loss of digits. If the eye is affected, blindness can occur.

Risk Factors:

It is more common in warmer climates, in countries such as Latin America and southeast Asia. The incidence is higher in families in close contact with an individual with lepromatous leprosy.

Caution and Recommendations to Therapists:

Not all clients with this condition are infectious. The risk of infection even in untreated clients is very low. In most clients, the symptoms are due to the residual effects of the disease on the nervous system and skin. The Therapist who is motivated to treat these individuals who are generally stigmatized, requires a thorough knowledge about the disease and its course. It is also important to work as part of a team which should include Physiotherapists, Occupational Therapists, Orthopedic Surgeons, Nurses and Social Workers among others. Refer to Appendix B: Strategies for infection prevention and safe practice for some useful guidelines. Also see Appendix D for organizations and support groups.

release of contractures are some of the surgical procedures that may have to be used.

Patient education can prevent the occurrence of many of the deformities.

Early detection by periodic screening of close contacts and prompt treatment can help control spread.

For more details see Appendix C: Painkillers; Antipyretics; Antimicrobial - antibacterial agents; Antiinflammatories - non steroidal drugs; Organ transplantation.

References

Morello JA, Mizer HE, Wilson ME, Granato PA. Microbiology in patient care. 6th ed. New York: McGraw-Hill; 1998. p. 434-436.

Hastings, RC, Opremolla DV, editors. Leprosy. In: Medicine in the tropics. New York: Churchill Livingstone; 1994.

Leukemia

A cancerous multiplication of white blood cells in the bone marrow and lymph tissue with abnormally large number of white blood cells in the blood.

Cause:

Notes

Leukemias are generally treated with chemotherapy and/or radiation. Bone marrow transplantation may be considered for specific patients. Administration of blood products and antibiotics may be required to treat associated problems. Wearing of face masks and meticulous hand washing while in contact with clients, isolation of those with severe depletion of immune cells are some of the supportive measures.

Immunotherapy, where antibodies against antigens located on the leukemic cells are used, is a newer treatment option under exploration.

For more details see Appendix C: Chemotherapy; Radiation therapy; Organ transplantation; Blood transfusion; Immunotherapy.

It may be due to certain viruses. But family history, exposure to radiation and certain chemicals have also been associated with this disease. The immature white blood cells seem to multiply abnormally in the area of origin: lymphatic tissue - lymphocytes and bone marrow - other white blood cells. They then spill over into the blood and other organs affecting their normal function.

Leukemias are classified according to the speed of onset as *acute* or *chronic leukemias*. The type with increase in lymphocytes is called *lymphoblastic/ lymphocytic leukemia*. The type with increase in other white blood cells is called *myeloblastic leukemia*. Those producing increase in monocytes are called *monocytic/monoblastic leukemias*. Thus there could be an acute or chronic type of each of the above. The age group they affect and the progress of each of the types vary.

Signs and Symptoms:

It may present as a sudden onset of fever and abnormal bleeding from the nose, gums or other regions. The individual is also more prone to bruise easily (due to reduced platelets). There may be mild fever, weight loss, and fatigue lasting for a number of days. Even though the number of white blood cells are increased they are immature with lowered function, so there is a tendency to have repeated infections. The rapid multiplication in the bones may also produce bone pain. Most types of leukemia result in enlargement of the spleen and liver. There may be associated enlargement of lymph nodes.

Risk Factors:

Family history, Down's syndrome, exposure to radiation and occupations involving exposure to benzene are all predisposing factors. Though certain viruses have been implicated, the common leukemias are not contagious and the incidence is not increased in those in close contact.

Caution and Recommendations to Therapists:

References

Scheinberg DA, Golde DW. The Leukemias. In: Isselbacher KJ et al, editors. Harrison's principles of internal medicine. 13th ed. New York: McGraw-Hill Inc; 1994. p. 1764-1774.

Do not massage a client diagnosed with leukemia without consulting the treating Physician. However, since the problem is in the circulating blood and tissues producing blood cells, there is little chance of spreading the condition to other areas by massaging. These clients are more prone to infection due to the lowered immunity. Even if the Physician approves a massage, do not treat clients if you have even a mild infection. Ensure that they are scheduled for a time when they are unlikely to come in contact with infected individuals. These clients also bruise easily and have a tendency to bleed. Do not use excess pressure. Use ice packs in areas that have bled or bleed. There may be enlargement of spleen or liver. Avoid massaging the upper abdominal region ie. over the liver and spleen. Only a very gentle relaxation massage should be given. Avoid areas of radiation if the person is on radiation therapy. See Appendix D for organizations and support groups.

Lichen planus

An inflammatory skin disorder.

Cause:

The cause is unknown.

Signs and Symptoms:

Lichen planus (Greek: tree moss) presents as itchy, small, papular lesions that appear like tree moss in the wrist, ankles and trunk. It may affect the mucous membranes. The eruptions glisten and appear as white lines or spots. See Appendix A: page 353.

Risk Factors:

It may be associated with drugs and chemicals like arsenic, bismuth and gold. It is more common between the ages of 30-60.

Caution and Recommendations to Therapists:

It is not contagious. Chemicals in the oil used may make the condition worse so unadulterated oil should be used while massaging such clients. Avoid massaging over lesions.

Notes

The lesions may disappear spontaneously. It is treated symptomatically and drugs are given to relieve the itching. Sometimes steroids or ultraviolet radiations are used.

For more details see Appendix C: Antihistamines; Antiinflammatories - steroidal drugs.

References

Fitzpatrick TB et al. editors. Dermatology in general medicine. 3rd ed. New York: McGraw-Hill; 1987.

Liver failure (Hepatic failure)

A condition when the liver is unable to cope up with the demands made.

Cause:

Any condition that extensively damages the hepatic tissue leads to liver failure. Only 10% of the liver is required for it to function.

Signs and Symptoms:

These are related to the various functions that the liver performs. Due to the lack of clotting factors, the person bleeds easily and anemia results. The congestion of the portal circulation can lead to fluid in the peritoneal cavity (ascites), edema and varicosities of esophageal and rectal vessels - potential sites of fatal bleeding (see Esophageal varices). Spider Nevi - superficial spiderlike, dilatation of blood vessels are common in individuals with liver failure. (See Appendix A: page 357).

The inadequate metabolism of steroid hormones is reflected as menstrual irregularities, impotence and sterility. There is atrophy of the testis and abnormal

Notes

Treatment is largely supportive and aims to remove conditions that perpetuate the problem.

Liver transplant is one of the newer treatment options. Those who have had transplants are required to be on immunosuppressants to prevent the body from rejecting the donor tissue. Hence these individuals are prone to infections.

For more details see Appendix C: Immunosuppressants; Organ transplantation.

a Handbook for Massage Therapists

enlargement of breasts in men. Jaundice is also present. The increase in toxins in the blood can affect the nervous system causing lack of mental alertness, confusion, coma and convulsions.

Risk Factors:

Hepatitis, cirrhosis and ingestion of drugs toxic to the liver, alcoholism and prolonged obstruction to the bile ducts can predispose to liver failure.

Caution and Recommendations to Therapists:

The cause of the liver failure should be determined before proceeding. Get clearance from the treating Physician. It is important to know the functions of the liver as the symptoms are directly related to the functions. Treatment is altered according to the cause. See Hepatitis, Cirrhosis and Portal hypertension for specific recommendations. See Appendix D for organizations and support groups.

References

Isselbacher KJ, Podolsky DK. Approach to the patient with liver disease. In: Isselbacher KJ et al, editors. Harrison's principles of internal medicine. 13ᵗʰ ed. New York: McGraw-Hill Inc; 1994. p. 1437-1504.

Respiratory system

Lung abscess

A lung infection associated with accumulation of pus.

Cause:

It may be caused by different types of bacteria. Rarely, lung abscess may be due to amoebic or fungal infection. Lung abscess may occur as a complication of bronchopneumonia and other lung infections. It is also associated with aspiration of contents of the mouth and pharynx.

Signs and Symptoms:

Cough with foul-smelling or blood-tinged sputum, chest pain produced by breathing movements, difficulty in breathing, fever and weight loss are the classical symptoms.

Risk Factors:

The incidence is higher in people with poor oral hygiene ie. those with dental or gum diseases. Coma, general anaesthesia, repeated vomiting, bronchial obstruction by tumors or thick secretions, chronic upper respiratory tract infections, individuals with difficulty in swallowing as a result of muscle weakness or cranial nerve damage are all predisposing factors.

Caution and Recommendations to Therapists:

Individuals with lung abscess have to be on antibiotic treatment often lasting for months. Consult Physician before treating. Do not massage during the acute stage. Postural drainage is beneficial (see Bronchiectasis). Tapotement, chest hacking and vibration movements help with drainage of pus. Deep breathing exercises also help. Steam inhalation before commencing treatment in a person recovering from lung abscess may be beneficial. Refer to Appendix B: Strategies

Notes

It is treated with potent antibiotics. Surgery is required only rarely, when there is a neoplasm or large volume of blood in sputum. Oxygen and other supportive measures to help with drainage may be given.

For more details see Appendix C: Antimicrobial - antibacterial therapy; Oxygen therapy.

References

Levison ME. Pneumonia, including necrotizing pulmonary infections (lung abscess). In: Isselbacher KJ et al. editors. Harrison's principles of internal medicine. 13ᵗʰ ed. New York: McGraw-Hill Inc; 1994. p. 1186.

for infection prevention and safe practice for some useful guidelines. Also see Appendix D for organizations and support groups.

Lyme disease (Lyme arthritis)

An inflammatory infectious disease transmitted by ticks that affects many systems.

Nervous, Cardiovascular, Musculoskeletal, Integumentary systems

Cause:

This disease is caused by a bacteria carried by ticks. The life cycle of the tick spans over two years and has three stages - larvae, nymph and adult. In North America, the mouse carries the larvae and nymph and the white-tailed deer, the adult tick. All three stages can feed on humans and transmit the bacteria. It is necessary for the infected tick to be attached to the human body for 24 hours for the infection to be transmitted.

Signs and Symptoms:

Within an few days or a month after the tick bite, the bacteria moves to the surface of the skin producing a circular, ring-like rash that has red borders with central clearing. The person has flu-like symptoms - fever, headache, fatigue and enlargement of lymph nodes. If it is not treated, the bacteria migrate to the other systems through the lymph or blood. Complications like meningitis and arthritis may result.

Risk Factors:

It is common in North America, Europe and Asia.

Caution and Recommendations to Therapists:

This disease spreads only by tick bites and there is no danger of spread through massage. Since the disease is chronic - lasting for months to years, the massage treatment has to be individualized according to symptoms. Encourage client to see Physician and take the full course of antibiotics prescribed. Refer to Appendix B: Strategies for infection prevention and safe practice for some useful guidelines. Also see Appendix D for organizations and support groups.

Notes

Avoiding tick-infested areas from May to October can prevent this disease. While moving through heavily wooded areas, exposure of the skin should be reduced by suitable clothing.

Application of insect repellent and removal of ticks within a few hours of attachment prevents the disease.

References

Morello JA, Mizer HE, Wilson ME, Granato PA. Microbiology in patient care. 6th ed. New York: McGraw-Hill; 1998. p. 485-486.

Marbit MD, Willis E. Lyme disease: Implications for health educators. Health Educ. 1990; 22(2): 41-43.

Silverstein DB. Lyme disease: Easy to treat, easy to miss. J Am Acad Nurse Pract 1989; 1(3): 73-76.

Lymphangitis

Inflammation of lymphatic vessels.

Lymphatic system

Cause:

It is usually caused by the streptococci bacteria.

Signs and Symptoms:

There is pain and swelling of the affected area accompanied by enlargement of lymph nodes, inflammation of the lymph vessels and fever. The inflamed vessels appear as red streaks on the skin.

Notes

It is treated with suitable antibiotics and antiinflammatory drugs. For more details see Appendix C: Antimicrobial-antibacterial agents; Antiinflammatories - non steroidal drugs.

Risk Factors:

It usually spreads from infection in other areas.

Caution and Recommendations to Therapists:

If open wounds are present the Therapist can get infected by contact. Massage is contraindicated. Massage can exacerbate the illness and also help spread the infection to other areas or to the rest of the body (septicemia). Advice clients to see a Physician if not seeing one already. Encourage client to take the full course of antibiotics. Refer to the section on Strategies for infection prevention and safe practice (Appendix B).

References

Mosby's medical, nursing, & allied health dictionary. 4ᵗʰ ed. Philadelphia: Mosby-Year book Inc; 1994.

Gastrointestinal system

Malabsorption syndrome

The spectrum of symptoms and signs seen when there is failure to absorb nutrients from the intestinal tract.

Cause:

Notes

Malabsorption syndrome is treated with supplements that are given intravenously.

This can be caused by reduced or no secretion of enzymes required for digestion and absorption of a specific type of food; or defect in the mucosa which transports the digested food from the lumen of the intestine to the blood for distribution or due to lymphatic obstruction in the gut. Reduced secretion occurs if the glands like the pancreas, liver etc. are dysfunctional. It can also occur if the normal growth of the bacteria in the gut have been disturbed.

No absorption occurs through the mucosa if there are lesions in it as in Crohn's disease or if a large portion of the gut has been removed by surgery. This may also occur if the intestinal villi are atrophied as in a condition called *celiac sprue* (*Celiac Disease*). Sprue is due to an immunological reaction to a certain protein called gluten contained in barley, wheat and rye.

Since the lymphatics transport fat in the gut, fat absorption is disturbed if the lymphatics are obstructed as in trauma, infections or cancer.

Signs and Symptoms:

These individuals present with diarrhea, fatty, foul-smelling stools that float in the toilet and are difficult to flush, abdominal pain, bloated abdomen and flatulence (passage of gas). There is weight loss in spite of a normal intake of food. Other signs seen are due to the lack of absorption of vitamins (see Nutritional deficiencies).

Risk Factors:

Celiac sprue has a genetic predisposition and is more common in Caucasians.

Caution and Recommendations to Therapists:

Due to the lack of vitamins, the skin is dry and scaly. The oil used for massage is therefore beneficial. Due to the lack of vitamin K, the individuals bruise very easily and moderate pressure can cause bleeding under the skin (see Appendix A: page 355). So very light pressure should be used. The lack of vitamin D makes them prone to osteoporosis - reiterating the use of only mild pressure during massage. Lack of vitamin B can produce alteration in sensations especially in the distal parts of the limbs - so the client may not be able to give adequate feedback. Protein deficiency can produce edema. Lymphatic drainage techniques may be used if edema is present. Gentle abdominal massage can help relieve the gas that produces the distension and discomfort. See Appendix D for organizations and support groups.

References

Greenberger NJ, Isselbacher KJ. Disorders of absorption. In: Isselbacher KJ et al, editors. Harrison's principles of internal medicine. 13th ed. New York: McGraw-Hill Inc; 1994. p. 1390-1403.

Malaria

Cardiovascular system

A parasitic disease spread by the bite of mosquitos.

Cause:

It is due to the transmission of the protozoa *Plasmodium*. There are many species of Plasmodium - *P. ovale, P. vivax, P. malariae, P. falciparum,* each of which cause different forms of the disease.

When a female Anopheles mosquito carrying sporozoites (early form of the malarial parasite) bites a human being, the sporozoites residing in the salivary glands of the mosquito enter the blood stream. The sporozoites reach the liver and enter the cells there to multipy and be transformed into another form - merozoites that enter the blood again. In some malarial species, the sporozoites remain dormant in the liver cells for a long time and are the cause of relapses of malaria. In the blood, the merozoites infect red blood cells where they multiply further. When the red cell ruptures, they are released into the blood to infect more red cells. Some of the merozoites in the red cells transform into a male or female gametocyte.

When a mosquito bites the infected individual, the gametocytes enter the gut of the mosquito where they fuse and after further transformation, produce many sporozoites that reside in the salivary gland ready to be injected into another human being and the cycle repeats.

Malaria may be transmitted by transfusion of infected blood or sharing needles between infected intravenous drug users.

Signs and Symptoms:

The signs and symptoms are due to the effects of the merozoites on red blood cells and the reaction of the body to the infection. The merozoites in the red blood cell produce changes in the red cell membrane. They also destroy the proteins inside the red blood cell. The red cell eventually ruptures. In some types of malaria, the infected red cells adhere to one another affecting circulation in the capillaries. When a person is infected, the presence of the parasite triggers an immune response.

Notes

Prevention of spread of infection plays an important part in endemic areas. Spraying of insecticides in breeding sites, use of mosquito nets - especially nets treated with insecticides (eg. permethrin), avoiding exposure to mosquitoes at peak feeding times (which is usually between dusk to dawn), using insect repellents, wearing clothes that cover skin, sleeping in rooms with screened windows are some forms of prevention.

Infected individuals are treated with drugs such as chloroquine, mefloquine etc. The drug that is used depends on the species of parasite and the drug resistance pattern in the area. Specific drugs may be given to travellers going to endemic areas. Since the pattern of drug resistance changes, and is different from one area to another, it is important for individuals to obtain updated malaria information before travelling. People who originally lived in an endemic area and have been away for many years loose their immunity and need to take prophylactic treatment before returning to the country of origin.

Severe malaria has to be treated as a medical emergency and carefully monitored in intensive care units.

For more details see Appendix C: Antimalarial drugs.

The spleen is activated and both infected and non-infected red cells are removed.

Typically, the person first presents with headache, fatigue, abdominal discomfort and muscle aches. This is followed by high fever with chills. If not treated promptly, fever patterns typical for individual parasite species is noted. The fever may spike daily, every 2 days, 3 days etc. according to the infecting species. Anemia and jaundice may be seen.

In some severe cases (P. falciparum infection) other organs may be affected. If the brain is affected, *cerebral malaria* results. The person may be delirious or go into coma. Generalized convulsions may be seen. Hypoglycemia may occur due to failure of the infected liver cells to produce adequate glucose. Acidosis due to accumulation of lactic acid may occur if circulation to tissue is blocked by adhering red cells. Renal impairment, pulmonary edema, severe anemia are other symptoms seen in some forms of infection. Many of these complications may be seen if a pregnant woman is infected.

In many infected individuals living in endemic areas, the spleen and liver are massively enlarged.

Risk Factors:

Malaria is common in the tropical regions. The incidence of malaria in a region is related to the genetic and immunological makeup of the population, the species of parasite and the type of mosquito in the region. The environmental conditions affect the life cycle of the mosquito. Therefore, the amount of rainfall, the temperature, the distribution of the mosquito breeding sites and malaria control measures taken all play a part.

People with the genetic disorders such as sickle cell anemia, thalassemia and glucose-6-phosphate deficiency are less prone to malaria due to some form of protection conferred by the genetic disorder.

Caution and Recommendations to Therapists:

Malaria does not spread by contact and the Therapist cannot get the disease from contact with clients who give a history of having had malaria. Encourage clients who intend to travel to endemic areas to seek help and information from a local travel clinic on strategies to prevent malaria.

If living in an endemic area, ensure that the clinic is "insect proofed". In many individuals living in endemic areas, the liver and spleen are enlarged. Do not massage the abdomen in these cases as excessive pressure can rupture the enlarged organs. Refer to Appendix B: Strategies for infection prevention and safe practice for some useful guidelines. Also see Appendix D for organizations and support groups.

References

Morello JA, Mizer HE, Wilson ME, Granato PA. Microbiology in patient care. 6th ed. New York: McGraw-Hill; 1998.p. 496-498.

Hawking, F. The clock of the malaria parasite. Sci Am 1970; 222(6): 123. Friedman MJ, Trager W. The biochemistry of resistance to malaria. Sci Am 1981; 244(3): 154-165.

Malignant lymphomas (Non-Hodgkin's Lymphoma; Lymphosarcoma)

Lymphatic system

A cancer originating in the lymph nodes and other lymphoid tissues.

Cause:

The cause is unknown. It may be due to a virus.

Signs and Symptoms:

Initially, it presents as swelling of the lymph nodes, tonsils, adenoids, liver or spleen. The swelling is painless and the nodes feel rubbery. As the swelling increases in size it produces symptoms by pressure on surrounding areas accompanied by anemia, weight loss, fever, lethargy and fatigue.

Risk Factors:

It is more common in males and occurs in all age groups.

Caution and Recommendations to Therapists:

Advice the client to consult a Physician if you notice an abnormally large painless lymph node enlargement. Do not massage clients diagnosed with Lymphoma without consulting the treating Physician. Individuals with lymphoma have a lowered immunity and very prone to infections. See Appendix D for organizations and support groups.

Notes

Lymphoma is treated with radiation and/or chemotherapy. For more details see Appendix C: Radiation therapy; Cancer chemotherapy.

References

Premkumar K. The massage connection: Anatomy, Physiology and Pathology. Calgary: VanPub Books; 1998. p. N8-N12.

Freedman AS, Nadler LM. Malignant lymphomas. In: Isselbacher KJ et al, editors. Harrison's principles of internal medicine. 13th ed. New York: McGraw-Hill Inc; 1994. p. 1774-1784

Ferrell-Torry AT, Glick OJ. The use of therapeutic massage as a nursing intervention to modify anxiety and the perception of cancer pain. Cancer Nursing. 1993; 16(2):93-101.

McNamara P. Massage for people with cancer. London: Wandsworth Cancer Support Center; 1993.

Chamness A. Massage therapy and persons living with cancer. Massage Therapy Journal 32(3): 53-65.

MacDonald G. Massage for cancer patients: a review of nursing research. Massage Therapy Journal.34(3): 53-56.

Malnutrition (Protein energy malnutrition; Protein-calorie malnutrition)

Gastrointestinal, Integumentary systems

A condition that results from insufficient availability of energy or protein to meet the metabolic demands of the body.

Cause:

Protein energy malnutrition is classified as primary when it is caused by inadequate intake of protein or intake of dietary protein of poor quality (inadequate essential amino acids). The cause is termed secondary if it is due to increased metabolic demands or increased nutrient loss. Pregnancy, lactation and growth periods (infancy, childhood, adolescence), chronic infections and trauma are some states where the metabolic demand is increased. Increased nutrient loss may occur in malabsorption syndromes, inflammatory bowel disease, AIDS and renal problems. Fasting practices and starvation are states where there is inadequate intake.

Signs and Symptoms:

The best indicator of this condition is body weight. Standard tables of adequate

Notes

The cause of the condition has to be identified and treated. All the symptoms and signs can be reversed by proper nutrition.

body weight that are available may be used. There is a decrease in subcutaneous fat. This may be visually assessed or by using a skin-fold caliper. In children there is a reduction in physical development. Puberty may be delayed. Since protein is mobilised from the skeletal muscle, strength is diminished. Immunity is also lowered with increased susceptibility to infections. Pregnant women with this condition may deliver babies with a lowered birth weight.

In severe malnutrition, skin changes occur. The skin is wrinkled and prone to infections. Pressure ulcers are common. The skin may appear shiny and red with areas of hyperpigmentation and scaling. Hair is sparse, dry and tends to change colour (dull brown or red). There may be generalized edema due to the loss of protein. This presentation is termed *kwashiorkor*. Protein energy malnutrition without edema is termed as *marasmus*.

Changes are produced in various other organs. In the gastrointestinal tract, the cells atrophy due to lack of stimulation by ingested nutrients. As a result malabsorption may occur. Various hormonal secretions are affected. Stoppage of menstruation and infertility is common. The heart atrophies and conduction defects may result. The heart is unable to cope when increased demands are made. The respiratory muscles are atrophied, reducing the capacity to inspire and expire larger volumes of air. Wound healing is delayed due to the decrease in collagen formation.

Risk Factors:

Pre-school children are more prone as they depend on others for the quality and quantity of food intake. Associated gastrointestinal infection in this age group increases the risk. Malnutrition may be seen in hospital patients where the nutritional intake is not carefully monitored.

Caution and Recommendations to Therapists:

Advice client to get medical help if their body weight is abnormally low. Only a gentle massage should be attempted in these clients as the skin is fragile and they tend to bruise easily. The immunity is also low making these individuals prone to infection. Some may present with edema but massage is unlikely to be beneficial in these clients as it is due to reduced availability of protein. Get clearance from the treating Physician if necessary.

References

Mason JB, Rosenberg IH. Protein-energy malnutrition. In: Isselbacher KJ et al, editors. Harrison's principles of internal medicine. 13ᵗʰ ed. New York: McGraw-Hill Inc; 1994. p. 440-446.

Marfan's syndrome

Musculoskeletal, Cardiovascular systems

An inherited disorder producing abnormal development of elastin and collagen of the connective tissue.

Cause:

It is inherited from either of the parents and the child exhibits symptoms of the disease to varying degrees even if one parent is normal ie. it is a dominant trait. In 15% of the cases, it may be due to a fresh mutation ie. there is no family history.

Notes

There is no specific treatment. Drugs (vasoconstrictors) may be given to reduce aortic dilatation and aneurysm. Supportive therapy such as bracing and

Signs and Symptoms:

Most commonly, these individuals are very tall with an arm span that is longer than the height of the person. The ligaments, tendons and joint capsules are weak resulting in hyperextensibility of joints. The joints tend to get dislocated easily. Marfan's syndrome also affects the eye causing detachment of the lens and increased pressure of the ocular fluid. Bone deformities are also seen with development of pigeon chest. If the cardiovascular system is affected, the weak walls of the aorta dilate and bulge resulting in aneurysm formation with potential for rupture.

Risk Factors:

See Cause.

Caution and Recommendations to Therapists:

Gentle massage is recommended. If the client has cardiovascular abnormalities get clearance from the Physician. Do not use pressure or manipulative and mobilization techniques as the ligaments are lax and joints hyperextensible. Encourage client to take genetic counselling. Refer to local support groups, if available. See Appendix D for resources.

physiotherapy are given if bony deformities are present.

For more details see Appendix C: Genetic testing / counselling; Vasoconstrictors.

References

Pyeritz RE. The Marfan syndrome. In: Royce PM, Steinmann B, editors. Connective tissue and its heritable disorders. New York: Wiley-Liss; 1993. p. 437.

Measles (Rubeola)

A virus infection that produces rashes in the skin.

Integumentary, Respiratory systems

Cause:

It is caused by the measles virus. The virus is spread by air borne and droplet contact. The incubation period ranges from 1-3 weeks. The virus enters the respiratory tract and then gains access to the blood via the lymphatic system.

Signs and Symptoms:

It presents as fever, cough, watering of the eyes and congestion of the nose, 2-3 days before the development of the rash. Small, irregular, reddish spots blue-white centers (*Koplik's spots*) tend to appear in the mucous membrane of the mouth a few days before the appearance of the rash. The rash appears over the face and head as small reddish spots. Within a day the rash spreads to the arms, trunk and back. Soon, the rashes join together and present as large reddish

Notes

No treatment is required after symptoms are seen. However, the client should be monitored for superinfections and other complications.

Measles vaccines are available. The newer vaccines have minimal side effects and are very effective in preventing the disease. For more details see Appendix C: Immunization.

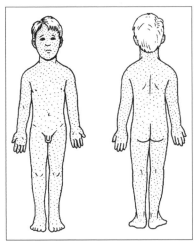

Distribution of rash

areas. Some of the complications of measles include pneumonia, hepatitis, glomerulonephritis, myocarditis and encephalitis.

Risk Factors:

Contact with an infected individual increases the risk. The virus is very contagious and a person with the infection may transmit the virus 5 days after exposure to 5 days after the skin lesions appear.

Caution and Recommendations to Therapists:

Although measles is one of the milder forms of diseases, it can have serious consequences in an individual whose immunity is low. Infected individuals should refrain from work for 5-21 days after exposure, or at least 7 days after the rash appears to ensure that they do not spread the disease. Refer to Appendix B: Strategies for infection prevention and safe practice for some useful guidelines. Also see Appendix D for organizations and support groups.

References

Morello JA, Mizer HE, Wilson ME, Granato PA. Microbiology in patient care. 6th ed. New York: McGraw-Hill; 1998.p. 285-288.

Wood PJ. Measles, mumps, and mud: Childhood epidemics at the turn of the century. Nurs Prac NZ 1993; 8(3): 21-29.

Musculoskeletal system

Medial tibial stress syndrome (Tibial periostitis)

The inflammation of the periosteum in the distal posteromedial aspect of the tibia.

Notes

Rest, support and avoidance of movement that aggravate the pain and painkillers are used. This may be followed by physiotherapy.

For more details see Appendix C: Painkillers.

Cause:

It is caused by excessive use of the posterior tibialis and soleus muscle.

Signs and Symptoms:

This condition is similar to shin splints, but the pain is localized to the distal third of the tibia in the posteromedial aspect. The pain is felt over a discrete area about 3-6 cms in this region. The pain is increased on plantar flexing and turning the foot inwards.

Risk Factors:

Exercises involving plantar flexion and inversion of foot can predispose to this condition.

Caution and Recommendations to Therapists:

In acute cases, the limb is rested for 2-3 days. Apply icepacks, and elevate limb to reduce swelling and inflammation. Later use friction massage, to increase blood flow and prevent adhesions. Gentle stretching also helps. Refer to Physiotherapist for strengthening exercises.

References

Adams JC, Hamblen DL. Outline of orthopaedics. 11th ed. London: Churchill Livingstone; 1990.

Pathology A to Z -

Meningitis

An inflammation of the meninges (the covering of the brain and spinal cord - pia, arachnoid and dura mater).

Cause:

It is usually caused by a bacterial infection but can be due to virus or tuberculosis. The infection often spreads from foci in other regions of the body and may follow pneumonia, osteomyelitis, ear infection, sinusitis etc. Infection may also follow fracture of the skull or invasive procedures such as lumbar puncture or neurosurgery.

Signs and Symptoms:

The person has fever with chills - the generalized symptoms of infection. Due to the inflammation in the intracranial cavity, the pressure of the cerebrospinal fluid is increased producing headache and vomiting. The person resists any movement that tends to stretch the meninges. Hence there is resistance on passively raising the leg of a person with meningitis (*Kernig's sign*). If the neck is flexed passively that too is resisted (*Brudzinski's sign*). Other symptoms include irritability, double vision, drowsiness, convulsions, confusion, delirium and coma.

Risk Factors:

Prolonged untreated or inadequately treated infection in other areas of the body may predispose to meningitis. Bacterial meningitis is more common in children and the elderly.

Caution and Recommendations to Therapists:

Suspect meningitis as the cause of headache if there is a history of sudden onset of headache associated with fever and neck stiffness in a person who has never experienced such a headache before. Do not massage, but refer to a Physician. Viral meningitis can occur as a seasonal epidemic. The virus spreads through the secretions of infected individuals. Scrupulous hand washing prevents spread of disease. Be fully informed of epidemics in your area. Refer to Appendix B: Strategies for infection prevention and safe practice for some useful guidelines. Also see Appendix D for organizations and support groups.

Notes

Meningitis is treated with antibiotics, if bacterial. Other forms of treatment are supportive and include painkillers, bed rest and monitoring of fluid and electrolyte balance. The complications of meningitis may be cranial nerve damage, blockage of flow of the cerebrospinal fluid leading to hydrocephalus.

For more details see Appendix C: Antimicrobial - antibacterial agents; Painkillers.

References

Morello JA, Mizer HE, Wilson ME, Granato PA. Microbiology in patient care. 6th ed. New York: McGraw-Hill; 1998. p. 322-326.

Molluscum contagiosum (Acne varioliformis)

A viral disease of the skin.

Cause:

This is a mildly contagious disease of the skin caused by a virus. It can be transmitted by skin-to-skin contact, fomites or by self-inoculation. The incubation period ranges from 1 week to 6 months.

For more details see Appendix C: Sclerosing agents.

Signs and Symptoms:

Crops of semi-globular, pinhead sized, waxy, pinkish yellow painless growths are seen on the surface of the skin. Typically, each papule has a central depression through which a cheesy secretion can be expressed (see Appendix A: page 354). The papule slowly grows in size and may persist for months or years. Secondary infection may occur. Often, patients do not seek treatment, as the condition is painless.

Risk Factors:

It tends to be more common in those who are immunocompromised.

Caution and Recommendations to Therapists:

It can spread by direct contact. Avoid the area, or cover the lesions with a bandage before massaging. Since the treatment is a simple procedure, advice the client to seek a Physician's help. Refer to Appendix B: Strategies for infection prevention and safe practice for some useful guidelines. Also see Appendix D for organizations and support groups.

References

Morello JA, Mizer HE, Wilson ME, Granato PA. Microbiology in patient care. 6th ed. New York: McGraw-Hill; 1998.

Multiple myeloma (Malignant plasmacytoma; Plasma cell myeloma; Myelomatosis)

Musculoskeletal system

An abnormal and uncontrolled multiplication of plasma cells (type of B-lymphocytes).

Cause:

Notes

It is treated with chemotherapy, radiation and painkillers. For more details see Appendix C: Cancer chemotherapy; Radiation therapy; Painkillers.

The cause is unknown. There is abnormal multiplication of the plasma cells in the bone marrow. The tumor cells infiltrate the skeleton making them prone to pathological fractures. Later other organs of the body are infiltrated.

Signs and Symptoms:

It usually begins as a severe low back pain. Bone pain, and joint swelling may be present. Other signs are found when the weakened vertebra collapses. In late stages, symptoms related to other systems such as the renal and respiratory systems are seen.

Risk Factors:

It is more common in men above the age of 40.

Caution and Recommendations to Therapists:

References

Longo DL. Plasma cell disorders. In: Isselbacher KJ et al, editors. Harrison's principles of internal medicine. 13th ed. New York: McGraw-Hill Inc; 1994. p. 1621-1624.

The disease is often diagnosed after it is wide spread. Consult Physician before massage. These clients are prone to fractures due to the demineralization of bones. Only very light, superficial massage, range of motion and breathing exercises should be considered. If the client is bedridden look for pressure ulcers and avoid area. See Appendix D for organizations and support groups.

Multiple Sclerosis (MS)

A disorder that progressively affects the myelin sheath of the neurons in the brain and spinal cord.

Nervous system

Cause:

The cause is unknown. It may be due to a slow acting viral infection or due to an autoimmune response. Due to the higher prevalence in certain geographical areas, an environmental factor has been implicated. The presence of lymphocytes in the affected neurons suggests an abnormal immunological response. The white matter of the brain - where the myelin is present, is the area affected. The peripheral nervous system is spared. Chronic inflammation, loss of myelin and scarring are characteristics of the disease. Conduction across the affected neuron is slowed and may be altered by changes in body temperature and metabolic environment, explaining the characteristic changes in function from hour to hour.

Signs and Symptoms:

The symptoms vary according to the area and extent of the brain and spinal cord affected. There is exacerbation and remission of the disease with the person symptom-free between the spells in the early stages of the disease. The symptoms last from hours to weeks. It initially presents as numbness and tingling sensations in different regions. Double vision and blurred vision are some of the other symptoms. Weaknesses, muscle paralysis affecting one or more limbs, tremors, gait problems, increased tone of muscles and exaggerated reflexes are other symptoms. Mood swings, irritability and depression may be present. In some, there may be difficulty in speech and swallowing.

Risk Factors:

Studies have shown that if a person moves from an area of greater risk to a lower risk area before the age of 15, the incidence is as in the lower risk area. However, if the migration was after the age of 15, the high risk still prevails. There is also a genetic link as people in the same family are at higher risk. It is more common between the ages of 20-40 and affects more women than men. It affects Caucasians more frequently and the incidence is higher in the higher socioeconomic, urban population. Cold, damp climate increase the risk of MS. Stress, emotional upset and extremes of temperature can precipitate an attack.

The incidence of MS decreases with decreasing latitude - ie. incidence is higher closer to the poles.

Caution and Recommendations to Therapists:

Take time to assess the client thoroughly during every visit as the symptoms vary and progress unpredictability. The symptoms may change from day to day. The aim is to shorten exacerbations, relax the individual, decrease the tone in muscles which are rigid, prevent joint stiffness and contractures. Since hot or cold temperatures can make the symptoms worse, avoid using high heat or cold

Notes

More than 100 treatment options are available. In general, treatment is aimed towards arresting the disease process and to manage the symptoms.

In order to arrest the disease process, drugs to suppress the immune reaction may be given. Glucocorticoids may be given to reduce inflammation. Since it may be due to a chronic viral infection, some options for treatment aim to stimulate the immune system.

Yoga, tai chi, massage are other alternatives that have been found to be beneficial. Drugs to reduce pain, spasticity and depression may be used.

The progress of the disease is variable. In most cases, there is a relapsing and remitting course with complete or partial recovery between relapses. In some cases the course is progressive and chronic with slow continual degradation. In others, it is acute and traumatic with severe disability within a few years.

For more details see Appendix C: Antiinflammatories - steroidal drugs; Painkillers; Antidepressants.

References

Mathews WB et al. McAlpine's multiple sclerosis. New York: Churchill Livingston; 1991.

therapy. Mild heat helps improve circulation and decrease spasticity. Perform range of motion exercises of all joints. Use relaxing strokes while massaging rigid muscles. The strokes should be repetitive and rhythmic. Abdominal massage helps relieve constipation, which is a common problem.

These clients tire easily so the duration of each session should be short in general and should be adjusted according to individual clients. Two half hour sessions per week are recommended but the treatment needs to be ongoing. Moderate exercise programs have been found to be beneficial. Since any kind of infection can precipitate an attack, and since these clients may be on corticosteroids which depresses immunity, avoid treating clients with MS when you have any kind of infection. Encourage clients to join a local support group. See Appendix D for resources.

Mumps

Gastrointestinal system

A viral infection resulting in painful enlargement of the parotid gland (one of the salivary glands).

Notes

There is no specific treatment. Mouth care, use of bland diet and analgesics are beneficial. Vaccines are available to prevent disease.

For more details see Appendix C: Painkillers; Immunization.

Cause:

It is caused by a *paramyxo virus*. The virus is transmitted in salivary secretions of infected individuals. The virus may be secreted in the saliva as early as six days before the onset of symptoms. The virus has been isolated in urine, suggesting that it may spread through this route too. In some patients, the virus has been shown to be present up to 3 weeks after the onset of symptoms. The person is most infective one or two days before symptoms to 5 days after.

The virus enters a person via the respiratory tract and replicates in the upper respiratory tract for about 12-25 days. From here it is distributed via the blood to target organs like the parotid gland, meninges, testis etc.

Signs and Symptoms:

There is a sudden onset of swelling and pain of the parotid gland located near the angle of the jaw. Loss of appetite, fever, and sore throat may follow. If the testis is affected, there is swelling and pain over the area. If the pancreas is inflamed, there may be abdominal pain and tenderness.

Risk Factors:

The incidence is higher in spring.

Caution and Recommendations to Therapists:

Do not treat individuals with mumps, as this is an infectious disease. Therapists who have mumps should stay away from work till all symptoms disappear. Refer to Appendix B: Strategies for infection prevention and safe practice for some useful guidelines. Also see Appendix D for organizations and support groups.

References

Morello JA, Mizer HE, Wilson ME, Granato PA. Microbiology in patient care. 6th ed. New York: McGraw-Hill; 1998. p. 284-285.

Wood PJ. Measles, mumps, and mud: Childhood epidemics at the turn of the century. Nurs Prac NZ 1993; 8(3): 21-29.

Muscular dystrophy (Duchenne's muscular dystrophy; Becker muscular dystrophy; Landouzy-Dejerine dystrophy; Limb-girdle dystrophy)

Musculoskeletal system

A group of congenital disorders that produce symmetrical wasting of skeletal muscles. There is no loss of sensation or neural activity.

Cause:

It is a genetic disorder where there is a decrease/lack of a muscle protein called dystrophin. *Duchenne's* and *Becker's types* are due to defects in the X chromosome.

Signs and Symptoms:

The degree of severity and onset of disease vary according to the type. Duchenne's begins between 3 and 5 years of age and the child may be confined to a wheelchair by age 10. The weakness of muscle starts in the leg and pelvic region. This affects the gait and posture. The muscles may give a false appearance of strength due to the bulk. The bulk is produced by replacement of muscle tissue by fibrous tissue and fat. Becker's type presents as Duchenne's, but progresses more slowly. The *Facio-scapulo-humeral* or *Landouzy-Dejerine dystrophy* weakens the muscles of the face, shoulders and upper arms initially, and then progresses to all muscles. The lips are weak and the patient has difficulty whistling or puckering the mouth. The lack of control over the facial muscles gives the patient a masklike appearance. The *limb-girdle type* starts early (age 6) but progresses slowly, first affecting the upper arm and pelvis. The weakness may spread to the involuntary muscles and produce cardiac failure, constipation etc.

Risk Factors:

Duchenne's and Becker's affect males; the other two types affect both males and females equally.

Caution and Recommendations to Therapists:

There is no cure for the disease. Move all joints actively and passively. Massage helps slow down muscle atrophy. Abdominal massage may help with the constipation that these clients suffer due to the effect of the disorder on the involuntary muscles. Clients with this disorder take a longer time to accomplish every day tasks. Be patient with client while the client climbs on and off table. Keep telephone number and address of local Muscular Dystrophy Associations to refer client for emotional support and genetic counseling. (see Appendix D for resources)

Notes

Steroids have been shown to slow down the progress of Duchenne type. Supportive treatment in the form of orthoses, passive and active stretching to improve range of motion is used on an individual basis.

For more details see Appendix C: Antiinflammatories - steroidal drugs.

References

Mendell JR, Griggs RC. Inherited, metabolism endocrine and toxic myopathies. In: Isselbacher KJ et al, editors. Harrison's principles of internal medicine. 13th ed. New York: McGraw-Hill Inc; 1994. p. 2383-2387.

Myasthenia gravis

An autoimmune, neuromuscular disorder with weakness and fatigability of muscles.

Cause:

It is caused by reduced availability of acetylcholine receptors at the neuromuscular junction. The receptors present in the muscle cell membrane combine with the chemical acetylcholine released by the nerve terminals. This in turn enables the nerve impulses to be propagated into muscle to produce contraction. In this condition, the number of receptors available on the muscle membrane is reduced resulting in decreased efficiency of transmission of impulses.

The abnormality is due to an autoimmune response. It is not known why the response is triggered. It is believed that it is due to an abnormality in the lymphatic organ - thymus.

Signs and Symptoms:

Myasthenia gravis presents as weakness and fatigability of muscles. Initially, the muscles located in the head are affected. Weakness of muscles of the eyelids and eyes is common. Drooping of the eyelids (ptosis), and double vision (diplopia) is present in this case. Difficulty in swallowing, speech and facial weakness are other symptoms that may be present if other muscles are affected. If the weakness is more generalised the respiratory muscles may be affected leading to serious complications. The symptoms may present as exacerbations and remissions and is improved by sleep.

There is no loss of sensation and muscle reflexes are normal.

Risk Factors:

It is more common in women.

Caution and Recommendations to Therapists:

Massage may be helpful in reducing the fatigue in the muscles by increasing circulation and lymph drainage. Stimulatory massage may help improve weakness. If the client is on steroids, they may exhibit the side effects of the

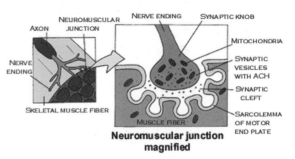

Neuromuscular junction magnified

drug such as lowering of immunity and increased susceptibility to infections. Suitable precautions have to be taken. Encourage the client to take medications. See Appendix D for organizations and support groups.

References

Drachman DB. Myasthenia gravis. In: Isselbacher KJ et al, editors. Harrison's principles of internal medicine. 13th ed. New York: McGraw-Hill Inc; 1994. p.

Myositis ossificans

Musculoskeletal system

Ossification in a muscle.

Cause:

The cause is usually trauma to a muscle followed by bleeding, inflammation and fibrosis. Deposition of bone-forming tissue in the muscle can result in calcification producing this condition. The osteoblasts (bone forming cells) may originate from the injured periosteum adjacent to the injured muscle or could be by transformation of cells in the injured tissue. The ossified tissue, apart from restricting movement serves as a constant source of irritation to the surrounding soft tissue.

Signs and Symptoms:

The individual gives a history of fracture or trauma which is followed by reduced movement, pain and swelling in the local area. A hard mass may be felt in the injured region.

Risk Factors:

The brachialis muscle is a common site for myositis ossificans. The incidence is higher after a supracondylar fracture and posterior dislocation of the elbow. Some believe that the risk is higher if a fractured part is mobilized too soon, too vigorously.

Caution and Recommendations to Therapists:

Do not forcibly mobilize joints especially the elbow, if there is restriction to extension. Consult Physician regarding the cause of the restriction before embarking on mobilization techniques. Tenderness, signs of inflammation (swelling, increase in temperature etc.) in an injured muscle especially in the brachialis should be treated with great caution. Massage should be avoided in and around the area.

References

Adams JC, Hamblen DL. Outline of orthopaedics. 11 Ed. New York: Churchill Livingstone; 1990. p. 52.

Nasal polyps

Respiratory system

A rounded growth arising from the mucosa of the nose or sinus.

Cause:

They are thought to be a result of allergy and infection. Due to recurrent infection and allergic reaction there is edema of the nasal or sinus mucosa

Notes

Medical treatment is the same as that for allergic rhinitis. Steroid nasal sprays may be used to reduce the inflammatory reaction. Surgery is done to remove the polyp. However, recurrences are common.

For more details see Appendix C: Antihistamines; Antiinflammatories - steroidal drugs; Nose drops/nasal decongestants.

References

Maran AGD, editor. Logan Turner's diseases of the nose, throat and ear. 10th ed. London: Wright; 1988. p. 54-55.

causing it to protrude as a rounded, smooth, soft, glistening mass with a narrow neck. Polyps commonly arise from the ethmoid sinuses. Rarely, it arises from the mucosa of the maxillary sinus. Cystic fibrosis may cause polyp formation.

Signs and Symptoms:

Depending on the size of the polyp, the person has nasal block and increased nasal secretion. In some cases, the polyp may be visible through the nostril.

Risk Factors:

Repeated upper respiratory infection and allergic rhinitis predispose to polyp formation.

Caution and Recommenations to Therapists:

Often these individuals have a history of allergy. Ensure that there are no allergens in the clinic that may trigger an allergic reaction.

Necrotizing fasciitis (Hemolytic streptococcal gangrene; Flesh eating disease)

Musculoskeletal system

A bacterial infection involving the fascia surrounding the muscles.

Cause:

Notes

Once diagnosed, the condition has to be treated aggressively by exploratory surgery. The area has to be drained and dead tissue removed. Antibiotic treatment is also necessary. For more details see Appendix C: Antimicrobial - antibacterial agents.

References

Morello JA, Mizer HE, Wilson ME, Granato PA. Microbiology in patient care. 6th ed. New York: McGraw-Hill; 1998.

Wessels MR. Streptococcal infections. In: Isselbacher KJ et al, editors. Harrison's principles of internal medicine. 13th ed. New York: McGraw-Hill Inc; 1994. p. 620.

The source of infection is varied. Organisms in the skin may be introduced into the deep tissue by trauma. Sometimes the organisms are part of the bacterial flora located in the gut, which have been disseminated during abdominal surgery. They may also be from abscesses located deep in the body.

Signs and Symptoms:

There is severe pain at the site of infection accompanied by fever and chills. There may be redness of skin over the site. The infection progresses in a matter of hours and edema is seen. There may be loss of sensation if the inflammation has spread to local nerves.

Risk Factors:

See Cause.

Caution and Recommendations to Therapists:

It is a serious, infectious condition. Be informed about cases diagnosed in your area. Refer to Appendix B: Strategies for infection prevention and safe practice for some useful guidelines. Also see Appendix D for organizations and support groups.

Nephrotic syndrome

Collection of symptoms that result from leaky glomeruli that allow plasma protein to be filtered.

Renal system

Cause:

It can be a result of chronic glomerular disease. Diabetes mellitus and systemic lupus erythematosus are other disorders that result in increased permeability of the glomeruli.

Signs and Symptoms:

The loss of protein in the urine along with the retention of sodium and water causes extensive generalized edema. The loss of antibodies (immunoglobulins) makes the individual susceptible to infections. Loss of blood factors (also plasma proteins) that inhibit coagulation makes the person prone to thrombus formation. The increased level of lipids in the blood that results, makes the individual prone to atherosclerosis. The blood pressure is elevated.

Risk Factors:

See Cause.

Caution and Recommendations to Therapists:

A very light, soothing massage of short duration can be given. If the symptoms are severe, get clearance from the treating Physician. Do not try to reduce the edema that is present as it may overload the heart. Encourage client to be active as it can help reduce the chances of thrombus formation. These individuals are susceptible to infections as they may be on steroids. Avoid treating if harboring any infection. See Appendix D for organizations and support groups.

Notes

This condition is treated supportively. Diet restriction and antibiotics, diuretics and corticosteroids form part of the treatment regime. For more details see Appendix C: Antimicrobial - antibacterial agents; Antiinflammatories - steroidal drugs; Diuretics.

References

Glassock RJ, Brenner BM. The major glomerulopathies. In: Isselbacher KJ et al, editors. Harrison's principles of internal medicine. 13th ed. London: McGraw-Hill Co; 1994. p. 1299-1308.

Nerve entrapment syndromes (Entrapment neuropathies)

Includes conditions that result in continuous or intermittent compression of peripheral nerves.

Musculoskeletal, Nervous systems

Cause:

Some peripheral nerves are especially prone to compression as they pass through specific regions that do not allow them to escape the effects of pressure from surrounding areas.

Signs and Symptoms:

The symptoms and signs vary with the degree of compression and whether it is continuous or intermittent. Pain and loss of sensation may be present along the distribution of the nerve that is trapped. Muscles supplied by the nerve are atrophied and weak.

Notes

Most often, the symptoms and signs are reversed once the cause of the compression has been identified and treated.

One of the common nerve entrapment syndromes is *Carpal tunnel syndrome* (see Carpal tunnel syndrome) where the median nerve is 'entrapped'. The ulnar nerve may be trapped at the elbow (*delayed* or *tardy ulnar palsy, cubital tunnel syndrome*) as it passes through a groove behind the medial epicondyle. In this case, the patient complains of pain and loss of sensation along the distribution of the ulnar nerve (medial aspect of forearm). The radial nerve may be compressed at the axilla (*crutch palsy*). Here the patient may experience pain and loss of

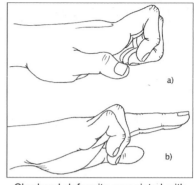

Clawhand deformity associated with
a) Ulnar nerve palsy
b) Median nerve and Ulnar nerve palsy

sensation along the distribution of the radial nerve. The extensor muscles of the finger and wrist are affected.

The brachial plexus may be entrapped at the thoracic outlet (*scalenus syndrome*). The signs and symptoms depend on the nerve affected. The tibial nerve, a branch of the sciatic nerve, may be injured as it passes over the popliteus and under the soleus muscle. This is known as the *popliteal entrapment syndrome.* At the ankle the nerve may be compressed as it passes through the tarsal tunnel. The tarsal tunnel is formed by the medial malleolus, calcaneus and talus on one side and the tibiocalcaneal ligament on the other. This is known as the *tarsal tunnel syndrome.* Sometimes,

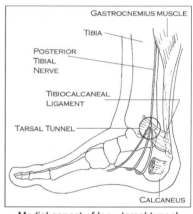

Medial aspect of leg - tarsal tunnel

the digital nerves of the foot may be compressed (*Morton's metatarsalgia*). This is more common in women who wear excessively tight shoes.

Risk Factors:

See Cause, Signs and Symptoms.

Caution and Recommendations to Therapists:

Knowledge of the distribution of the nerve that is entrapped is required. The Therapist has to familiarize with the area of skin from which the nerve carries sensations and the muscles supplied by the motor component of the nerve. Knowledge of the origin, insertion and action of the muscles affected as well as the synergists and antagonists to this movement is required to effectively treat

Pathology A to Z -

the specific nerve entrapment syndrome.

In general, the soft tissue along the path of the nerve affected should be gently stretched in a direction perpendicular to the direction of nerve, without direct pressure on the nerve. The muscles supplied by the nerve are weak and tend to atrophy. The aim should be to stimulate these muscles and strengthen them. On the other hand, the muscles that are synergists are overloaded with increased tone. The strokes used on these muscles should aim to relax them. Care should be taken not to use excessive pressure in areas of skin where the sensation is affected. Vibration and tapotement may be used to stimulate the sensory nerves.

See under Carpal tunnel syndrome and Cubital tunnel syndrome for specific details on treatment. The radial nerve descends on the posterior aspect of the arm, lying medial to the humerus in the upper 2/3rds before going to the lateral side and behind the elbow. It travels posteriorly on the lateral aspect of the radius to reach the hand at the base of the thumb. Entrapment of this nerve at the axilla results in loss of sensation on the dorsal surface of the 1st to 3rd fingers and half of the 4th finger up to the proximal interphalangeal joints. Depending on the location of injury, sensations may be lost on the posterior aspect of the arm. The client has difficulty extending and abducting the thumb and the proximal phalanges of the other fingers. 'Wristdrop hand' where the client is unable to lift the fingers or hand, and difficulty in extending the elbow may be present.

References:

Turchaninov R, Cox CA. Medical massage. Scottsdale: Stress Less publishing Inc; 1998. p. 228-281.

Hackwood RA. Conservative treatment plan for carpal tunnel syndrome. BC Massage Practitioner 1997; Fall 17 (1):19-22.

Neurofibromatosis (NF; Von Recklinghausen's disease; Neurofibroma; Neurofibromata; Multiple neuroma; Neuromatosis)

Musculoskeletal, Integumentary, Nervous, Endocrine, Renal systems

An inherited disorder affecting many systems characterized by formation of soft, multiple tumors along peripheral nerves.

Cause:

It is caused by defects in chromosome 17 or 22. It is inherited from an affected parent and there is 50% chance of the child inheriting the defective gene, regardless of sex. Since it is a dominant trait the disease is seen in an affected child even if one parent is normal. In 50% of cases, it is caused by a new mutation ie. a new defect in the chromosome. The symptoms are caused by abnormal multiplication of tissue - Schwann cells and fibroblasts, that surrounds peripheral nerves.

Signs and Symptoms:

It is characterized by multiple, soft growths of varying sizes along the nerves. There may be uniformly darkened, large, flat lesions on the skin. The skin lesions are known as *café au lait spots*. The symptoms usually appear in childhood or adolescence and may stop as the child matures. The growths may produce additional symptoms by compressing surrounding tissues. Compression of nerves inside the skull or spinal column can produce neurological problems like blindness, seizures, mental deficiency etc. In addition, other

Notes

There is no specific treatment. Patient education and genetic counselling are important aspects. For more details see Appendix C: Genetic testing / Counselling.

systems may be involved. Skeletal involvement can produce scoliosis, kyphosis and vertebral column defects. It can also affect the endocrine system resulting in hyper or hyposecretion of various glands. Renal failure may result if the kidney is affected.

Risk Factors:

See Cause.

Caution and Recommendations to Therapists:

References

Caviness VS. Neurocutaneous syndromes and other developmental disorders of the central nervous system. In: Isselbacher KJ et al, editors. Harrison's principles of internal medicine. 13th ed. New York: McGraw-Hill Inc; 1994. p. 2330.

This is a genetic condition, and not infective, though the skin and tumors may look unsightly. It is important for the Therapist to provide emotional support to the client who may be marginalized by society because of the appearance of the skin. A detailed history should be taken to assess the extent of the disease and massage treatment individualized accordingly. There is no danger of spreading the tumors by massage. Refer client to local support groups and for genetic counselling if in the reproductive age group (see Appendix D for resources).

Respiratory, Cardiovascular, Nervous, Gastrointestinal systems

Nicotine addiction

A compulsive use of cigarettes, with signs of tolerance, physical and psychological dependence.

Cause:

The cause of nicotine addiction is multifactorial and complex. Personal and environmental factors play an important role.

Notes

More than 80% of ex-smokers quit "cold turkey". Some may benefit from cessation programs that are available. Prevention in the pediatric and adolescent age group is most effective.

The composition of smoke from the combustion of tobacco leaf is responsible for the varying short term and long term effects of cigarette smoking. More than 4000 substances have been identified in the smoke. Many of the constituents of smoke are carcinogenic (produce cancer). Some reduce the activity of the cilia in the respiratory tract and irritate the mucosa with resultant increase in mucus secretion. Nicotine produces its effects by increasing catecholamine release - resulting in signs of sympathetic nervous system stimulation. Carbon monoxide, which is one of the constituents, affects the transport of oxygen to the tissues.

Signs and Symptoms:

Those with nicotine addiction use cigarettes compulsively, exhibiting signs of tolerance and physical and psychological dependence.

Large population studies have shown the association between smoking and diseases such as atherosclerosis; angina pectoris; myocardial infarction; cerebrovascular disease (eg. stroke); thromboangiitis obliterans; hypertension; chronic obstructive pulmonary disease (eg. emphysema, bronchitis) and cancer. Peptic ulcers are more common in smokers. Many cancers such as lung cancer are associated with smoking. Adverse effects are seen in the fetus when women smoke during pregnancy.

Involuntary smoke inhalation has also been associated with many of these disorders.

Risk Factors:

The risk of becoming addicted to smoking is very complex and is affected by personal and environmental factors.

Caution and Recommendations to Therapists:

It may be advisable to have a 'No smoking' sign in the clinic as smoking may discourage non-smokers from using your services. Also, smoke in the air may provoke symptoms in clients with lung disorders. Never smoke in the clinic if you are a smoker. Ensure that there is no trace of smoke on your body during a session as it is offensive to some individuals.

Since smoking is the leading cause of many disorders, the Therapist should encourage clients to give up smoking. Making information about the harmful effects of smoking available in the clinic may be the first step.

References

Fiore MC, editor. Cigarette smoking : A clinical guide to assessment and treatment. Med Clinic North Am 1992; 76: 289.

U.S. Department of Health and Human Services: The health benefits of smoking cessation. A report of the Surgeon General. DHHS(CDC) Publication no 90-8416, 1990.

Nutritional deficiencies - Vitamin A

Gastrointestinal system

The deficiency of Vitamin A which is one of the fat-soluble vitamins.

Cause:

It is usually caused by inadequate intake of foodstuff high in this vitamin. High levels of vitamin A is present in liver, kidney, butter, milk, cream, cheese, fortified margarine, green leafy vegetables, egg yolk, yellow and orange fruits. Since this vitamin is fat soluble, deficiency states are also found in those who have difficulty in absorbing fats. Fat absorption is altered in people with liver disorders, malabsorption syndromes etc.

Notes

The recommended dietary allowance is 1,400 IU (children); 4000-5000 IU (adults); 6000 IU (lactating women).

Signs and Symptoms:

Since vitamin A participates in the functioning of the receptors in the eye, as well as in the formation of epithelium and bone growth, symptoms are associated with these sites. The first symptom is *night blindness*- difficulty in seeing in dark places. Drying of the conjunctiva with thickened gray colored spots in the conjunctiva are other symptoms. Untreated, this can lead to blindness. The skin is dry and scaly. The hardening and drying of the mucous membranes makes them prone to infections.

Risk Factors:

See Cause.

Caution and Recommendations to Therapists:

Encourage clients to eat green leafy vegetables and fruits along with adequate intake of dairy products. Those with problems in absorption may require Vitamin A in the form of injections. Advice clients on the harmful effects of

References

Wilson JD. Vitamin deficiency and excess. In: Isselbacher KJ et al, editors.Harrison's principles of internal medicine. 13th ed. New York: McGraw-Hill Inc; 1994. p. 472-479.

excessive intake of vitamin supplements (see Hypervitaminosis). Use oil liberally while massaging clients with dry skin. Refer clients complaining of night-blindness to a Physician.

Nutritional deficiencies – Vitamin B

The deficiency of Vitamin B complex - a group of water-soluble vitamins.

Cause:

It usually results from inadequate intake or malabsorption of the vitamins.

Vitamin B1 - thiamine deficiency is seen in those whose staple diet is unenriched rice or wheat. Malnourishment, alcoholism and pregnancy are other conditions that can predispose to thiamine deficiency.

Vitamin B2 - riboflavin deficiency results when the intake of milk, meat, fish, green leafy vegetables are inadequate. Absorption of this vitamin is reduced in alcoholics and in those with prolonged diarrhea.

Niacin - another of the B complex vitamins, is seen in those whose diet lacks animal protein or whose staple food is corn.

Pyridoxine (B6) deficiency is usually a side effect of those taking drugs such as isoniazid (antituberculosis) which are pyridoxine antagonists.

Cobalamin - vitamin B12 deficiency usually results in those with difficulty in absorption of Vitamin B12. Vitamin B12 requires a factor - called *intrinsic factor* that is secreted by the stomach, for proper absorption in the ileum. Those who lack this intrinsic factor or those who have had surgery where the stomach or ileum has been removed can show signs of cobalamin deficiency.

Signs and Symptoms:

These vitamins are required for cell growth, bone formation and normal breakdown of food products.

Vitamin B1 deficiency - Beriberi, mainly affects the nervous system. Irritability, mental disturbances, gait abnormalities are some of the symptoms. It can also be a cause of edema. Abdominal pain, vomiting, convulsions are other symptoms. It also affects the cardiovascular system producing enlargement of the heart, rapid heart rate and cardiac failure.

Riboflavin deficiency produces cracking of the lips and corners of the mouth, sore throat, inflammation of the tongue. The skin appears dry and scaly. In children the growth may be slowed.

Niacin deficiency produces vague symptoms such as fatigue, loss of appetite, muscle weakness, weight loss, indigestion etc. In advanced stages (*pellagra*), the skin becomes darkened and scaly. (See Appendix A: page 354).The mouth, tongue and lips become sore. The central nervous system may be affected with confusion and other mental disturbances. It is also called the "*3-D syndrome*" - Dementia, Diarrhea and Dermatitis. Pyridoxine deficiency resembles that of niacin deficiency.

B12 deficiency affects the development of red blood cells and results in anemia. Anemia produced by B12 deficiency is known as *Pernicious anemia*. Associated symptoms include loss of weight, constipation, diarrhea, inflammation of the tongue and nervous disorders like spasticity of the muscles and gait abnormalities.

Risk Factors:

See Cause.

Caution and Recommendations to Therapists:

Use oil liberally in those with dry scaly skin. Encourage clients to take a well balanced diet. While vitamin supplements do have a role to play, there is no substitute for a well balanced diet.

References

Wilson JD. Vitamin deficiency and excess. In: Isselbacher KJ et al, editors. Harrison's principles of internal medicine. 13th ed. New York: McGraw-Hill Inc; 1994. p. 472-479.

Nutritional deficiencies - Vitamin C

(Scurvy)

Integumentary, Cardiovascular, Gastrointestinal systems

A condition where there is a deficiency of ascorbic acid - vitamin C, a water-soluble vitamin.

Cause:

It is usually due to the deficient intake of vitamin C in the diet. Vitamin C is destroyed by overcooking and on overexposure to air. So deficiency may result if the cooking process destroys it.

Signs and Symptoms:

Since vitamin C is required for the production of collagen - a component of connective tissue that helps bind cells of teeth, bones and capillaries together, deficiency of it presents as abnormalities in these tissues. The capillaries become fragile and break easily. Small spots of bleeding (*purpura* and *petechiae*) under the skin are seen. (See Appendix A: page 355). The person is anemic, with loss of appetite, limb and joint pain. The gums become swollen and bleed easily. Wounds take a longer time to heal. Irritability and depression are some of the psychological problems. This disease is potentially fatal.

Risk Factors:

See Cause.

Caution and Recommendations to Therapists:

Encourage client to drink fresh orange juice. Advice client on the harm of taking too much vitamin C. Excess Vitamin C causes, vomiting, diarrhea and formation of stone in the kidney. Do not use excessive pressure, as the client tends to bleed easily.

Notes

Citrus fruits, tomatoes, cabbage, broccoli, spinach and berries are some of the food rich in vitamin C.

About 100-200mg of vitamin C is required per day. The vitamin has to be replenished every day, as it cannot be stored.

References

Wilson JD. Vitamin deficiency and excess. In: Isselbacher KJ et al, editors. Harrison's principles of internal medicine. 13th ed. New York: McGraw-Hill Inc; 1994. p. 472-479.

Nutritional deficiencies - Vitamin D

(Rickets; Osteomalacia)

A condition due to the deficiency of Vitamin D - calciferol, a fat-soluble vitamin.

Cause:

Notes

Injection of Vitamin D is required for those with deficiency due to malabsorption. Recommended dietary allowance: 400 IU daily.

Vitamin D can result from inadequate intake, malabsorption in the gut or low exposure to sunlight. Rarely, it occurs as an inherited disorder where there is excessive loss of phosphates in the urine. Vitamin D being fat-soluble is not absorbed in gastrointestinal disorders that affect fat absorption - liver disease, malabsorption syndrome, obstruction to the bile duct etc. Since vitamin D requires normal secretion of parathormone from the parathyroid gland, and is altered to its active form in the kidney and liver, diseases of parathyroid gland, liver or kidney can also result in deficiency states.

Signs and Symptoms:

Vitamin D is required for normal bone formation as it participates in the absorption and regulation of calcium and phosphorus and its lack present as bone deformities. Early symptoms are excessive sweating, restlessness and irritability. The bones become soft resulting in bow legs, knock knees, pigeon chest, enlargement of the wrist and ankles and thickening of the costochondral junction. These deformities can produce problems in walking, climbing stairs etc.

Risk Factors:

Breast-fed infants who do not have supplements are prone to this problem. It is more common in overcrowded urban areas.

References

Wilson JD. Vitamin deficiency and excess. In: Isselbacher KJ et al, editors.Harrison's principles of internal medicine. 13th ed. New York: McGraw-Hill Inc; 1994. p. 472-479.

Caution and Recommendations to Therapists:

The bones are prone to fracture easily. Only light pressure should be used while massaging these individuals. Encourage clients to increase intake of vitamin rich foodstuff such as cod liver oil, herring, liver, egg yolk, and fortified milk. Exposure to the sun should also be encouraged.

Nutritional deficiencies - Vitamin E

Deficiency of vitamin E - tocopherol, a fat-soluble vitamin.

Cause:

It is usually caused by malabsorption of fat from the gut as in malabsorption syndrome, liver disease, bile duct blockage etc. Vitamin E is required for normal metabolism of fatty acids and other lipids inside the cells. Rarely, low intake of vitamin E causes this problem. Deficiency may also result in people whose diet includes high consumption of polyunsaturated fatty acids. Diets rich in Vitamin E are vegetable oils, green leafy vegetables, nuts and legumes.

Signs and Symptoms:

Deficiency of vitamin E is difficult to recognize. It can present with edema, red raised skin lesions that slowly peels, or muscle weakness. In newborn children it can present as anemia.

Risk Factors:

See Cause.

Caution and Recommendations to Therapists:

Encourage client to take a well balanced diet.

References

Wilson JD. Vitamin deficiency and excess. In: Isselbacher KJ et al, editors.Harrison's principles of internal medicine. 13th ed. New York: McGraw-Hill Inc; 1994. p. 472-479.

Nutritional deficiencies - Vitamin K

Deficiency of Vitamin K, a fat-soluble vitamin - one of the components required for normal coagulation of blood.

Cardiovascular, Gastrointestinal systems

Cause:

Vitamin K is normally produced by the organisms present in the intestines. Drugs such as antibiotics that destroy these organisms in the gut can lead to vitamin K deficiency. The anticoagulant dicoumarol that is given to people with venous thrombosis, reduces thrombus formation by antagonizing vitamin K. Therefore, in a person on prolonged treatment with anticoagulants, vitamin K deficiency occurs. In those with difficulty in the digestion and absorption of fat, this deficiency may result. Liver disease, bile duct obstruction, malabsorption syndrome are some of the other conditions that can lead to such a state. Rarely, it may due to inadequate intake of vitamin K.

Notes

Replacement therapy is required if the vitamin is deficient. Injections have to be given if the deficiency is due to inadequate absorption.

Signs and Symptoms:

The main symptom is a tendency to bleed easily and an increase in time for clotting to occur (see Appendix A: page 355; Purpura). The bleeding can be severe and fatal.

Risk Factors:

See Cause.

Caution and Recommendations to Therapists:

A proper history is required from a client who is on anticoagulant therapy. Since there is a tendency to bleed, pressure can cause tiny bleeding spots under the skin. A very gentle and light massage is all that should be attempted in such clients. Vitamin K deficiency can be treated very easily and it may be best to postpone a massage till adequate treatment has been taken. If the deficiency has resulted in a client on treatment for venous thrombosis, consult Physician before scheduling a massage.

References

Wilson JD. Vitamin deficiency and excess. In: Isselbacher KJ et al, editors.Harrison's principles of internal medicine. 13th ed. New York: McGraw-Hill Inc; 1994. p. 472-479.

Obesity

An increase in adipose tissue that imparts a health risk. It has been shown that weights exceeding 20% of the expected weight for that age, sex and height is a definite health risk.

Notes

If obesity is secondary to some other disease, the underlying disease has to be treated.

For most people, obesity is an eating disorder and the causes of overeating have to be understood for long-term effect of treatment. In primary obesity, measures are taken to reduce weight. One of the methods is to alter the diet.

In general, a deficit of 7700 kcal results in the loss of approximately 1kg fat. Many different types of diets are available in the market. They are to be taken under medical supervision as these diets may be harmful if a person has associated conditions where such diets are contraindicated.

Another measure that is used for weight reduction is behaviour modification, where abnormal patterns of eating behaviour are targeted. Incorporation of exercise regimes along with the diet and behaviour modification improves the chance of maintaining the weight loss.

Drugs used for weight loss have an effect on the hypothalamus. They are effective on a short-term basis and may complicate the situation further by habituation, addiction etc.

References

Olefsky JM. Obesity. In: Isselbacher KJ et al, editors. Harrison's principles of internal medicine. 13th ed. New York: McGraw-Hill Inc; 1994. p. 446-452.

Obesity: Basic aspects and clinical implications. Med Clin North Am 1989; 73:1.

Foster DW. Eating disorders: Obesity and anorexia nervosa. In: JD Wilson,

Foster DW, editors. Williams' textbook of Endocrinology. Philadelphia: Saunders; 1992. p. 1335.

Cause:

It is caused by intake of nutrients more than the expenditure or when the expenditure is less than the intake. Many factors influence the intake. There are feeding centers and satiety centers located in the hypothalamus that regulate the intake in accordance to the glucose/insulin levels in the blood. These centers also sense the distention of the stomach and the amount of body fat. In addition, the centers are sensitive to catecholamine levels. This explains the weight loosing effect of the drug amphetamine. However, ultimately the cerebral cortex controls the eating behavior. Thus psychological, social and genetic factors have an effect on weight.

Obesity may be secondary to other diseases like Hypothyroidism, Cushing's disease and hypothalamic disorders, among others.

To be accurate, obesity is determined by measuring the thickness of the skin in various areas of the body like the skin over the triceps or below the scapula.

Signs and Symptoms:

Obesity is associated with an increase in the incidence of many diseases. The incidence of Diabetes mellitus is higher. This may be due to the resistance of tissues in obese individuals to insulin. The increased levels of cholesterol in the bile make these individuals prone for developing gallstones. The excess mechanical and physical stress on various body-systems result in disorders like osteoarthritis, sciatica, varicose veins, thromboembolism and hernias. Hypertension, atherosclerosis are also common increasing the risk of angina and stroke.

Risk Factors:

See Cause.

Caution and Recommendations to Therapists:

Most obese individuals have a low self-esteem so Therapists have to be sensitive to the needs of these individuals. Excessive pressure may be needed to massage even the superficial muscles. Ensure that the massage table is sufficiently steady. After a good rapport has been established, encourage client to lose weight by altering dietary intake, behavior modification and lifestyle. See Appendix D for organizations and support groups.

Osteochondrosis (Osgood-Schlatter disease)

A painful, incomplete separation of the epiphysis of the tibial tubercle from the tibial shaft and/or tendinitis of the patellar tendon at its insertion to the tibial tubercle.

Musculoskeletal system

Cause:

Trauma to the area before the fusion of the tibial epiphysis before adulthood is the most common cause. The trauma may be a single episode or repeated knee flexion against an unyielding quadriceps. It affects single or both knees.

Signs and Symptoms:

It presents as a constant ache, pain and tenderness below the patella, which is worsened on climbing stairs, squatting or any activity involving flexion of knee. Signs of inflammation - heat, swelling and tenderness may be present.

Risk Factors:

It is more common in active adolescent boys. Genetic factors are also associated.

Caution and Recommendations to Therapists:

Ice massage and rest are recommended in the initial stages. This condition used to be treated by immobilization for 6-8 weeks, but recently rehabilitative exercises are used. Stretching with ankle dorsiflexion and strengthening of leg muscles should be resorted to if weakness is found. Patellar support also helps. Use friction massage around the knee to stretch collagen fibres and reduce adhesions.

Notes

The inefficient use of the extensors is targeted by rehabilitative exercises. Stretching and strengthening exercises are useful. Support to the knee is also beneficial.

References

Adams JC, Hamblen DL. Outline of orthopaedics. 11 Ed. New York: Churchill Livingstone; 1990

Osteogenesis imperfecta

(Brittle bones; Fragilitas ossium)

Musculoskeletal system

An inherited disorder that affects the development of connective tissue and bones.

Cause:

It is transmitted to a child from an affected parent, regardless of sex, usually as a dominant trait.

Signs and Symptoms:

The signs and symptoms vary according to whether it is of mild, moderate or severe type. It is characterized by thin and underdeveloped bones that are prone to fracture with the most trivial trauma. In a child, the face appears triangular due to the soft and prominent forehead. The person is short in stature, with thin skin, blue sclera, hypotonic muscles and loose-jointedness.

Risk Factors:

See Cause.

Notes

There is no effective treatment. Physical therapy and surgical management of fractures are some forms of treatment that may be required. For more details see Appendix C: Genetic testing / Counselling.

a Handbook for Massage Therapists

References

Adams JC, Hamblen DL. Outline of orthopaedics. 11 Ed. New York: Churchill Livingstone; 1990. p. 44.

Caution and Recommendations to Therapists:

Do not massage a client with this condition, as they are very prone to fractures.

Musculoskeletal system	# Osteomyelitis
	A bone infection.

Cause:

Notes

It is treated with long term antibiotics and surgery to remove dead tissue or foreign bodies like metal plates etc. For more details see Appendix C: Antimicrobial - antibacterial agents.

Osteomyelitis (*osteo* - bone; *myelo* - bone marrow) can be caused iatrogenically - ie. as a complication after surgical or other treatment. Infection can also be spread to the bone through the blood from another infected site. Direct contamination as in gun shot wound, trauma, open fracture, or by spreading from an adjacent infection are other causes. Infection persisting beyond 6-8 weeks is considered to be chronic osteomyelitis. This is usually due to inadequately treated acute osteomyelitis.

Signs and Symptoms:

Symptoms vary according to whether it is acute or chronic. In acute osteomyelitis, the tibia, femur, humerus or radius are affected more frequently. The patient has fever along with pain, redness and swelling over the bone. In chronic osteomyelitis, there may be shortening or lengthening of the limb due to overgrowth caused by increased blood flow to the area. If the joints are affected, deformity, stiffening and dislocation may occur.

Risk Factors:

Open fracture, gunshot wounds, extensive tissue injury with contamination, complication of surgery involving bones and joints are all risk factors. Osteomyelitis is more common in those below 20 years of age.

Caution and Recommendations to Therapists:

References

Adams JC, Hamblen DL. Outline of orthopaedics. 11 Ed. New York: Churchill Livingstone; 1990. p. 66-71.

In clients with unhealed or recently healed wounds keep the area covered with bandage and avoid local massage. In clients who have been healed, the aim is to help restore the strength of muscles around the affected area and improve movement in stiff joints if not ankylosed. Use friction strokes and vibration around adherent scars. Olive oil can be used to help soften the fibrous tissue. If there are signs of inflammation or pus discharge from an old scar it indicates reinfection. Stop treatment and refer to Physician. Refer to Appendix B: Strategies for infection prevention and safe practice for some useful guidelines. Also see Appendix D for organizations and support groups.

Osteoporosis

A disorder where bone resorption is greater than bone formation.

Cause:

It occurs as part of the aging process and begins around the age of 25. It can also result from endocrine disorders or malignancy. In this condition both the organic as well as the mineral content of bone is reduced.

Signs and Symptoms:

The bone is fragile and brittle and fractures easily with minimal stress. Bone pain and stress fractures are usually the first symptoms.

Risk Factors:

Osteoporosis is more common in postmenopausal women. The progress is also faster in women as compared to men. Reduced sex hormone levels in the blood have been shown to speed up resorption of bone. Caucasians are affected more often. Poor nutrition, decrease in intestinal absorption of calcium and a sedentary lifestyle are some of the predisposing factors. It may also be caused by excessive exercise. Osteoporosis is common in people with endocrine disorders such as hyperthyroidism, hyperparathyroidism, Cushing's syndrome, diabetes mellitus and with prolonged use of corticosteroids. Aluminium containing antacids that increase calcium excretion and anticonvulsants are some of the drugs that increase the risk of osteoporosis.

Cigarette smoking, high protein diet, alcoholism and family history of osteoporosis are other known risk factors. Prolonged immobilization of a limb increases resorption of bone and osteoporosis. It is also seen in people with rheumatoid arthritis.

Caution and Recommendations to Therapists:

Encourage clients to exercise. Use gentle massage avoiding undue pressure over bones in all postmenopausal and geriatric clients.

Notes

Osteoporosis is detected by gauging the density of bones. It is best treated by elimination of risk factors and adequate dietary intake of calcium. The normal requirement of calcium in an adult is 800 mg per day. The requirement is more during pregnancy and nursing. Good calcium supplements are available in the form of calcium gluconate or calcium citrate.

Postmenopausal women are treated with estrogen therapy to slow down the process. However, estrogen therapy may predispose to some forms of uterine cancer.

For more details see Appendix C: Hormone therapy / replacement; Cancer chemotherapy.

References

Porth CM, editor. Pathophysiology – concepts of altered health states. 4th ed Philadelphia:. JB Lippincott Co; 1994. p. 1233-1235.

Otitis media

An inflammation of the middle ear.

Cause:

It is usually caused by dysfunction of the Eustachian tube. The Eustachian tube connects the pharynx to the middle ear and equalises the pressure between the middle and external ear. Inflammation in the pharynx due to upper respiratory tract infection or influenza, sinusitis, allergic rhinitis etc. can cause blockage of the tube and otitis media.

Notes

The cause has to be treated. Nasal decongestants and antihistamines are some forms of treatment. Antibiotics may be needed if it is due to bacterial infection. In chronic otitis media, surgery may be required to close the abnormal opening in the tympanic membrane.

For more details see Appendix C:
Antimicrobial - antibacterial agents;
Antihistamines; Nose drops / nasal
decongestants.

Signs and Symptoms:

The person complains of difficulty in hearing, popping of the ears and a feeling of pressure. Other symptoms of upper respiratory infection may be present. If the condition is chronic, there may be a discharge through the external ear or ringing in the ear (tinnitus).

Rarely, the infection may spread to surrounding areas and produce complications. Complications include mastoiditis (spread to the mastoid), labyrinthitis (spread to the inner ear), facial nerve paralysis (the facial nerve is in close proximity before it exits the skull), meningitis and brain abscess (if it spreads into the cranium) among others.

Risk Factors:

See Cause. It is more common in children as the Eustachian tube is shorter and the lumen smaller.

Caution and Recommendations to Therapists:

References

Maran AGD, editor. Logan Turner's
diseases of the nose, throat and ear. 10th
ed. London: Wright; 1988. p. 278-281,283-
293.

Avoid massage if the symptoms are acute and the person has concurrent upper respiratory tract infection. For those with chronic otitis media, ensure that the ears are plugged with cotton and discharge from the ears do not contaminate the linen as the position of the client is changed.

Reproductive system	# Ovarian cysts
	Fluid-filled cavities in the ovary.

Cause:

Notes

Ovarian cysts usually disappear
spontaneously and do not require
treatment. In some, it is treated with
hormones like progesterone that cause
the cysts to regress. Surgery may be
done for abnormally large cysts, or those
that show malignant changes.

For more details see Appendix C:
Hormone therapy/ replacement.

Ovarian cysts are usually formed by the persistence of follicles that mature during every menstrual cycle. The cysts may be single or multiple.

Signs and Symptoms:

It is usually asymptomatic. In some, a dull aching pain may be felt on the affected side. If the cyst gets twisted or ruptures, the person will have severe abdominal pain. Since the ovaries also secrete the hormones that are responsible for the menstrual cycle, the cycles may be irregular. In those with multiple cysts, infertility is common.

Risk Factors:

It is common in women between puberty and menopause.

References

Hillard PA. Benign diseases of the female
reproductive tract. In: Berek JS. Novak's
gynecology. 12th ed. Philadelphia:
Williams & Wilkins; 1996. p. 362-363.

Caution and Recommendations to Therapists:

Do not massage the abdomen if a client has been diagnosed with a cyst. Pressure on the cyst can rupture it and cause severe pain in the individual.

Paget's disease (Osteitis deformans)

A progressive metabolic disease of bone.

Cause:

The cause is unknown. It may be due to a virus that can absorb bone. It is theorized that previous viral infections like mumps may cause a dormant skeletal infection that presents later as Paget's disease.

Signs and Symptoms:

The disease begins slowly and progresses over many years. There is an imbalance in the destruction, resorption and regrowth of bone. As a result the affected bone is replaced by fibrous tissue which gives the bone a rough and pitted outer surface. The symptoms depend on the area affected. Most people are asymptomatic. Lesions of the skull could result in headaches, ringing of the ears, dizziness and hearing loss. If the spine is affected, kyphosis may occur. If the long bones of the legs are affected, bow legs or knock-knees may be seen. The gait may be waddling as a result. Pathological fractures may occur with the slightest injury as the disease makes the bones fragile and weak. Bone pain may be present in the affected area. One of the rare, but dreaded complications of Paget's disease is the development of osteogenic sarcoma.

Risk Factors:

It affects people over the age of 40 and more men are affected than women.

Caution and Recommendations to Therapists:

These clients are likely to be on painkillers and antiinflammatory drugs. Hence the feedback from the clients may be inadequate during massage. Massage gives symptomatic relief only. Do not use excessive pressure, as they are prone for pathological fractures. See Appendix D for organizations and support groups.

Notes

In most people no treatment is warranted as it is localised or does not cause symptoms. Those people requiring treatment may be given painkillers and hormones like calcitonin to decrease bone resorption.

For more details see Appendix C: Painkillers; Hormone therapy / replacement.

References

Adams JC, Hamblen DL. Outline of orthopaedics. 11 Ed. New York: Churchill Livingstone; 1990. p. 47-50.

Pancreatitis

An inflammation of the pancreas.

Cause:

The common causes are disease of the bile ducts and alcoholism. The bile duct disease causes back flow of bile into the pancreas. This occurs as the secretions of the pancreas and the bile flow into the duodenum through a common opening. The reflux of the bile activates the protein and fat digesting enzymes of the pancreas causing autodigestion of the pancreas and surrounding tissue.

Alcohol is a direct stimulant of pancreatic secretion. The increased secretion along with bile reflux may be the cause of pancreatitis in alcoholics.

Notes

In most people acute pancreatitis subsides by itself in 3-7 days. The treatment aims to give the pancreas "rest". Painkillers, intravenous fluids, nasogastric suction to prevent secretions from entering the duodenum and no oral food (initially) are some forms of treatment. In severe cases, surgery with removal of dead tissue may be done.

Treatment of chronic pancreatitis aims to reduce pain and deal with malabsorption.

Enzyme replacement therapy may be required. For more details see Appendix C: Painkillers; Nasogastric suction.

Signs and Symptoms:

Acute onset of pancreatitis typically occurs after intake of a heavy, fatty meal and alcohol. There is severe pain radiating to the back. The intensity of pain increases on lying down and is reduced on bending forward. There is abdominal distention accompanied by low-grade fever, cold and sweaty palms. If the endocrine part of the pancreas is also damaged, diabetes mellitus results.

In chronic pancreatitis, as seen in alcoholics, the pancreas is slowly destroyed with reduced secretion of enzymes. The symptoms are that of malabsorption syndrome in this case. Recurrent and persistent pain localized to the upper left quadrant of the abdomen and below the sternum is present.

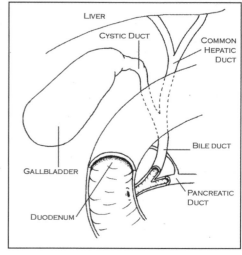

Pancreatitis may be complicated by formation of abscesses, cysts and super infection. Malabsorption of vitamins, diabetes, intestinal bleeding, jaundice (due to inflamed pancreas obstructing the bile duct) are other complications.

Risk Factors:

Alcohol intake, high fatty diet, drugs such as corticosteroids, certain diuretics and antibiotics can predispose to pancreatitis.

Caution and Recommendations to Therapists:

Acute pancreatitis is a medical emergency and could be fatal. Avoid abdominal massage in those with chronic pancreatitis. Encourage client to take a low fat diet. Refer to local support groups if an alcoholic. Refer to Appendix D for resources.

References

Yeo CJ, Cameron JL. The pancreas. In: Sabiston DC, editor. Textbook of Surgery 14th ed. Philadelphia: WB Saunders Company; 1991. p. 1080-1088.

Panic disorder

Nervous system

A condition where sudden, unexpected attacks of feelings of terror and impending doom occur.

Cause:

The cause is uncertain and is believed to be due to both psychological and biological determinants. Some suggest that hyperactivity of the neurons in the

Notes

It is important to rule out all other conditions and use of medications that

brainstem that secrete noradrenaline as neurotransmitters may be responsible. There may be a genetic predisposition.

can produce such anxiety. It is treated with specific medications for anxiety and by psychotherapy.

Signs and Symptoms:

The person has a sudden attack of panic while involved in a non-threatening activity. The feelings are similar to that felt in a life-threatening situation. The person feels lightheaded and sweaty. It is associated with palpitation, chest pain and choking sensation. The feelings peak in less than 10 minutes and disappear in 20-30 minutes. Since the attacks repeat, the patient tends to associate and avoid situations when they had previous attacks. Depression and substance abuse are some complications of the disorder.

Specific criteria exist for diagnosing this disorder. Some of the criteria are: the attacks are unexpected and occur when the person is not the focus of attention; at least four attacks occur within a 4-week period or the attacks are followed by a period of at least one month where the person fears another attack.

Risk Factors:

It is more common in teenagers and those in their early twenties. Panic disorder tends to be familial.

Caution and Recommendations to Therapists:

Massage helps to reduce stress and calm the individuals. By stimulating the parasympathetic nervous system and inhibiting the sympathetic system, massage can reduce tension in muscles, lower blood pressure and reduce heart rate. The Therapist should be prepared with strategies to deal with the client if an attack occurs in the clinic. It is important to have the address and telephone number of a contact person and the treating Physician.

References

Briton KT. Anxiety disorders in a medical setting. In: Isselbacher KJ et al, editors. Harrison's principles of internal medicine. 13th ed. New York: McGraw-Hill Inc; 1994. p. 2409-2411.

Parkinson's disease (Shaking palsy; Paralysis agitans; Parkinsonism)

Nervous system

A chronic, progressive disorder affecting the motor system.

Cause:

It is produced by a deficiency of the neurotransmitter dopamine in the basal ganglia of the brain. It may also be due to overactivity of acetylcholine in the same area. Since the basal ganglia participates in muscle coordination and plays an inhibitory part in motor function, the symptoms are typically related to the motor system.

Signs and Symptoms:

The symptoms may begin slowly and the disease may progress at different rates in each individual. There is muscle rigidity (increased tone on passively stretching a muscle), typically called *lead pipe rigidity* as the rigidity is present

Notes

The disease is progressive and chronic and treatment - at present, is to slow down or stop the progress of the disease. These individuals are treated with levo-dopa - a drug that increases the level of dopamine in the brain. Anticholinergics that reduce acetylcholine levels in the area are also used. In some individuals surgery may be resorted to. Research is underway to explore the possibilities of transplant. Alternative therapies include water exercises like swimming, yoga, tai chi and aerobic exercises within tolerable levels. To reduce constipation, high fibre diet is recommended.

For more details see Appendix C:
Anticholinergic drugs; Organ
transplantation.

throughout the range of motion. The rigidity results in alterations in posture and gait. The person is bent forward from the hips and stands with the knees and hips flexed. The head is also flexed. Tremors at rest - typically a pill-rolling movement of the fingers are present. The tremor is exaggerated when stressed and is reduced on performing a purposeful movement or during sleep.

The gait is abnormal and is shuffling or hurrying in type. On walking, the person seems to be trying to catch his/her center of gravity with a tendency to walk faster and faster with shorter steps. The natural swinging of the arm is absent with walking. The face is mask-like - lacking in expression and the tone of the voice is monotonous. The general coordination is difficult and there is difficulty in eating, swallowing, speaking and writing. However, the intellect is normal. There is no sensory loss but the person may suffer from cramps and aches. There may be sudden sensations of heat, and increased sweating in certain areas of the body. Constipation and loss of bladder control is also common. These individuals are prone to depression.

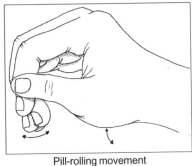

Pill-rolling movement

Risk Factors:

It is more common in men. It occurs more frequently between the age of 50-60. Rarely, Parkinsonism is seen after carbon monoxide poisoning, cerebrovascular accidents (stroke), tumors in the region of the basal ganglia, drug treatment for schizophrenia and other psychiatric disorders.

Caution and Recommendations to Therapists:

The aim of treatment is to reduce the rigidity and maintain bowel movements. The client may find it difficult getting on and off the table because of the motor dysfunction and the Therapist should address these issues.

A full body relaxation massage definitely reduces the symptoms, though temporarily. Use gentle, slow to moderate speed, repetitive, rhythmic strokes starting with the back - the least rigid area, before moving on to the shoulder, neck and upper limbs. Use effleurage and light to moderate pressure friction. Passively move all joints after the massage - but do not use force. Massage in a prone position helps to counteract the flexing effect of the disease - but elderly clients may feel uncomfortable in this position.

Abdominal massage helps relieve constipation in these individuals. Use clockwise movements - along the direction of movement in the colon. Special vibration techniques called "pushing" along with effleurage have been found to be useful. The total duration of the massage should be short lasting for about half an hour with equal time spent in all areas. Some Massage Therapists have found treatment schedules that include a total of 15 sessions, two to three

References

Meisler D. Parkinson's disease and massage therapy. Massage Therapy Journal 1996; 35(1): 34-37.

Mueller JN. Elderly Parkinson's patient – feeling good. Massage Therapy Journal 1996; 35(1): 28-42.

Standaert DG, Stern MB. Update on the management of Parkinson's disease. Med Clin North Am 1993;77:169.

times per week followed by a break for one to two months with repetition of the same sequence, to be beneficial to the client. Encourage the clients to be as active as possible. Refer the client to local support groups. See Appendix D for organizations and support groups.

Paronychia

An acute or chronic infection of the nail folds on the finger.

Cause:

It is usually caused by the bacteria *Staphylococcus aureus*.

Signs and Symptoms:

In acute lesions the nail fold appears swollen and tender and pus may be expressed after gentle pressure. In chronic lesions pain and swelling may be mild. See Appendix A: page 354.

Risk Factors:

It is common in individuals whose fingers are subjected to repeated immersion in water or foodstuffs. It may be a superinfection of eczema affecting the area. Aggressive manicuring may predispose to this condition. Finger sucking and nail biting may predispose to chronic infections.

Caution and Recommendations to Therapists:

Avoid local area while massaging.

To prevent the occurrence of paronychia, the Therapist should avoid prolonged immersion of hands and feet in water. The nail folds should be carefully dried after washing.

Notes

Mild cases are treated with immersion in warm saline water and application of antibiotic agents. If the infection is severe, the pus has to be drained and the client treated with oral antibiotics. For more details see Appendix C: Antimicrobial - antibacterial agents.

References

Daniel CR, Scher RK. The nail. In: Sams WM, Lynch PJ, editors. Principles and practice of Dermatology. 2nd ed. New York: Churchill Livingstone; 1996. p. 770-771.

Pediculosis (Lice infestation)

An infestation with lice - wingless insects that feed on human and animal blood.

Cause:

Three types of lice infect man - body lice (*pediculus humanus corporis*), pubic lice (*pediculus pubis* or *crabs*) and head lice (*pediculus humanus capitis*). The lice go through different stages - egg (*nit*) laid along the hair shaft, moult stage and adult stage. The egg incubates for 6-10 days. From the time the egg is laid, head and body lice develop into adults in 19-25 days. The life span of a louse is between 30 to 50 days. An adult louse is as big as a pinhead, light grey or brown in color.

Notes

Head lice can be treated with anti-lice shampoo/cream. The hair is washed, toweled dry and the cream applied to coat the hair and scalp. The cream is left on for about 10 minutes and washed away. A second treatment may be required after 7-10 days. It may be wise to treat the whole family simultaneously. To remove adult lice from clothing and other linen, they have to be machine washed and dried using the hot cycle or laundered using hot water. Clothing that cannot be washed may have to be dry-cleaned. Combs and brushes may be washed in hot water for 10-20 minutes. Vacuuming other areas may help remove hair with viable eggs attached to them.

In the case of body/pubic lice, only those infested and sexual contacts need to be treated.

The body lice can survive for 10 to 14 days in bedding, seams of clothes etc., unlike the head lice that die within a day outside the body. The pubic lice can live away from the body for up to two days.

Signs and Symptoms:

If affected with *body* lice, the patient will complain of itching especially in the shoulder, back and buttock area. Itchy, reddened and raised areas may be seen on the body.

In *head* lice, nits may be found in the hair. Nits are pearl-gray or brown, oval structures found on the hair shaft close to the scalp. The scalp may appear red and raw due to scratching. Rarely, an adult louse may be sighted.

Some of the diseases that are louse-borne are epidemic typhus, relapsing fever and trench fever.

Risk Factors:

Living in a crowded environment in contact with an infected individual, sharing towels, brushes, combs and hats of those infected puts a person at risk. Pubic lice are transmitted by sexual contact.

Caution and Recommendations to Therapists:

The social stigma attached to lice infestation can ruin the prospects of a clinic if a client contracts lice after a visit. Lice spread from close contact with an infested person. Massage is contraindicated. In body lice infestation, since the lice can survive without the host for a long time, the bedding and linen should be washed in boiling water and steam pressed or dry cleaned if a client has been massaged inadvertently. Clothes can also be disinfected by keeping them in airtight bags for two weeks or more. Special shampoos and body lotions with malathion or pyrethrum are available. Mattresses and upholstery should be vacuumed and disinfected. Similar treatment is given for pubic and head lice infestations. Nits from hair can be removed using a fine toothed comb. If a shampoo is used, the treatment should be repeated after a week to kill newly hatched lice.

Reer to Appendix B: Strategies for infection prevention and safe practice for some useful guidelines.

References

Orkin M, Maibach H. Mite infestations and Pediculosis. In: Sams WM, Lynch PJ, editors. Principles and practice of Dermatology. 2ⁿᵈ ed. New York: Churchill Livingstone; 1996. p. 209-212.

Reproductive system

Pelvic Inflammatory Disease (PID)

Any inflammation of the organs in the female pelvis. It includes inflammation of the fallopian tubes, ovaries, uterus and supporting tissues.

Cause:

Notes

A full course of antibiotics for 14 days is required to control the disease. If inadequately treated, adhesions can form between the organs in the pelvis, or the tubes may become blocked leading to

It is usually caused by bacteria (*Chlamydia*) normally found in the vagina, or which has been transmitted sexually.

Signs and Symptoms:

Fever, lower abdominal pain and tenderness, pain on having intercourse (*dyspareunia*) and white discharge from the vagina are the common symptoms.

Risk Factors:

It is more common in women with multiple sexual partners, between the ages of 16-24 years. The risk is increased with the use of intrauterine devices for contraception.

Caution and Recommendations to Therapists:

Encourage client to take the full course of the prescribed antibiotics. Educate the client that sexual partners may also have to be treated to prevent reinfection. Avoid abdominal area while massaging the client. The client may feel more comfortable in a position with the head and knee raised with pillows. There is no scope for the transmission of infection as it is sexually transmitted. Ask client to keep underclothes on during massage. The standard precautions for any infection should be taken (see Appendix B: Strategies for infection prevention and safe practice).

complications such as infertility, ectopic pregnancy, or abscesses in the pelvis.

For more details see Appendix C: Antimicrobial - antibacterial agents.

References

Soper DE. Genitourinary infections and sexually transmitted diseases. In: Berek JS. Novak's gynecology. 12th ed. Philadelphia: Williams & Wilkins; 1996. p. 435-438.

Peptic ulcer

Ulcers in the mucosa of the esophagus, stomach (gastric), duodenum or jejunum.

Gastrointestinal system

Cause:

The most common cause is infection of the mucosa with *Helicobacter Pylori* (*Campylobacter pylori*). Use of nonsteroidal anti-inflammatory drugs and other conditions that increase the acid secretion of the stomach and/or breakdown the mucosal barrier that prevents the erosion of the stomach wall by the acid, cause peptic ulcer.

Signs and Symptoms:

It varies with the location of the ulcer. In gastric ulcer, there is indigestion and heartburn. The person may loose weight. There may be associated bleeding from the stomach resulting in blood in vomitus (*hematemesis*) or dark tarry stools (*melena*).

In duodenal ulcer, the pain produced is similar to that of gastric ulcer but is relieved by food. However, the pain comes on about two hours after ingestion of food. The picture may be complicated by formation of stricture in the intestinal end of the stomach - *pyloric stenosis*.

Risk Factors:

Ingestion of alcohol, smoking, intake of steroids or non-steroidal anti-inflammatory drugs in an empty stomach are all risk factors. It affects men more than women. Gastric ulcers are more common between 50 - 60 years of age. Stress and anxiety contribute to the formation of ulcers as they reduce the secretion of mucus in the walls of the duodenum. This mucus production,

Notes:

The treatment aims to relieve pain and accelerate healing of ulcers. Antacids help accelerate healing by neutralizing the acid. The most widely used antacids contain aluminium hydroxide and magnesium hydroxide. Histamine secreted in the stomach increase acid secretion. Drugs that block histamine (H2) receptors speed up the healing of ulcers and reduce recurrence. Other drugs such as sucralfate that coat the surface of the ulcer may be used. These coating agents speed up healing and reduce the injurious effects of acid on the ulcer. Some types of prostaglandins (those of the E series) that stimulate gastric mucus secretion, reduce acid secretion and mucosal healing are also used for treating ulcers. Antibiotics may be given to combat the bacterial infection.

Many different diet programs may be advocated. However, there is no evidence to show that milk and cream, bland diets, diets free of spices or fruit juices reduce acid secretion or speed up healing. But, if it is found that certain foods increaseing the symptoms, those foods should be avoided. Reduced intake of caffeine or caffeine containing drinks and alcohol intake, elimination of cigarette smoking may be advised as they affect gastric acid secretion.

In severe cases where complications such as hemorrhage, perforation etc. exist, surgical measures are taken to decrease acid secretion in the stomach.

For more details see Appendix C: Antacids; Antimicrobial - antibacterial agents.

References:

JE McGuigan. Peptic ulcer and gastritis. In: Isselbacher KJ et al, editors. Harrison's principles of internal medicine. 13ᵗʰ ed. New York: McGraw-Hill Inc; 1994. p. 1363-1378

which is inhibited by sympathetic stimulation, serves to protect the stomach lining.

Caution and Recommendations to Therapists:

Avoid massage to the upper abdominal area. Massage helps reduce stress - a predisposing factor to ulcers. Encourage clients to take the full course of antibiotics, avoid alcohol and to stop smoking if a smoker. See Appendix D for organizations and support groups.

Cardiovascular system

Pericarditis

Inflammation of the pericardium (the membranes surrounding the heart).

Cause:

There are many causes of pericarditis. It may be due to infection - viral, bacterial, tuberculosis or other infections. Pericarditis may follow myocardial infection or tumors; trauma or irradiation to the region. It may be related to hypersensitivity or autoimmune disease such as rheumatic fever, systemic lupus erythematosus, rheumatoid arthritis, scleroderma etc. Some drugs may induce inflammation of the pericardium. In some cases, the cause is unknown.

Signs and Symptoms:

Notes:

The patient with acute pericarditis is placed at bed rest till the pain disappears and is carefully monitored. If there are signs of cardiac tamponade, the fluid has to be removed from the pericardial cavity (*pericardiocentesis*) immediately. Anti-inflammatory drugs or steroids may be given to reduce inflammation and fibrous tissue formation.

Constrictive pericarditis is treated with surgery where the pericardium is removed. If the cause of pericarditis has been identified, it has to be treated.

For more details see Appendix C: Antiinflammatories - steroidal drugs; Antiinflammatories - non steroidal drugs.

Usually it presents as chest pain. The pain is located behind the sternum, over the left side of the chest, over the back or shoulder. When associated with inflammation of the pleura, the pain increases on inspiration. Typically, the pain may be reduced by sitting up or leaning forward. If the inflammation develops slowly, pain may be absent. High fever may be present especially if the condition is due to an infection. Pericarditis is often associated with fluid in the pericardial cavity - *pericardial effusion*. If the fluid accumulates rapidly, it can restrict relaxation of the heart and obstruct the inflow of blood into the ventricles. This condition is known as *cardiac tamponade*.

Sometimes, acute pericarditis may progress to a chronic form. Here, healing takes place with fibrosis, obliterating the pericardial cavity and restricting the movement of the heart (*constrictive pericarditis*). The pericardium becomes thick and rigid. In chronic pericarditis, there is loss of weight, appetite and the person feels weak and fatigued. Signs of cardiac failure (see Heart failure) are seen.

Risk Factors:

See Cause.

References

Braunwald E. Pericardial disease. In: Isselbacher KJ et al, editors. Harrison's principles of internal medicine. 13ᵗʰ ed. New York: McGraw-Hill Inc; 1994. p. 1094-1133.

Caution and Recommendations to Therapists:

Massage is contraindicated during the acute phase. In the chronic phase, after obtaining clearance from the treating Physician, a gentle relaxation massage may be given with the client seated on in a half-lying position.

Pathology A to Z -

Periodontitis

An inflammation of the oral mucosa around the teeth.

Cause:

Along with gingivitis, it is due to infections that result in accumulation of bacterial plaques that mineralize to form calculus.

Signs and Symptoms:

It starts as inflammation of the gums. The problem is painless, but bleeding may occur on brushing the teeth. The disease may spread to the surrounding areas like the ligaments and bone. Resorption of bone occurs with gaps being formed between the tooth and the bone leading to superinfection and abscess formation.

Risk Factors:

Poor oral hygiene is a predisposing factor.

Caution and Recommendations to Therapists:

If the Therapist has this condition, prompt treatment should be sought as it can have a detrimental effect on the "image" of the clinic.

Notes

It can be prevented by improved oral hygiene such as frequent brushing of teeth, flossing, antibacterial mouth rinses and the removal of impacted food. It is treated by removing plaques, calculus and administration of antibiotics against infective agents. Patient education is an important component.

For more details see Appendix C: Antimicrobial - antibacterial agents.

References

Genco et al. Contemporary Periodontics. St. Louis: Mosby; 1989.

Peripheral neuritis (Multiple neuritis; Peripheral

neuropathy; Polyneuritis)

A degenerative disorder of peripheral nerves especially those supplying the distal parts of the limbs (fingers and toes).

Cause:

It is a non-inflammatory degeneration of the sensory and motor nerves to the hand and toes. Many conditions have been associated with peripheral neuritis (see Risk factors).

Signs and Symptoms:

The symptoms appear slowly, with atrophy and flaccid paralysis of the small muscles of the hand and feet. The sensation is also diminished with the vibratory sense being affected first. Footdrop may be present. The muscles may be tender and hypersensitive to touch and pressure. There may be decreased sweating and the skin appears red and glossy.

Risk Factors:

It is more common in men between the ages of 30-50. Chronic alcoholism, lead poisoning, diabetes mellitus, gout, rheumatoid arthritis, Systemic Lupus Erythematous, vitamin deficiencies, excessive intake of sulphur containing drugs like sulphonamides have all been implicated. It has also been associated with

Notes

Although the treatment is supportive, the cause of the neuritis has to be established. High intake of vitamins especially vitamin B12 is required.

infections like tuberculosis, diphtheria, meningitis, mumps and Guillain-Barre syndrome.

Caution and Recommendations to Therapists:

Encourage clients with persistent symptoms of tingling and numbness to seek medical help.

The aim is to increase the tone, prevent contractures and joint stiffness and to relieve pain if present. Care should be taken to avoid undue pressure as the sensations are diminished. Some clients may be hypersensitive to touch, in which case avoid the areas. Perform range of motion exercises to all the joints of the hand, but do not use force to increase the range. Use lymphatic drainage techniques to reduce edema if present. Use strokes that are directed from distal to proximal areas. Look for pressure ulcers - especially if the client is wearing splints or braces. Avoid areas of ulcers and give a wide margin around the area. Enriched oils (with high Vitamin A or Vitamin E content) can be used while massaging the affected areas. See Appendix D for organizations and support groups.

References

Asbury AK. Diseases of the Peripheral nervous system. In: Isselbacher KJ et al, editors. Harrison's principles of internal medicine. 13th ed. New York: McGraw-Hill Inc; 1994. p. 2368-2379.

Dyck PJ et al, editors. Peripheral neuropathy. 3rd ed. Philadelphia: Saunders; 1987.

Peritonitis

Gastrointestinal system

An inflammation of the membrane (peritoneum) that lines the abdominal cavity and covers the organs in the abdomen.

Notes

The treatment is supportive. Fluid and electrolyte balance is maintained. Antibiotics are given to combat infection and painkillers to reduce pain. The cause of secondary peritonitis such as perforation of ulcers etc. may have to be treated surgically.

For more details see Appendix C: Painkillers; Antimicrobial - antibacterial agents.

Cause:

It can be caused by bacteria or by chemical irritation. Any condition that exposes the peritoneum to the contents of the intestine can cause Peritonitis. Chemical irritation most often occurs after abdominal surgery.

Signs and Symptoms:

Pain and tenderness are the common symptoms. The pain is increased on moving the abdomen and the person lies still. The breathing is shallow. The abdominal muscles go into a spasm and become boardlike. There are signs of dehydration as the inflammation of the peritoneum causes fluid to ooze into the abdominal cavity (ascites). The movements of the intestines are stopped reflexly. Fever may be present.

Risk Factors:

Peptic ulcer that has perforated, ruptured appendix or bowel, inflamed gall bladder, abdominal trauma and wounds can predispose to peritonitis. Peritonitis may occur spontaneously in people with cirrhosis of the liver.

Caution and Recommendations to Therapists:

Usually, the client will be too sick to be massaged. Gentle and soothing massage with minimal movement of the client, avoiding the abdomen, can be given in a hospital setting to reduce stress and pain, after clearance from a Physician.

References

Yamada T et al, editors. Textbook of Gastroenterology. Philadelphia: Lippincott; 1991.

Pheochromocytoma

A tumor of the adrenal medulla that secretes excess adrenaline and noradrenaline.

Endocrine system

Cause:

The cause of the tumor is not known. It may be due to defective genes transmitted from the parent.

Signs and Symptoms:

The adrenal medulla secretes adrenaline and noradrenaline - which are also secreted as neurotransmitters by the sympathetic nervous system. Hence the symptoms resemble that of hyperactivity of the sympathetic nervous system - fight-or-flight reaction. The person has persistent increase in blood pressure. The heart rate is rapid. Excessive sweating, headache, flushed and warm skin, anxiety, nervousness and rapid respiration are some of the symptoms. The person also has dizziness on changing posture (postural hypotension). The symptoms persist or come on suddenly many times a day. The symptoms may be precipitated by exercise, laughing, urination, or by any type of stress.

Risk Factors:

See Cause.

Caution and Recommendations to Therapists:

Do not massage an individual before treatment. If necessary, before treatment, massage should be undertaken only after Physician's approval. Although massage helps reduce stress, palpation of the abdomen or lower back can bring on an attack of symptoms by direct stimulation of the tumor. These individuals are prone for postural hypotension and it should be ensured that changes in posture like getting off the table are done slowly and with support.

Notes

It is treated by surgically removing the tumor.

References

JD Wilson, Foster DW, editors. Williams' textbook of Endocrinology.Philadelphia: Saunders; 1992.

Pityriasis rosea

An inflammatory skin disorder.

Integumentary system

Cause:

The cause is unknown. It may be of viral origin and close contact with an infected individual may spread this condition.

Signs and Symptoms:

It appears as a single macule or papule surrounded by redness in the neck or trunk. As it spreads the central area clears. The lesion fades in 2-10 days while a fresh crop begins to appear. The lesions disappear in 6-8 weeks. Some itching may be present.

Notes

Usually no treatment is required. If there is itching, antihistamines and local application of corticosteroids is resorted to. For more details see Appendix C: Antihistamines; Antiinflammatories - steroidal drugs.

Risk Factors:

It is common in spring and fall seasons. The incidence is higher in young adults.

Caution and Recommendations to Therapists:

Do not massage the local area, as it may be contagious. The immunity may be suppressed if the client is on oral corticosteroids. Ensure that you do not have any mild form of infection while treating these clients as it may present more seriously if spread to these immunocompromised individuals. Wash hands thoroughly and disinfect linen and bed after massage treatment to clients with this condition. See Appendix B: Strategies for infection prevention and safe practice.

References

Madison KC. Lichen Planus, Pityriasis Rosea, Pityriasis Rubra pilaris, and related disorders. In: Sams WM, Lynch PJ, editors. Principles and practice of Dermatology. 2nd ed. New York: Churchill Livingstone; 1996. p. 368-370.

Lymphatic, Gastrointestinal, Respiratory, Nervous systems

Plague

An acute infection caused by the bacillus Yersinia pestis and spread by rodents.

Notes

It is treated with antibiotics. Plague can be prevented by controlling the rodent population. Treatment of pets with flea repellent powders and use of insecticides are all methods that can be used. A vaccine is available against plague and those individuals working in high-risk occupations should consider taking it.

For more details see Appendix C: Antimicrobial - antibacterial agents; Immunization.

Cause:

The bacillus multiplies in infected rodent fleas and blocks its gut. When the flea takes its next blood meal, the bacillus is injected into the body. Humans acquire the disease when they are bitten by infected rodent fleas. Rats, ground squirrels and prairie dogs are potential carriers of fleas. The bacillus may persist in the soil of rodent burrows and remain infective for long periods of time. Sometimes, animals that eat rodents may spread the disease. The infection can be transmitted by contact of open wounds to infected tissue. Human lice and ticks are also capable of transmitting the bacillus.

Signs and Symptoms:

After being injected into the body through the skin, the bacillus migrates to the local lymph nodes. The lymph nodes become inflamed and enlarged (*bubo*). The lymph nodes may be as large as 10 cms. From the lymph nodes, the bacillus can enter the bloodstream and produce reactions in other organs such as the spleen, lungs and lymph nodes in other areas.

It takes about 2-7 days from the insect bite to the first symptoms. The person presents with fever, headache, abdominal pain and painful enlargement of lymph nodes. Loss of appetite, nausea, vomiting and diarrhea may accompany the abdominal pain. If the condition is left untreated, the toxins liberated by the bacilli and the presence of organisms in the blood can lead to serious illness and death. Thrombi formation is common and blockage of circulation can lead to gangrene formation.

If the lungs are involved, there are signs of pneumonia. The patient has cough, fever and rapid breathing. It may progress to respiratory failure and death. If the infection has spread to the meninges, signs of meningitis are seen.

Risk Factors:

Exposure to wild animals or rodents increases the risk.

Caution and Recommendations to Therapists:

Ensure that the clinic is insect and rodent proof. Refer to Appendix B: Strategies for infection prevention and safe practice.

References

Morello JA, Mizer HE, Wilson ME, Granato PA. Microbiology in patient care. 6th ed. New York: McGraw-Hill; 1998. p. 482-485.

McNeill WH. Plagues and peoples. New York: Anchor Press; 1976.

Plantar fasciitis

Musculoskeletal system

Inflammation of the plantar fascia and the surrounding structures.

Cause:

It is caused by excessive stress on the foot especially near the attachment of the fascia to the calcaneus bone. The stress causes calcium deposit in the site thus forming a spur.

Signs and Symptoms:

Notes

Non-steroidal anti-inflammatory drugs may be given to reduce the pain. The heel has to be protected by using cushions or insoles. In severe cases, corticosteroids may be injected into the tender area. Recovery is very slow in this condition. If all above fail, surgical detachment of the fascia and removal of bony spurs (if present) may be necessary. For more details see Appendix C: Antiinflammatories - non steroidal drugs.

The person complains of pain in the heel that is made worse on climbing stairs, walking or running. The pain is relieved by rest. There is tenderness near the attachment of the fascia to the calcaneus, medial aspect of the foot and in the abductor

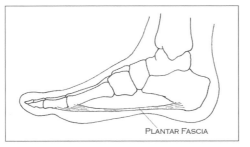

PLANTAR FASCIA

hallucis muscle. The pain is increased on stretching the plantar fascia by dorsiflexion. There is no loss of sensation. The plantar surface of the foot may be red and swollen.

Risk Factors:

It is more common in individuals with high arched feet and those over the age of 40. In the younger age group it can occur in those who are active in sports. People who are in occupations that involve prolonged standing or walking are also prone.

Caution and Recommendations to Therapists:

Ice massage and rest is used initially. In the subacute or chronic stage, friction massage at the origin of the calcaneus is given to reduce adhesions. Mobilize the joints of the foot, to reduce stiffness. Lymphatic massage and drainage techniques can be used in the leg and ankle. The muscles of the leg should be massaged thoroughly to increase circulation and reduce spasm and trigger points. Remedial exercises to stretch the gastrocnemius and the plantar fascia should also be done. The client may be on anti-inflammatory drugs, and this may prevent them from giving a proper feedback regarding pressure and otherwise painful techniques. Treatments lasting for half an hour, at a frequency of two to three times a week are recommended.

References

Mercier LR. Practical Orthopedics. 4th ed. St. Louis: Mosby Year book Inc; 1995. p. 243-244.

Turchaninov R, Cox CA. Medical Massage. Scottsdale: Stress Less publishing Inc; 1998. p. 385-387.

a Handbook for Massage Therapists

Pleural effusion

*Denotes an excess of fluid in the pleural space. Pleural space is the space
between the lungs and the thoracic wall lined by a thin membrane called pleura.*

Notes

If the fluid is excessive, it is treated in the
hospital setting by drainage with a tube in
the pleural cavity. If caused by infection,
antibiotics are administered. For more
details see Appendix C: Antimicrobial -
antibacterial agents.

Cause:

The cause is similar to that of edema. When the pressure in the lung capillaries
increase or when the osmotic pressure in the blood decreases, fluid from the blood
tends to collect in spaces outside the blood vessels of which the pleural space is
one. Such a situation can be produced in heart failure, liver disease, reduced
protein in the blood as in malnutrition or kidney failure. Pleural effusion can also
be produced when the capillaries become more permeable (leaky) as in
inflammatory conditions, lung infections like tuberculosis, lung cancer or trauma
to the chest.

Signs and Symptoms:

Difficulty in breathing is
present. The movement of
the chest wall is decreased
on the side of collection of
fluid. There may be chest
pain that is increased on
movements produced by
breathing. If there is pus
in the pleural cavity
(*empyema*) there may be
associated fever and
weakness. Sometimes the
fluid in the pleural cavity
may be bloody as in
lung cancers or trauma
(*hemothorax*). Rarely, the
fluid may be lymph
(*chylothorax*).

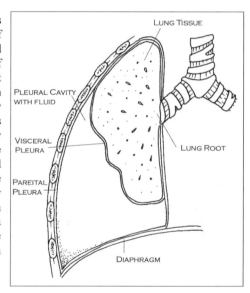

Risk Factors:

It may be seen in individuals with Systemic Lupus Erythematosus (SLE) and
Rheumatoid Arthritis.

Caution and Recommendations to Therapists:

Consult Physician regarding cause of effusion. If due to infection do not massage
till treated completely. If due to tuberculosis follow precautions given under
tuberculosis. The aim is to help with the absorption of fluid, prevent adhesions,
prevent permanent changes in posture and help with the ventilation. Avoid
areas of drainage tube if it is in place. These clients have a tendency to develop
scoliosis. The shoulder is lower and the hip higher on the affected side as
compared to the normal side, so the postural muscles should be addressed
while massaging.

References

Light RW. Disorders of the pleura,
mediastinum, and diaphragm. In:
Isselbacher KJ et al, editors. Harrison's
principles of internal medicine. 13th ed.
New York: McGraw-Hill Inc; 1994. p.
1229-1232

Pathology A to Z -

The treatments should be short - not more than fifteen minutes with more time spent to massage the arms, shoulder girdles and back. In chronic pleural effusion, massage with the client lying on the side with the normal side on the table helps to expand the affected lung. Ask client to push against your hand that is placed on the affected side, while breathing in. Deep breathing exercises are also helpful. The intercostal muscles can be stretched by using two fingers in the intercostal space and pressing inwards during expiration. Work in conjunction with a Physiotherapist. See Appendix D for organizations and support groups.

Pleurisy (Pleuritis)

An inflammation of the pleura.

Respiratory system

Cause:

Pleurisy develops as a complication of pneumonia, tuberculosis, Systemic Lupus Erythematosus, cancer or trauma to the chest. It is caused by bacterial infection.

Notes

The cause of the pleurisy has to be identified and treated.

Signs and Symptoms:

It presents as an intense, sharp stabbing pain over the chest on breathing deeply. There is difficulty in breathing and respiration is shallow and rapid. Fever is present and may be accompanied by a dry cough. The patient leans to the affected side to avoid pain.

Risk Factors:

See Cause.

Caution and Recommendations to Therapists:

Encourage client to breath deeply. Since it may be due to bacterial infection, massage should not be done until the cause has been identified. If due to other causes, a full body relaxation massage may be done with focus on the shoulder, back and arms. Encourage client to take bed rest. See Appendix D for organizations and support groups.

References

Light RW. Disorders of the pleura, mediastinum, and diaphragm. In: Isselbacher KJ et al, editors. Harrison's principles of internal medicine. 13th ed. New York: McGraw-Hill Inc; 1994. p. 1229-1232

Pneumoconiosis - Asbestosis

A progressive disease that produces diffuse fibrosis in the lung. One of the spectrum of diseases called pneumoconiosis that is a result of airborne pollutants that damage the lung.

Respiratory system

Cause:

It is caused by inhalation of asbestos fibers. The defence reaction of the body to the inhaled fibres causes thickening of the pleura, and diffuse fibrosis of lungs.

Notes

Treatment includes avoidance of exposure and other supportive measures.

Signs and Symptoms:

The individual has difficulty in breathing and has a dry cough. In advanced cases there is chest pain and recurrent respiratory infection. Asbestosis can predispose to lung cancer.

Risk Factors:

Workers involved in asbestos mines and mills, construction industry workers where asbestos is used for prefabrication, fireproofing and textile industries are more prone. Asbestos is used in paints, plastics, pipe and broiler insulations, brake and clutch linings. Families of asbestos workers are prone as a result of asbestos fibres shaken off the clothing of the worker. Others are at risk through inhalation of asbestos fibres from the waste piles of neighboring asbestos plants.

Caution and Recommendations to Therapists:

These clients are prone to respiratory infections. Schedule them at a time when they are unlikely to be exposed to other clients who may have respiratory infection. Do not massage them when you have a respiratory infection. There is a high incidence of tuberculosis in people with silicosis. Ensure that it is not so with the client you are treating. Encourage client to stop smoking, if smoker, as it speeds up the progress of the disease. Do a whole body relaxation massage using hacking, clapping and vibration strokes over the chest. The latter helps to drain secretions better. Steam inhalation before start of treatment may be beneficial. Keep room at higher humidity and warmth. See Appendix D for organizations and support groups.

References

Porth CM, editor. Pathophysiology – concepts of altered health states. 4th ed Philadelphia:. JB Lippincott Co; 1994. p. 552-553.

Pneumoconiosis - Berylliosis (Beryllium poisoning;

Respiratory, Cardiovascular, Renal, Gastrointestinal, Integumentary systems

Beryllium disease)

One of the spectrum of diseases called pneumoconiosis that is a result of airborne pollutants that damage the lung. It is a progressive disease that predominantly affects the lungs.

Cause:

Notes

Avoidance of the causative agent and supportive treatment are beneficial.

It is caused by inhalation of beryllium dusts, fumes, and mists. Beryllium may also be absorbed through the skin. The mechanism by which it produces the effects is not known.

Signs and Symptoms:

If absorbed through the skin, beryllium produces itching, a rash and later an ulcer at the site. If inhaled, it produces swelling and ulceration of the mucosa of the nose. It may lead to perforation of the nasal septum. It may also be associated with a dry cough, pain below the sternum and difficulty in breathing. It may progress to right heart failure due to the increased resistance in the lungs to blood flow. Enlargement of the liver and spleen may result.

Pathology A to Z -

Risk Factors:

Beryllium alloy workers, cathode ray tube makers (cathode ray tube is used in television/computer monitors), gas mantle makers, missile technicians, nuclear reactor workers are all at risk. Families of beryllium workers exposed to it by dust shaken off the clothes of workers; individuals exposed to it through neighboring plants are also at risk.

Caution and Recommendations to Therapists:

These clients are prone to respiratory infections. Schedule them at a time when they are unlikely to be exposed to other clients who may have respiratory infection. Do not massage them when you have a respiratory infection. There is a high incidence of tuberculosis in people with silicosis. Ensure that it is not so with the client you are treating. Encourage client to stop smoking, if smoker, as it speeds up the progress of the disease. Do a whole body relaxation massage using hacking, clapping and vibration strokes over the chest. The latter helps to drain secretions better. Steam inhalation before start of treatment may be beneficial. Keep room at higher humidity and warmth. See Appendix D for organizations and support groups.

References

Porth CM, editor. Pathophysiology – concepts of altered health states. 4ᵗʰ ed Philadelphia:. JB Lippincott Co; 1994. p. 552-553.

Pneumoconiosis - Coal Worker's (Black lung disease; Coal miner's disease; Miner's asthma; Anthracosis; Anthracosilicosis)

Respiratory system

A progressive disease that produces nodules and fibrosis in the lung. One of the spectrum of diseases called pneumoconiosis that is a result of airborne pollutants that damage the lung.

Cause:

It is due to chronic inhalation of coal dust - especially particles that are smaller than 5 microns in diameter. The body's defense mechanisms in the form of macrophages engulf the coal dust, but are unable to process it. The macrophages die with release of enzymes into the surrounding tissue. This produces a local inflammatory reaction that heals by fibrosis, affecting the lung structure and function.

Notes

Supportive treatment and avoidance of the precipitating agent is required.

Signs and Symptoms:

It begins asymptomatically. Depending on the duration and intensity of exposure, presence of silica in addition to the coal dust, and the susceptibility of the individual, the symptoms progress to difficulty in breathing, fatigue, cough with black sputum and recurrent respiratory tract infection.

Risk Factors:

Smoking speeds up the progress of the disease. Coal miners or others working with coal are susceptible.

Caution and Recommendations to Therapists:

These clients are prone to respiratory infections. Schedule them at a time when they are unlikely to be exposed to other clients who may have respiratory infection. Do not massage them when you have a respiratory infection. There is a high incidence of tuberculosis in people with silicosis. Ensure that it is not so with the client you are treating. Encourage client to stop smoking, if smoker, as it speeds up the progress of the disease. Do a whole body relaxation massage using hacking, clapping and vibration strokes over the chest. The latter helps to drain secretions better. Steam inhalation before start of treatment may be beneficial. Keep room at higher humidity and warmth. See Appendix D for organizations and support groups.

References

Porth CM, editor. Pathophysiology – concepts of altered health states. 4th ed Philadelphia:. JB Lippincott Co; 1994. p. 552-553.

Pneumoconiosis - Silicosis

Respiratory system

A progressive disease that produces nodules and fibrosis in the lung. One of the spectrum of diseases called pneumoconiosis that is a result of airborne pollutants that damage the lung.

Cause:

Notes

Avoidance of the offending agent and supportive treatment are given.

It is caused by chronic inhalation and deposition of crystals of silica dust in the lungs. The body's defense mechanisms in the form of macrophages engulf the silica but are unable to process it. The macrophages die with release of enzymes into the surrounding tissue. This produces a local inflammatory reaction that heals by fibrosis. This in turn affects lung function.

Signs and Symptoms:

Initially this condition is asymptomatic. Later, there is difficulty in breathing, dry cough, chest pain and recurrent respiratory infection. There is a high incidence of tuberculosis in these individuals.

Risk Factors:

Individuals working in industries or areas that are a source of silica such as ceramic (flint) manufacturers, cement, building materials like sandstone are prone. Silica is found in paints, porcelain, scouring soaps, wood fillers, mines of gold, coal, lead, zinc or iron. Foundry workers, boiler scalers and stone cutters are others exposed to silica dust.

Caution and Recommendations to Therapists:

These clients are prone to respiratory infections. Schedule them at a time when they are unlikely to be exposed to other clients who may have respiratory infection. Do not massage them when you have a respiratory infection. There is a high incidence of tuberculosis in people with silicosis. Ensure that it is not so with the client you are treating. Encourage client to stop smoking, if smoker, as it speeds up the progress of the disease. Do a whole body relaxation massage using hacking, clapping and vibration strokes over the chest. The latter helps to

References

Porth CM, editor. Pathophysiology – concepts of altered health states. 4th ed Philadelphia:. JB Lippincott Co; 1994. p. 552-553.

drain secretions better. Steam inhalation before start of treatment may be beneficial. Keep room at higher humidity and warmth. See Appendix D for organizations and support groups.

Pneumonia

An acute infection of the lung tissue that can affect the exchange of gas.

Cause:

Notes

It is treated with antibiotics. For more details see Appendix C: Antimicrobial - antibacterial agents.

Pneumonia could be due to virus (chicken pox, measles, influenza), bacteria (streptococcus, staphylococcus), fungus, protozoa, mycobacteria, mycoplasma or rickettsia. The pneumonia may affect the bronchus and alveoli - *bronchopneumonia*, affect part of a lobe - *lobular pneumonia*, or an entire lobe - *lobar pneumonia*. The infection produces inflammation in the lung with increased blood flow and fluid moving into the alveoli. Slowly, this is resolved by reabsorption of fluid into the blood and by expulsion as sputum.

Signs and Symptoms:

Cough with sputum, chest pain that increases with the movement of the chest accompanied by fever and chills are classical symptoms. The breathing may be noisy and difficult.

Risk Factors:

Individuals with chronic illness such as cancer, asthma, other chronic obstructive pulmonary diseases, bronchiectasis and cystic fibrosis are prone. Smoking, malnutrition, alcoholism are other risk factors. Inhalation of toxic chemicals that damage the lung, nasogastric tubes, tracheostomies, thoracic or abdominal surgery, coma, immune deficiency and immunosuppressive treatment also predispose to this condition. Individuals on antibiotics that kill the normal respiratory flora can put an individual at risk.

Caution and Recommendations to Therapists:

Do not massage in the acute stage. During recovery, massage may be given with the client in a half lying position with the upper body propped up with pillows. Ask client to breathe deeply while offering mild resistance to the expansion of the chest by placing your hand flat on the side of the chest. This helps to re-expand the lung tissue. Tapotement over the chest helps drain secretions. Massage the muscles of posture to increase tone and blood flow, as Pneumonia tends to cause scoliosis. Passively move joints and massage the lower limbs vigorously to prevent disuse atrophy of muscles from the prolonged bed rest. Ensure that you do not come in contact with the respiratory secretions. Place tissues used by client in a leak proof bag before disposal. Refer to Appendix B: Strategies for infection prevention and safe practice for some useful guidelines. Also see Appendix D for organizations and support groups.

References

Levison ME. Pneumonia, including necrotizing pulmonary infections (lung abscess). In: Isselbacher KJ et al, editors. Harrison's principles of internal medicine. 13th ed. New York: McGraw-Hill Inc; 1994. p. 1184-1191.

Pneumothorax

A condition where there is accumulation of air in the pleural space.

Cause:

It may be due to abnormalities of the lung structure. In some individuals the lung tissue is weak and tends to give way to the pressure inside the lungs. There is escape of air into the pleural space as a result. This may happen in tuberculosis and emphysema. Trauma to the chest is another cause. Sometimes the opening is such that it allows air to enter but not leave the pleural cavity. This leads to *tension pneumothorax* and requires immediate assistance.

Signs and Symptoms:

The symptoms are produced by the pressure of the air in the pleura on the lung tissue and blood vessels. There is sudden, sharp pain that increases on movements produced by breathing. The chest wall moves unequally on both sides. Difficulty in breathing is experienced.

Risk Factors:

Emphysema and tuberculosis increase the risk. Rarely there is a family history.

Caution and Recommendations to Therapists:

Consult Physician. Do not massage unless cleared by Physician.

Notes

A wide bore needle may be used to drain out the excessive air in a hospital setting. It is treated with bed rest. Tension Pneumothorax is a surgical emergency.

References

Light RW. Disorders of the pleura, mediastinum, and diaphragm. In: Isselbacher KJ et al, editors. Harrison's principles of internal medicine. 13th ed. New York: McGraw-Hill Inc; 1994. p. 1229-1232.

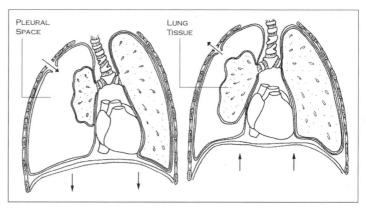

PLEURAL SPACE

LUNG TISSUE

Trauma to the chest wall resulting in pneumothorax

Poliomyelitis (Polio; Infantile paralysis)

An acute viral infection which causes paralysis.

Cause:

It is caused by the poliovirus, which are of many types. The virus is transmitted from person to person by direct contact with infected saliva, droplets from the nose and throat or feco-oral contamination. The incubation period is 5 - 35 days. The virus enters the body through the gut, multiplying in the pharynx and then spreading to the lymph nodes and blood. The virus specifically affects the neurons in the anterior horn - the motor neurons that supply muscles.

Polio can be spread by "carriers" or during the incubation period and early signs of infection. Care should be taken to contain the spread.

Signs and Symptoms:

Ninety-five percent of infections do not produce any symptoms. Four to eight percent of cases subside after sore throat, vomiting and fever lasting for 2-3 days. Others present with symptoms of the nervous system.

In the non-paralytic form, the person is irritable and has fever, headache, vomiting and generalized pain and stiffness. This may last for a week or two and the person is normal again. In the paralytic form, in addition to the symptoms of nonparalytic form, the person has weakness of various groups of muscles, with loss of reflexes. The individual may be hypersensitive to touch. Loss of bladder control and constipation may be present. If the cranial nerves are affected, the facial muscles may be weak. There may be difficulty in swallowing. Polio affecting the brainstem region may result in difficulty in breathing. There is no loss of sensation or mental function.

Following the acute infectious stage, there may be improvement due to the recovery of undamaged neurons that had been compressed by the edema produced by inflammation. Neurons that are damaged result in chronic signs of muscle atrophy and paralysis.

The loss of function of muscles can slow down the growth of bone in children producing shortening of a limb. Disuse of the joint and soft tissue in the affected limb can lead to joint stiffness and contractures of the soft tissue.

Some patients develop weakness about 20-30 years later. This condition is known as *postpoliomyelitis neuromuscular atrophy* or *postpolio syndrome*. Some of the symptoms include muscle pain, weakness, involuntary movements and atrophy. If the respiratory muscles or muscles of the pharynx and larynx are affected the person may have difficulty breathing and swallowing. Food may enter the respiratory tract and complicate the situation. It is believed that it is due to slow disintegration of the motor neurons. In some patients, this syndrome may be due to the reactivation of polio virus lying dormant in the central nervous system.

Notes

Treatment is largely supportive during the acute stage. The vital signs have to be carefully monitored.

For those in the chronic non-infective stage of the disease, the aim is to retain joint mobility and prevent contractures. Physical therapy is important.

Polio vaccines are given as oral drops and it is 90% effective in preventing the disease. However, the vaccine should be avoided in people with lowered immunity.

For more details see Appendix C: Immunization.

Risk Factors:

The chances of paralysis after infection is increased during pregnancy, old age, excessive physical exertion, tonsillectomy, tooth extraction or vaccination - all factors that tend to lower the immunity or ease the entry of the virus into the blood and lymph.

Caution and Recommendations to Therapists:

Polio can be spread by "carriers" or during the incubation period and early signs of infection. Massage should be avoided at all costs during the acute stages of the disease. Massage Therapists are more likely to encounter adults in the chronic non-infective stage of the disease. The aim is to retain joint mobility and prevent contractures. Position the affected area of the client in a neutral position. You may need to support the area with pillows. The paralysis of one group of muscles results in overactivity of the antagonist muscle and increased tone. The increased tone in turn, results in excessive stretch and scarring of the affected group.

Passively move joints through the full range of motion. Use transverse friction movements over joints and atrophied muscle. Strokes like effleurage and pétrissage can increase the circulation in these unused areas. Remember that the loss of motor function is permanent. The loss of nerve supply to the area may be associated with dryness and fragility of skin. Do not use vigorous massage or excessive pressure. Edema may be present in the affected limb. Keep the limb elevated and use lymphatic drainage techniques. Concentrate massage strokes on muscles that are stressed by the alteration of posture to compensate for the paralyzed muscle groups. Look for pressure ulcers and skin changes in people who wear braces or use crutches. Avoid massaging these areas.

Reer to Appendix B: Strategies for infection prevention and safe practice for some useful guidelines. Also see Appendix D for organizations and support groups.

References

Morello JA, Mizer HE, Wilson ME, Granato PA. Microbiology in patient care. 6th ed. New York: McGraw-Hill; 1998. p. 364-369.

Melnick JL. Current status of poliovirus infections. Clin Microbiol Rev 1996; 9(3): 293-300.

Renal system

Polycystic renal disease (Polycystic kidneys)

An inherited disorder where multiple cysts are found in the kidney/s.

Cause:

Notes

The individual should avoid situations that can precipitate renal failure such as dehydration, reduced intake of salt, intake of certain drugs (eg. analgesics) etc. Hypertension, if present, should be treated. In severe cases where the symptoms due to the cysts are extensive, the kidney may be removed (nephrectomy).

For more details see Appendix C: Painkillers; Antihypertensives.

The condition is transmitted to the offspring from parents. Both the cortex and medulla of the kidney have numerous fluid-filled cysts of varying sizes.

Signs and Symptoms:

Due to the presence of cysts, the kidney/s are larger in size and in some patients it may be palpable in the abdomen. Often, the condition is detected only at autopsies. Symptoms usually occur in middle age. The cysts compress the nephrons and cause localized obstruction. Infection, lumbar pain and blood in urine (hematuria) - especially after trauma are some of the symptoms.

Hypertension, kidney stones and renal failure may develop in some patients.

Risk Factors:

It is often associated with cysts in the liver and other organs. In some cases, the condition is associated with aneurysms in the brain.

Caution and Recommendations to Therapists:

Avoid abdominal massage in clients who have been diagnosed with polycystic renal disease as the cysts can be ruptured by pressure resulting in severe abdominal pain. Bleeding may also occur as a result.

References

Coe FL, Kathpalia S. Hereditary tubular disorders. In: Isselbacher KJ et al, editors. Harrison's principles of internal medicine. 13th ed. New York: McGraw-Hill Inc; 1994. p. 1323-1325.

Polycythemia

Cardiovascular system

An increase in the number of red blood cells above normal levels.

Cause:

There are many causes of polycythemia. Polycythemia is considered to be *relative* if it is due to a reduction in plasma and concentration of red blood cells, as may occur in dehydration and burn injury. It is considered to be *absolute* if it is due to some other cause. If absolute polycythemia is produced by a known stimulus it is termed *erythrocytosis* and if it is due to an unknown cause it is termed *erythremia*. *Polycythemia vera* is an example of erythremia.

Erythrocytosis may be due to increases in the hormone erythropoietin that stimulates formation of red blood cells. This may occur in certain types of neoplasms or may be familial. Erythropoietin may increase secondary to hypoxia. Living in high altitudes, lung disorders, shunting of blood from the right to left side of the heart and abnormal hemoglobin function (eg. carboxyhemoglobin) are examples. Certain hormones such as steroids and androgens can stimulate formation of red blood cells and polycythemia.

Signs and Symptoms:

Patients with polycythemia appear cyanosed. They may complain of dizziness and headache. Thrombi are easily formed and symptoms may be due to blockage of blood vessels supplying specific tissues.

Risk Factors:

Smoking increases the level of carboxyhemoglobin and can cause polycythemia.

Caution and Recommendations to Therapists:

Avoid massage or get clearance from treating Physician, as there is a tendency to form clots.

Notes

It is important to identify and avoid precipitating factors. Blood transfusions may be required. For more details see Appendix C: Blood transfusion.

References

Braunwald E. Hypoxia, polycythemia, and cyanosis. In: Isselbacher KJ et al, editors. Harrison's principles of internal medicine. 13th ed. New York: McGraw-Hill Inc; 1994. p. 179-181.

Erslev AJ. Erythrocytosis. In: WJ Williams et al, editors. Hematology. 4th ed. New York: McGraw-Hill; 1990. p. 705.

Polyps (Polyposis)

Any lesion that projects into the lumen (usually the gut) is known as a polyp.

Cause:

Polyps may be single or multiple. Only microscopic examination can determine if it is benign or malignant. Hyperplastic polyps are commonly seen in the colon. They are thought to occur due to failure of the multiplying cells to slough off from the mucosa. Juvenile polyps are usually 1-2 cms in size with a short neck and found more often in the rectum. Many other types of polyps have been identified in the gut, some of which are hereditary. Adenomatosis polyposis is said to be present when there are more than 100 adenomas in the large intestine. Adenomas are benign tumors arising from the gastrointestinal epithelium.

Signs and Symptoms:

Hyperplastic polyps do not produce any symptoms and may be discovered accidentally. Juvenile polyps undergo torsion easily and may present with rectal bleeding and abdominal pain.

Risk Factors:

Hyperplastic polyps may predispose to cancer of the colon. Juvenile polyps are seen in the first five years of life and are often familial.

Caution and Recommendations to Therapists:

References

Sabiston DC, editor. Textbook of Surgery 14th ed. Philadelphia: WB Saunders Company; 1991.

Avoid abdominal massage in those diagnosed with polyps. If in doubt, get clearance from the treating Physician. See Appendix D for organizations and support groups.

Porphyria

Disorders of specific enzymes required for synthesis of the heme component of hemoglobin.

Cause:

This condition may be inherited or acquired. The deficiency of specific enzymes result in accumulation of precursors of heme - porphyrin. Depending on where the precursors accumulate, porphyria is classified as hepatic or erythropoietic.

Signs and Symptoms:

The symptoms can be precipitated by drugs, diet and steroid hormones. Often, the symptoms are seen only in adolescence. The symptoms vary according to the enzyme that is deficient. *Hepatic porphyrias* present with abdominal pain, peripheral neuropathy and mental disturbances. There is degeneration of the axons, especially of the motor neurons. The muscles of the shoulders and arms are affected first. The person may have symptoms such as anxiety, loss of sleep, depression, hallucination, convulsions etc. Nausea and vomiting may be present. The symptoms are vague and diagnosis is often delayed.

Erythropoietic porphyrias usually present as skin sensitivity to the sun. This is because ultraviolet light reacts with the excess porphyrins in the skin leading to scarring and deformation. Fluid-filled vesicles may develop on the surfaces exposed to the sun. The skin is easily injured and heals slowly. The skin heals by fibrosis and is thickened with scar formation.

Risk Factors:

Excess alcohol, iron, certain drugs and steroid hormones are precipitating factors.

Caution and Recommendations to Therapists:

Since the symptoms vary, the client has to be carefully assessed and treatment planned accordingly.

References

Desnick RJ. Porphyrias. In: Isselbacher KJ et al, editors. Harrison's principles of internal medicine. 13th ed. New York: McGraw-Hill Inc; 1994. p. 2073-2079.

Portal hypertension

Gastrointestinal system

An abnormal increase of pressure in the portal circulation.

Cause:

The portal circulation is responsible for carrying blood from the abdominal organs into the liver before it flows into the inferior vena cava and the right side of the heart.

Any condition that blocks or obstructs the flow of blood in the portal or hepatic veins can cause this. The portal vein can be occluded by structures around it like enlarged lymph nodes or tumors. Thrombosis in the vein can also cause obstruction. The most common cause of portal hypertension is cirrhosis of the liver where the fibrous bands formed distort the hepatic blood vessels. In severe right heart failure, there is damming of blood in the veins leading to this condition.

Notes

The primary concern is to avoid bleeding from the dilated collateral veins. Sclerosing agents are used to occlude the veins in the esophagus, which are prone to hemorrhage extensively. Surgery to shunt the blood from the portal vein, bypassing the obstruction is also resorted to.

For more details see Appendix C: Sclerosing agents.

Signs and Symptoms:

The signs and symptoms are produced by the damming of blood in the veins of the abdomen. The increase in pressure forces fluid from the abdominal capillaries into the peritoneal cavity (ascites). It also results in the blood seeking alternate routes to reach the heart. Dilatation of collateral vessels in the lower end of the esophagus, around the umbilicus and rectum occurs. Rupture and bleeding of these dilated and tortuous vessels can be fatal (see Esophageal varices). Portal hypertension also causes the spleen to enlarge.

Risk Factors:

Risk factors of thrombus formation, chronic alcohol intake and any condition that causes cirrhosis predisposes an individual to portal hypertension.

References

Podolsky DK, Isselbacher KJ. Alcohol-related liver disease and cirrhosis. In: Isselbacher KJ et al, editors. Harrison's principles of internal medicine. 13th ed. McGraw-Hill Co; 1994. p. 1483-1495

Musculoskeletal system

Posterior compartment syndrome

A collection of signs and symptoms produced by increased pressure and consequent reduced blood flow to a closed muscle compartment in the leg.

Notes

The condition is diagnosed by measuring the pressure in the compartment. If the symptoms are chronic or severe, surgery may be done to reduce the pressure. If left untreated, the muscle tissue dies and is replaced by fibrous tissue leading to contractures.

Cause:

In the calf ie. in the region posterior to the tibia and fibula, the muscles are compartmentalized into two by a thick fascia (connective tissue sheath). This sheath separates the gastrocnemius and soleus muscles into a superficial compartment, and the tibialis posterior, flexor hallucis longus and flexor digitorum longus into a deeper compartment.

Any condition that increases the pressure in either of these compartments compromises the blood flow to the soft tissue. The ischemia, inflammation and swelling in the compartment produce the characteristic symptoms.

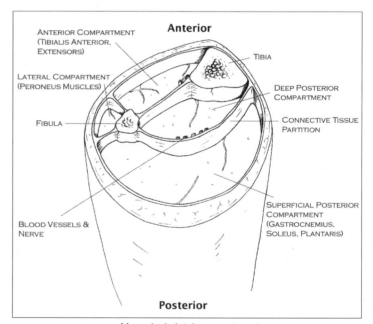

Musculoskeletal compartments

Pathology A to Z -

Signs and Symptoms:

There is a gradual onset of pain in the calf. The pain increases on using the limb and comes on after the same amount of exertion every time. Often, both legs are affected. If there is compression of nerves passing through the compartment, paralysis and changes in sensation may be present. Occlusion of blood vessels in the compartment may lead to pallor, coolness of the skin and swelling of the foot.

Risk Factors:

Overuse and repetitive use of the muscles in the compartment result in this condition.

Caution and Recommendations to Therapists:

The limb should be placed in level with the heart. Elevation may reduce the blood flow to the already compromised tissue. Placing the limb in a dependent position may increase the venous congestion due to the effect of gravity. In the acute stage, measures to reduce the inflammation and swelling are helpful. Rest and ice application have been found to be beneficial. The thighs should be massaged well, using broad strokes like effleurage and pétrissage to increase venous and lymphatic drainage. In the subacute stage, heat can be applied to soften the connective tissue. Suitable strokes such as cross fibre friction are used to stretch the tight fascia. However, such techniques should be avoided if it is too painful. In those with lowered sensation, care should be taken not to use excessive pressure, as the feedback from the client is likely to be inadequate.

References

Mercier LR, editor. Practical orthopedics. 4th ed. New York: Mosby-Year book Inc; 1995.p. 305-306.

Postpolio syndrome

(Postpoliomyelitis neuromuscular atrophy)

Musculoskeletal system

A complication of poliomyelitis that results in progressive muscle weakness.

Cause:

It is due to slow degeneration of motor neurons with resultant loss of nerve supply to muscles.

Notes

Treatment is supportive.

Signs and Symptoms:

There is progressive muscle weakness in some patients who have had poliomyelitis 20 to 30 years earlier. There may be slow deterioration of muscle function with muscle pain, fatigue, weakness, atrophy and involuntary movements. Usually the limbs are affected. In some cases, respiratory muscles, among others may be affected leading to difficulty in swallowing, choking, entry of food into the larynx and sleep apnea.

Risk Factors:

History of poliomyelitis infection at an earlier age.

References

Ray G. Enterovirus and reoviruses. In: Isselbacher KJ et al, editors. Harrison's principles of internal medicine. 13th ed. New York: McGraw-Hill Inc; 1994. p. 823, 1236.

Caution and Recommendations to Therapists:

Since it is sequelae to polio, this condition is not infective. The aim of the Therapist should be to reduce muscle pain, slow down atrophy and weakness of the muscles. See Appendix D for organizations and support groups.

Premenstrual syndrome

Reproductive system

(PMS; Premenstrual dysphoria disorder)

The physical and psychological symptoms perceived 3-14 days prior to the onset of menstruation.

Cause:

Notes

PMS is treated symptomatically with painkillers, regular exercise and dietary changes. Diets low in simple sugars, high in lean meat, avoidance of caffeine are some dietary measures used. In severe cases, hormones are given. Some benefit from vitamin B6 administration.

For more details see Appendix C: Painkillers; Hormone therapy/ replacement.

The cause has been attributed to a complex interaction between various factors. Excess levels of estrogen, prolactin, changes in estrogen-progesterone ratio, stress, hypoglycemia are some of the factors. Increased levels of aldosterone, decreased levels of dopamine and serotonin, deficiency of vitamin B12 have also been implicated.

Signs and Symptoms:

The breasts are painful and swollen. Headache, backache, changes in coordination, abdominal pain and a bloated feeling are other symptoms. The person may have craving for sweets. Psychologically, the individual may become depressed, irritable, and anxious with inability to concentrate. Other behavioral changes may also be seen. The symptoms and signs are different from woman to woman and from cycle to cycle in the same person.

Risk Factors:

It is more common in women above the age of 30.

Caution and Recommendations to Therapists:

References

Readers digest family guide to Alternative medicine. New York: Readers Digest Association Ltd; 1991, p. 274-275.

Berek JS. Novak's gynecology. 12th ed. Philadelphia: Williams & Wilkins; 1996. p. 306-307.

Since the exact cause of PMS is not known a variety of treatments are available, of which relaxation techniques is one. A relaxing and gentle whole body massage is indicated. Use of essential oils like lavender, chamomile, rose in a 5% dilution are recommended by some. Warm compresses to the back and lower abdomen helps reduce pain and tenderness. Some Therapists advocate breast massage. This should be done only after obtaining an informed consent from the client and only if the Therapist is comfortable and has had training in this area. Cold towel breast wraps, which reduce congestion by vasoconstriction of the blood vessels, are also used. Lymphatic drainage techniques with strokes directed towards the axillary lymph nodes are additional techniques used to reduce congestion and breast tenderness. Rhythmic, slow strokes using broad surface techniques like palmar kneading are used to massage the pectoralis major and minor muscles underlying the breast.

Pathology A to Z -

Prostatic hyperplasia

A benign enlargement of the prostate.

Cause:

It is caused by changes in the level of hormones with age.

Signs and Symptoms:

The symptoms are due to narrowing of the urethra as the middle lobe of the prostate enlarges and compresses the urethra. The person has urgency and difficulty in passing urine.

Risk Factors:

It is common with aging.

Caution and Recommendations to Therapists:

The prostate is more deeply placed and cannot be approached from the surface of the body. A light, soothing full body massage helps. Encourage client to take the full course of antibiotics prescribed.

Notes

This condition causes stagnation of urine making the urinary bladder, urethra and kidneys more susceptible to infection. Benign prostatic hyperplasia is treated with surgery (transurethral prostatectomy). Sometimes drugs are given to block the action of the sympathetics. For more details see Appendix C: Sympatholytic drugs.

References

Weinerth JL. The male genital system. In: Sabiston DC, editor. Textbook of Surgery - the biological basis of modern surgical practice. 14th ed. London: WB Saunders Co; 1991. p. 1468-1470.

Prostatitis

An inflammation of the prostate.

Cause:

It is usually caused by bacteria. However, the inflammation may occur after catheterization or using an instrument in the area.

Signs and Symptoms:

High fever with chills, muscle and joint pain are common. There is frequency and urgency on passing urine. The urine may be cloudy. A dull ache may be present in the low back and perineal area.

Risk Factors:

Catheterizations, use of instruments in the area are all predisposing factors. It is more common in males with diabetes mellitus.

Caution and Recommendations to Therapists:

The prostate cannot be accessed from the exterior of the body. A full body massage is given for general relaxation. Encourage client to seek medical help.

Notes

It is treated with antibiotics. For more details see Appendix C: Antimicrobial - antibacterial agents.

References

Weinerth JL. The male genital system. In: Sabiston DC, editor. Textbook of Surgery- the biological basis of modern surgical practice. 14th ed. WB Saunders Co; 1991. p. 1467-1468.

Psoriasis

A chronic, relapsing, inflammatory disease of the skin.

Cause:

The cause is unknown. The rate at which the keratinocytes (from the basal layer of the skin) migrate to the superficial layer is faster than normal in these individuals.

Signs and Symptoms:

The patients present with patches of different sizes with whitish or yellowish scales that loosely adhere to the epidermis of the skin. There is redness around these patches. The patches give the appearance of drops of mortar on the skin. The patches may persist throughout life with periods of remission and exacerbation. There are many forms of Psoriasis. In the more common form - *psoriasis vulgaris*, the patches are typically seen in the elbow, knee and scalp. In *eruptive psoriasis* the patches are smaller and seen in the trunk and limbs. In *pustular psoriasis*, the lesions have pustules and there is generalized fever. These patches occur even in the soles of feet and the palms. *Oval* or *annular psoriasis* is a rare form. It is not contagious. See Appendix A: page 355.

Risk Factors:

It commonly occurs in adults above 30 years of age. There is also a genetic predisposition. In individuals who are predisposed, skin trauma or alcohol consumption, may precipitate an attack. Psoriasis is usually worse in winter perhaps due to lower indoor humidity and relative lack of sunlight.

Caution and Recommendations to Therapists:

Psoriasis, although unsightly, is not contagious and massage can be beneficial. The scales that are loosely adherent may dislodge with massage and be a nuisance to the Therapist. Since there is no known cure for psoriasis the clients may be on varied treatment regimens. Some clients may be on topical corticosteroid treatment that makes the local area susceptible to superinfection by bacteria. Take care to wash hands thoroughly before massaging such individuals. Other treatment regimens used such as methotrexate or cyclosporine suppress the general immunity of the individuals and make them susceptible to infection. Do not massage such clients when you harbor a cold, cough or any other mild form of infection. Schedule their appointment at a time when they are unlikely to come in contact with other clients who may have an infection. See Appendix D for organizations and support groups.

Notes

Treatment options vary from patient to patient and the extent and location of lesions. Three categories of treatment exist. Topical application (daily application of lubricants, corticosteroids, coal tar solution, vitamin D3 etc), phototherapy (ultraviolet radiation) and systemic therapy (oral/intravenous drugs). For more details see Appendix C: Antiinflammatories - steroidal drugs; Phototherapy.

References

Zanolli MD. Psoriasis and Reiter's syndrome. In: Sams WM, Lynch PJ, editors. Principles and practice of Dermatology. 2nd ed. New York: Churchill Livingstone; 1996. p. 341-359.

Pulmonary edema

An accumulation of fluid in the lungs.

Cause:

Any condition that results in an increase in the pulmonary venous pressure can result in pulmonary edema. When the outflow from the left ventricle is reduced, there is damming of blood in the lungs and edema can result. Mitral stenosis, and left ventricular failure are some examples. Reduced protein levels in the blood (hypoalbuminemia) can cause movement of fluid into the interstitial tissue and edema. In some cases, the permeability of the capillaries and alveoli is increased. Pneumonia, inhalation of toxins and radiation are some examples of conditions that affect permeability. The cause of edema is unknown in some cases eg. high altitude pulmonary edema; pulmonary embolism etc.

Signs and Symptoms:

The person presents with rapid breathing (tachypnea) and dyspnea. If the edema is severe, the person may have associated anxiety. Cough is present and the sputum is frothy and blood-tinged. If not treated, gas exchange is markedly affected and it may lead to respiratory arrest and death.

Risk Factors:

See Cause.

Caution and Recommendations to Therapists:

Clearance from the treating Physician has to be obtained. A gentle massage of short duration may be given in a seated position with a focus on the tired respiratory muscles with an aim to relax and calm the individual. See Appendix D for organizations and support groups.

Notes

The cause of the edema has to be identified and treated. The venous return can be reduced by changing the posture of the patient to a sitting position. Oxygen administration is beneficial. Diuretics can be given to reduce blood volume and thereby the venous return. However, the systolic pressure has to be maintained to ensure adequate perfusion of tissues.

For more details see Appendix C: Diuretics; Oxygen treatment.

References

Ingram RH, Braunwald E. Dyspnea and pulmonary edema. In: Isselbacher KJ et al, editors. Harrison's principles of internal medicine. 13th ed. New York: McGraw-Hill Inc; 1994. p. 177-178

Pulmonary embolism

A blockage of a pulmonary artery by thrombus or a foreign substance.

Cause:

It is usually caused by a thrombus that has been dislodged from a leg vein. However, thrombus can be from other veins too. Rarely, the thrombus can be fat, air or tumor cells. Prolonged blockage can lead to death of lung tissue (*pulmonary infarction*).

Signs and Symptoms:

Large emboli that occlude the artery totally can be fatal. Smaller emboli produce difficulty in breathing, cough with blood-tinged sputum and chest pain. Low-grade fever may be present. Depending on the size of the emboli, the symptoms vary. Blue coloration of fingers and toes may be seen indicating reduced

Notes

Small emboli are treated with oxygen and drugs to reduce coagulation (clotting) of blood.

Emboli can be prevented by screening high-risk patients for impedence to blood flow and using prophylactic treatment such as heparin to reduce the coagulability of blood, use of compressive devices to facilitate blood flow and early mobilisation after surgery.

For more details see Appendix C: Anticoagulants.

oxygenation of blood. The neck veins may appear prominent.

Risk Factors:

Conditions which tend to reduce flow of blood as in prolonged immobilization, heart failure, varicose veins, thrombophlebitis (infection/inflammation of veins) and obesity can predispose to embolism. Increased clotting tendencies of blood as during pregnancy and use of oral contraceptives make a person prone for emboli. Fat emboli can be a complication of surgery and fractures. Conditions that thicken the blood (polycythemia) such as severe burn injury can also speed up emboli formation. Emboli are more common in the older age group.

Caution and Recommendations to Therapists:

NEVER massage vigorously, the legs of individuals with moderate to severe varicose veins, or those who have been immobilized for a long time, or those pregnant. Vigorous massage in individuals who are predisposed may result in dislodgment of thrombi already formed. Those clients with a previous history of emboli are likely to be on anti-coagulant therapy and are prone to bleed easily. Do not use excess pressure while massaging these individuals. Early mobilization after surgery helps avoid thrombi and emboli formation. Encourage clients in plaster casts or those advised prolonged bed rest to passively or actively move joints that are not immobilized.

See Appendix D for organizations and support groups.

References

Moser KM. Pulmonary thromboembolism. In: Isselbacher KJ et al, edotors. Harrison's principles of internal medicine. 13th ed. New York: McGraw-Hill Inc; 1994. p.1214-1220.

Respiratory system

Pulmonary hypertension

An abnormal increase in blood pressure in the pulmonary circulation.

Notes

The patient is advised to avoid physical exertion. Diuretics may be beneficial. Vasodilator drugs may be given to lower the blood pressure. Since thrombus formation is common, anticoagulants may be given. Those not responding to any medical treatment may be considered for lung transplantation.

For more details see Appendix C: Diuretics; Bronchodilators; Anticoagulants; Organ transplantation.

Cause:

There may be many causes. *Primary pulmonary hypertension* is a condition where the cause is not known. Pulmonary hypertension may be *secondary* to other disorders such as congenital and valvular heart disease, pulmonary thrombosis, liver disease, obstructive lung disease etc.

Signs and Symptoms:

There is slow onset of shortness of breath, fatigue, chest pain, loss of consciousness and edema in other regions.

Risk Factors:

See Cause.

Caution and Recommendations to Therapists:

Clearance has to be obtained from the treating Physician. A gentle massage of short duration may be given in a seated position with a focus on the tired respiratory muscles with an aim to relax and calm the individual.

See Appendix D for organizations and support groups.

References

Rich S. Primary pulmonary hypertension. In: Isselbacher KJ et al, editors. Harrison's principles of internal medicine. 13th ed. New York: McGraw-Hill Inc; 1994. p. 1211-1214.

Pathology A to Z -

Q fever

An acute infection caused by the rickettsial organism Coxiella burnetii.

Gastrointestinal, Respiratory systems

Cause:

The infection is caused in humans by the inhalation of contaminated dust, by handling infected material or by drinking contaminated milk. The organism is transmitted in nature by infected ticks. The infected tick feces may contaminate cattle hides. Sheep, cows, goats and other wild and domestic animals can be infected and their milk and excretions can contain the organism. The incubation period of the organism is between 14-26 days.

Signs and Symptoms:

The condition presents with high fever, chills, loss of appetite, muscle pain and lethargy. Later, dry cough and chest pain develops. The liver may be inflamed (hepatitis) and jaundice is seen. Inflammation of the heart valves may occur leading to damage and blood flow-volume abnormalities. Usually, the entire course of the disease does not last for more than two weeks unless there are complications.

Risk Factors:

Laboratory workers, slaughterhouse workers and others in occupations that are likely to expose them to contaminated dust are at greater risk.

Caution and Recommendations to Therapists:

Ensure that the clinic is 'rodent proofed'. Check the ventilation of the clinic periodically. Refer to Appendix B: Strategies for infection prevention and safe practice for some useful guidelines. Also see Appendix D for organizations and support groups.

Notes

The condition is treated with antibiotics such as tetracycline. It can be prevented by giving vaccines to susceptible individuals and those at risk. Measures should be taken to prevent exposure to contaminated dust and milk from infected livestock should be boiled or pasteurized.

For more details see Appendix C: Antimicrobial - antibacterial agents; Immunization.

References

Morello JA, Mizer HE, Wilson ME, Granato PA. Microbiology in patient care. 6th ed. New York: McGraw-Hill; 1998. p. 251-253.

Rabies

A viral infection that affects the central nervous system and is transmitted by infected saliva.

Nervous system

Cause:

Usually, rabies is transmitted by the bite of an infected animal. Occasionally, it may be due to ingestion or inhalation of the virus or transplantation of infected tissue (eg. cornea). In urban areas, it is spread by unimmunized domestic dogs. In the wild, it is spread by infected wolves, skunks, foxes, raccoons, mongooses and bats. The incubation period of the virus is variable and ranges from 10 days to 1 year.

The virus is introduced into the body through the skin or mucous membrane. The virus multiplies in the skeletal muscle located in the local area and migrates

Notes

If rabies is suspected in an animal, it should be captured and killed. If a person has been bitten by a normal dog or cat the animal has to kept under observation for at least 10 days to see if it becomes ill. The wound produced by the bite of the animal should be thoroughly washed with soap, disinfectant and water. Antirabies vaccines are available and should be given as soon as possible after exposure. Five doses of vaccine are required.

Readily available antibodies (passive immunization) are also used. Rabies vaccine may be given as a preventive measure to those at risk because of their occupation. Other forms of supportive treatment are given to control symptoms.

For more details see Appendix C: Immunization.

References

Morello JA, Mizer HE, Wilson ME, Granato PA. Microbiology in patient care. 6th ed. New York: McGraw-Hill; 1998. p. 508-513.

Smith JS. New aspects of rabies with emphasis on epidemiology, diagnosis, and prevention of the disease in the United states. Clin Microbiol Rev 1996; 9(2): 166-176.

Kaplan MM, Koprowski H. Rabies. Sci Am. 1980; 242(1):120-134.

to the neuromuscular junction. From here, it ascends up the nerves to reach the central nervous system. From the central nervous system, the virus spreads to other tissues along the autonomic nerves. The disease can be spread through the saliva from infected salivary glands.

Signs and Symptoms:

Initially, the patient presents with fever, headache, malaise, body pain, fatigue, loss of appetite, nausea and vomiting. There may be loss of sensation at the site of the bite. Soon the person becomes excited and agitated. Confusion, mental disturbances, muscle spasms and convulsions are seen when the virus reaches the central nervous system. There is hypersensitivity to bright light, noise and touch. The person may become comatose. When the virus spreads to the autonomic nervous system, high temperature, irregular dilated pupils, excessive salivation, tearing, sweating and hypotension may be seen. Various cranial nerves may be paralysed. There may be painful, violent, involuntary contraction of the diaphragm and other muscles associated with swallowing fluids. If the respiratory center is involved, death may result from respiratory arrest.

Risk Factors:

See Cause.

Caution and Recommendations to Therapists:

Do not allow pets into the clinic except seeing eye dogs. Refer to Appendix B: Strategies for infection prevention and safe practice for some useful guidelines. Also see Appendix D for organizations and support groups.

Cardiovascular system

Raynaud's syndrome (Raynaud's phenomenon; Raynaud's disease)

Intense spasm of arteries and arterioles in the fingers or toes.

Cause:

The cause of primary Raynaud's syndrome is unknown, and may be precipitated by cold, strong emotions or stress. It is thought to be due to hyperactivity of the sympathetic nervous system. Some believe that it may be due to enhanced responsiveness of vascular smooth muscle to cold or other stimuli. Primary Raynaud's is known as Raynaud's disease. Secondary Raynaud's phenomenon can be associated with frost bite, occupations using heavy vibrating equipment or requiring frequent exposure of limbs to alternating temperatures of cold and warmth (eg. butchers, caterers), collagen disorders (eg. Systemic Lupus Erythematosus), neurological disorders and disorders which tend to occlude arteries.

Notes

Use of warm clothes and avoidance of unnecessary exposure to cold is advocated in mild cases. Drugs that produce vasodilation are used in severe cases. In some, surgical sympathectomy may be done.

For more details see Appendix C: Vasodilators; Surgical sympathectomy.

Signs and Symptoms:

The patient may present with slight swelling of fingers or toes. The reduced blood flow to these parts result in change of skin color - pale or cyanosed (blue). There may be loss of sensations, or tingling. Following the ischemia (reduced blood flow) the part may become pink (hyperemia). The nails may appear brittle and the skin of the fingers or toes may be thickened. In late stages, ulcers or gangrene may be seen.

Risk Factors:

Those in occupations using vibrating equipment or those requiring frequent exposure to alternating cold and heat are at higher risk. Smoking has been shown to be associated with this disease. Raynaud's disease is more common in women between the ages of 20 and 40.

Caution and Recommendations to Therapists:

Recurrent washing of hands with alternating cold and warm water should be avoided. Massage helps clients with Raynaud's by increasing blood flow to the periphery. By reducing stress, massage helps lower sympathetic stimulation and thereby relax the smooth muscles of blood vessels. Do not apply heat packs to affected areas during an attack of spasm.

See Appendix D for organizations and support groups.

References

Sams M. Temperature-dependent dermatoses. In: Sams WM, Lynch PJ, editors. Principles and practice of Dermatology. 2ⁿᵈ ed. New York: Churchill Livingstone; 1996. p. 575-576.

Relapsing fever

An acute spirochetal infection that results in recurrent bouts of fever.

Cardiovascular, Nervous systems

Cause:

The disease is caused by different species of the spirochete *Borrelia*. The organism may be transmitted by louse or tick. When the louse ingests blood from an infected person, the spirochetes enter its body and multiply there. The spirochetes are transmitted to another person when they are crushed and its body fluid enter the bloodstream through the bite site or skin injured by scratching. Infection can also be produced by entry through the conjunctiva or mucous membrane when a person with contaminated fingernails touches these areas.

Small rodents are hosts of ticks that carry the spirochetes causing tick-borne relapsing fever. The ticks feed at night and become infected when they take a blood meal from an infected rodent or human. The spirochetes multiply in the gut and migrate to the salivary gland and reproductive organs where they remain infective for years. Humans become infected by tick bite when the spirochetes are injected into the blood stream. Since the urine and milk of infected rodents also carry spirochetes, accidental contact of mucous membranes (eye, nose, mouth etc) with these secretions can cause this condition.

Signs and Symptoms:

As soon as the spirochetes enter the blood stream they multiply rapidly and

Notes

It is treated with antibiotics such as tetracycline. Relapsing fever can be prevented by taking measures to control lice (see Pediculosis) and ticks. In areas infested with infected ticks, spraying of insecticides is beneficial.

For more details see Appendix C: Antimicrobial - antibacterial agents.

the person presents with fever. The fever may be accompanied with chills, headaches, muscle and joint pain. Abdominal pain, nausea and vomiting are other symptoms. The fever is followed by profuse sweating and hypotension. The person may have a relapse of fever 5-10 days later experiencing no fever in between. There may be 5-20 relapses. The symptoms are seen about 3-12 days after entry of spirochetes.

The endothelium of the blood vessels are injured and blood can exude out through mucous membranes and skin and appear as multiple bleeding spots (petechiae) and patches (ecchymoses). Blood may be seen in the urine (hematuria) or sputum (hemoptysis). Intravascular coagulation is also triggered in the process. The spirochetes may enter the brain, heart and kidney resulting in inflammation, cell death and further complications. There may be enlargement of the spleen (splenomegaly) and liver (hepatomegaly). The spirochetes are also capable of crossing the placenta and may cause abortion.

Tick-borne relapsing fever tends to affect the nervous system and deafness, blindness and convulsions are some of the complications.

Risk Factors:

The louse-borne relapsing fever is more common in Central and East Africa, Peru and China. Tick-borne relapsing fever is more common in spring and summer when more time is spent outdoors.

Caution and Recommendations to Therapists:

Ensure that the clinic is "rodent and insect proofed". Massage is contraindicated till the full course of antibiotics has been taken and all symptoms have disappeared. Reer to Appendix B: Strategies for infection prevention and safe practice for some useful guidelines. Also see Appendix D for organizations and support groups.

References

Morello JA, Mizer HE, Wilson ME, Granato PA. Microbiology in patient care. 6th ed. New York: McGraw-Hill; 1998. p.486-487.

Renal failure (Kidney failure)

Renal system

A condition where the kidney is unable to fulfill its' function according to the demands made by the body.

Notes

Failure due to prerenal causes can be reversed by prompt correction of the abnormality in blood volume and flow. Postrenal failure can be corrected by removal of obstruction to urine flow. Failure due to renal causes is more difficult to treat and the aim is to prevent further problems and complications. It is important to monitor and maintain fluid and electrolyte balance. Dietary modification is an important aspect. In addition to the therapy advocated for acute renal failure, chronic renal failure may require dialysis or renal transplant.

Cause:

Renal failure could be *acute* (sudden onset) or *chronic* (occurs over a number of years). There are many causes of acute renal failure. The causes may be classified as those due to conditions other than the urinary tract - *prerenal*; those due to kidney disease - *renal*; and those due to problems with the drainage of urine from the kidney - *postrenal*.

Prerenal conditions affect the renal function by altering the blood flow to the kidney. Intrarenal conditions damage the kidney tissue. Postrenal causes are conditions that obstruct the outflow of urine and produce damage to the kidney by backpressure.

Chronic renal failure is caused by conditions that destroy the nephrons - the functional unit of the kidney. It may be a complication of untreated acute renal failure. Systemic diseases like diabetes mellitus, prolonged hypertension and hereditary defects of the kidney can lead to this.

For more details see Appendix C: Dialysis; Organ transplantation.

Signs and Symptoms:

The functions of the kidney are affected. The major functions of the kidney are to remove the end products of metabolism from the blood and to regulate the levels of fluid, electrolytes and thereby the pH of the body fluids. Other functions include secretion of hormones that regulate the formation of red blood cells (erythropoietin) and blood pressure (renin). It also plays a major role in the conversion of Vitamin D to an active form. Vitamin D participates in the regulation of calcium and phosphates.

Acute renal failure is usually reversible and can be treated effectively if diagnosed early. There is a sudden decrease in urine formation. The retention of fluid causes edema. The accumulation of urea, and other toxic substances, alteration in sodium, calcium and potassium levels have their own detrimental effects on the body.

Renal failure has effects on practically all systems. There is nausea, vomiting, diarrhea or constipation, bleeding from the gut (gastrointestinal system). Accumulation of fluid can cause pulmonary edema and difficulty in breathing (respiratory system). There is anemia, hypotension and finally heart failure (cardiovascular system). The skin is dry and pale, with a tendency to bruise easily. Itching is also present (integumentary system). The person is irritable and confused (nervous system). The bones are osteoporotic and prone to fracture easily (musculoskeletal system). Impotence, alterations in menstrual cycle and other sexual dysfunctions are common (reproductive system).

Risk Factors:

Prerenal: Dehydration (diarrhea, vomiting, and burn injury), loss of large quantities of blood, or heart failure can predispose to this type.

Renal: Exposure to drugs and chemicals that are toxic to the kidney eg. antibiotics like gentamycin, kanamycin and heavy metals like lead and mercury and autoimmune reactions like glomerulonephritis increase the risk.

Postrenal: Obstruction to the ureter by renal stones, prostatic hyperplasia and narrowing of the urethra can result in this type of failure.

Caution and Recommendations to Therapists:

Obtain a detailed history as to the cause of the renal failure and alter treatment accordingly. A light, soothing full body massage of short duration is recommended. The edema produced is a compensatory mechanism for the excess fluid that has been retained in the body. Therefore the massage should not be directed to reduce the edema. This may overload the heart that is already stressed by the fluid retention. The oil used helps reduce the dryness and itching of the skin. Only light pressure should be used as these individuals

References

Brady HR, Brenner BM. Acute renal failure. In: Isselbacher KJ et al, editors. Harrison's principles of internal medicine. 13th ed. New York: McGraw-Hill Inc; 1994. p. 1265-1274.

bruise easily. Also, the bones are fragile and may fracture even with moderate pressure. If the person is on dialysis, avoid massage over a wide area around the infusion site. Individuals who have had renal transplants may be on drugs that suppress immunity. Avoid massage if harboring even a mild form of infection. See Appendix D for organizations and support groups.

Renal system	**Renal stones** (Kidney stones; Renal calculi; Nephrolithiasis)
	Formation of solitary or multiple stones in the pelvis of the kidney.

Cause:

Stones are formed in the kidney when the urine is saturated with material that it normally excretes eg. calcium salts, uric acid, cystine, magnesium ammonium phosphate. This material tends to precipitate in the absence of substances that normally inhibit precipitation. A substance called nephrocalcin that has been recently identified is a natural inhibitor of precipitation. Precipitation is also promoted if organic material from the epithelium lining the tubules act as a nucleus or nidus for stone formation.

Signs and Symptoms:

Pain is the most common symptom. Excruciating, colicky pain in the upper outer quadrant of the abdomen and the flanks are common. The pain may be referred to the lower abdomen, scrotum/labia and inner thigh. It may be intense enough to cause nausea and vomiting. The skin may be cold and clammy. Small particles may be seen in the urine if the stone is excreted. The urine may be pink due to the presence of blood (hematuria).

Risk Factors:

Excessive bone resorption caused by immobility, bone disease and hyperparathyroidism predispose to calcium stones. Gout promotes formation of uric acid stones. Alkaline urine promotes formation of magnesium ammonium phosphate stones. A common cause of alkaline urine is bacterial infection. Any condition that predisposes to stagnation of urine also promotes stone formation.

Caution and Recommendations to Therapists:

Encourage the client to alter diet according to the type of stone identified by Physician and increase the intake of fluid. Massage is beneficial in reducing the pain, stress and muscle spasm. See Appendix D for organizations and support groups.

Notes

Dietary alterations can be made to prevent the recurrence of stone formation. To prevent calcium oxalate stones, diets rich in oxalate such as spinach, cocoa, chocolate, pecans, peanuts may be avoided. To prevent uric acid stones, high purine containing foods such as anchovies, liver, sardines, kidneys, sweetbreads, lentils and alcohol (especially beer and wine) should be avoided.

Urinary stones that are smaller than 5 mm are excreted in the urine spontaneously. Larger stones may have to be removed surgically. *Extracorporeal shock wave lithotripsy* - a procedure that uses shock waves to breakup the stones into tiny pieces small enough to be excreted in the urine is a popular form of treatment. Prevention of recurrence, however, should be the major goal.

For more details see Appendix C: Lithotripsy.

References

Coe FL, Favus MJ. Nephrolithiasis. In: Isselbacher KJ et al, editors. Harrison's principles of internal medicine. 13th ed. New York: McGraw-Hill Inc; 1994. p. 1329-1333.

Respiratory Distress Syndrome

(RDS; Hyaline membrane disease)

Respiratory system

A condition in infants, that produces difficulty in breathing due to the lack of a lipoprotein - surfactant, in the lungs.

Cause:

The normal lung produces a lipoprotein called surfactant that reduces the surface tension in the lung and allows the lung to expand easily on inspiration. In this condition, surfactant is lacking. This results in difficulty in inflating the lung and collapse of segments of lung (atelectasis).

Signs and Symptoms:

There is difficulty in breathing. The respiratory rate is rapid and labored and grunting may be present. If severe, the heart rate is rapid and cyanosis (blue coloration of the mucous membrane) may be seen.

Risk Factors:

Premature infants, infants born to diabetic mothers, infants delivered by Cesarean section are at risk.

Caution and Recommendations to Therapists:

Infants who have had this problem may take up to a year to recover - depending on the severity. Consult Pediatrician before massage.

Notes

Oxygen therapy and mechanical ventilatory support may be used. For more details see Appendix C: Oxygen treatment; Mechanical ventilation.

References

Fishman A, editor. Update: pulmonary diseases and disorders. New York: McGraw-Hill; 1992.

Rheumatic heart disease (Rheumatic fever)

Cardiovascular, Musculoskeletal systems

An inflammatory disease affecting many systems, following a streptococcal bacterial infection.

Cause:

It is due to the reaction of antibodies produced against the specific bacteria (viz. group A beta hemolytic streptococci), attacking other body tissues. The heart and the joints are most commonly affected.

Signs and Symptoms:

Typically, the person gives a history of sore throat a few days to 6 weeks before the onset of symptoms. There is fever and joint pain that seems to migrate from one large joint to another. Signs of inflammation - redness, swelling, loss of function, and warmth are seen in the affected joint. A rash may accompany these symptoms. Firm nodules (rounded masses) may be present under the skin. If the nervous system is affected, there may be symptoms of hyperirritability, inability to concentrate, abnormal writhing movements of the limb, among others. Often there is inflammation of the valves of the heart, which on resolving by fibrosis causes narrowing or leaky valves.

Notes

There is no specific cure for rheumatic fever. Supportive therapy can reduce the mortality and morbidity.

In the acute stage, it is treated with antibiotics and strict bed rest. Painkillers and anti-inflammatory drugs are given when arthritis is present. Corticosteroids may be used to treat carditis. Prolonged antibiotic treatment is used to prevent recurrence.

For more details see Appendix C: Painkillers; Antimicrobial - antibacterial agents; Antiinflammatories - sterodial drugs; Antiinflammatories - non steroidal drugs.

Risk Factors:

The incidence is higher in the lower socioeconomic group. It is more common in children between the ages of 5-15. Higher incidence is seen in the winter and early spring.

Caution and Recommendations to Therapists:

References

Stollerman GH. Rheumatic fever. In: Isselbacher KJ et al, editors. Harrison's principles of internal medicine. 13th ed. New York: McGraw-Hill Inc; 1994. p. 1046-1052.

A detailed history should be taken in order to ascertain the extent of the disease. In acute cases, massage is contraindicated. Measures to decrease pain and swelling in the joints may be taken. In chronic cases, treatment should be modified according to the extent of the disease. See Appendix D for organizations and support groups.

Integumentary system

Ringworm (Tinea; Dermatophytoses)

A fungal infection of the skin.

Cause:

Notes

Fungal infections can be treated, but require prolonged treatment sometimes lasting for six to twelve months. Usually topical agents are adequate and are used for 2-4 weeks.

For more details see Appendix C: Antimicrobial - antifungal agents.

A type of fungus - mold that has long, hollow, branching filaments, causes this disease. The fungus thrives on the cooler surface of the skin. Different fungi affect different areas. Fungal infection of the body is called *tinea corporis*, scalp - *tinea capitis*, hands - *tinea manus*, feet - *tinea pedis* (*athlete's foot*), nails - *tinea unguium*, groin and upper thighs - *tinea cruris* or *jock itch*, beard and moustache area - *tinea barbae*, face - *tinea faciei*. The infection is acquired by contact with an infected person, animal or infected soil. Infection may also occur through contact with infected surroundings such as clothes etc. Heat and humidity are conducive to the growth of fungi (see Appendix A: page 358).

Signs and Symptoms:

Tinea corporis appears as round or oval patches with a central clear area surrounded by a red border with pustules. Itching is pronounced. Many such lesions can be found all over the body.

Tinea capitis appears as painless, round, hairless patches on the scalp. Itching may be present. The lesion may appear red, with scaling.

Tinea pedis (athlete's foot) affect the spaces between the toes and appear as scaly lesions, or inflamed, oozing, painful lesions. Foul smells and itching may be present (see Appendix A: page 349).

In tinea unguium the nails become opaque or silvery, yellow or brown. The nails soon thicken and crack. In tinea manus, a blister appears in the palm of the hand or on the finger. Chronic lesions may appear dry and scaly.

Risk Factors:

Fungal infections are common in people with lowered immunity. Tinea pedis is more common in patients whose feet are constantly damp due to sweating or who wear occlusive shoes. Children are more prone to tinea capitis. Tinea corporis affects people of all ages and is transmitted from pet animals and other affected individuals.

Caution and Recommendations to Therapists:

Massage is contraindicated as the infection spreads by contact. Boil and steam press clothes, towels and bedding if contact has been made. Refer to Appendix B: Strategies for infection prevention and safe practice.

References

Morello JA, Mizer HE, Wilson ME, Granato PA. Microbiology in patient care. 6th ed. New York: McGraw-Hill; 1998. p. 302, 437.

Salpingitis

Reproductive system

An inflammation of the fallopian tubes.

Cause:

It is commonly caused by the organism *Chlamydia trachomatis* or *N. Gonorrhoeae*. The organisms are sexually transmitted. The infection reaches the fallopian tube via the vagina, cervix and endometrium.

Notes

It is treated with high doses of antibiotics for 14 days. Babies born to infected mothers may be infected and the organism can cause conjunctivitis in the babies. For more details see Appendix C: Antimicrobial - antibacterial agents.

Signs and Symptoms:

The person has lower abdominal pain, pain on passing urine, fever and white discharge from the vagina. The lower abdomen feels tender and rigid. There may be pain on having intercourse. The tube heals by fibrosis causing adhesions between organs in the pelvis and/or blockage of the tube - a common cause of infertility.

Risk Factors:

It is more common in sexually active women between the ages of 15-20. It is also common in those who use intrauterine devices for contraception or who have abnormal development of the reproductive organs. Oro-genital contact, vaginal or rectal intercourse with an infected person increases the risk of contracting the disease.

Caution and Recommendations to Therapists:

Encourage the client to take the full course of the prescribed antibiotics. Educate the client that sexual partners may also have to be treated to prevent reinfection. Avoid abdominal area while massaging the client. The client may feel more comfortable in a position with the head and knee raised with pillows. There is no scope for transmission of infection as it is sexually transmitted. Ask the client to keep underclothes on during massage. Refer to Appendix B: Strategies for infection prevention and safe practice.

References

Rapkin AJ. Pelvic pain and Dysmenorrhea.In: Berek JS, editor. Novak's gynecology. 12th ed. Philadelphia: Williams & Wilkins; 1996. p. 404-405.

Scabies

An itchy skin infection produced by mites.

Cause:

Notes

Topical agents are used. The agent should be applied thoroughly to all areas of the body, left on for a few hours and then washed off. Clothing, linen and towels should be machine-washed and dried using the hot cycle. Family members at high risk should also be treated.

Scabies is a disease that is caused by a mite - *Sarcoptes scabiei*. The mite burrows into the epidermis and these burrows along with the fecal matter of the mite are responsible for the itching. The females lay eggs in the burrows. The eggs hatch in 3-5 days thus restarting the cycle again.

Signs and Symptoms:

The patient presents with severe itching especially between the fingers, flexor surface of the wrist, axilla, gluteal creases, thigh, genital areas and other areas of the body. There may be secondary bacterial infection as a result of injury produced by scratching. Small reddish vesicles can be seen in these areas.

Risk Factors:

It affects people of all socioeconomic groups. It is transmitted by close skin to skin contact. Immunocompromised individuals are more prone.

Caution and Recommendations to Therapists:

Massage is contraindicated because scabies is contagious. However scabies is treatable. It is possible to contract scabies by sharing clothes, bedding or towels of an infected person. Do not massage a client even with a suspicion of scabies. If you have come in contact, apply the prescribed Lindane lotion or cream (Kwell) all over the body and wash after 12 hours. Repeat treatment if necessary. Wash all linen and clothes in boiling hot soapy water and detergent. Since scabies is very contagious, it is advisable to cancel all appointments for the day if you have treated an infected client inadvertently. Although the mite can survive outside the body for only a few hours, disinfect the furniture and all linen likely to have come in contact with the client with scabies. Refer to Appendix B: Strategies for infection prevention and safe practice for some useful guidelines.

References

Morello JA, Mizer HE, Wilson ME, Granato PA. Microbiology in patient care. 6ᵗʰ ed. New York: McGraw-Hill; 1998.

Sciatic nerve lesions (Sciatica)

A condition resulting from pressure or injury to the sciatic nerve.

Cause:

Notes

Treatment is modified according to the cause. Anti-inflammatory drugs, immobilization, soft-tissue mobilization techniques, massage, relaxation, traction, surgery and exercise among others, are some of the treatment options used. For more details see Appendix C: Antiinflammatories - non steroidal drugs.

This is usually caused by prolapse of the disc (herniated disc, slipped disc) with pressure on the nerve roots (L2, L5, S1, S2, S3) that give rise to the nerve. It may also be caused by narrowing of the intervertebral canal due to hypertrophy of the vertebral facets. Congenital abnormality of the vertebrae can also produce this. Trauma, gunshot wounds, fracture vertebrae are other causes. The sciatic nerve can also be injured or compressed after it exits from the spinal cord as in

Pathology A to Z -

spasm of the piriformis muscle that lies over the nerve. Improper administration of injections in the gluteal region can injure the sciatic nerve.

The nerve can also be injured anywhere along its long course as it travels from the gluteal region, behind the thigh, behind the knee in the popliteal fossa and as it divides into the common peroneal nerve (that goes around the neck of the fibula to the anterior compartment) and the tibial nerve (which descends in the calf region to the plantar aspect of the foot).

Signs and Symptoms:

The signs and symptoms vary according to the location of the lesion. If the sciatic nerve is injured close to the spinal cord then the person has difficulty in voluntarily flexing the knee (supply to the hamstrings affected), dorsiflexion and plantar flexion of the ankle (loss of nerve supply to the tibialis anterior, peroneal muscles, gastrocnemius and soleus). Movement of toes are also affected (nerve supply to the extensor and flexor muscles of the toes lost). The extension and abduction of the hip is weak.

The muscles supplied by the nerve are atrophic and have decreased tone. The person tends to swing the foot up and bring it with a slap onto the ground due to the tendency of the foot to drop (*footdrop*). Sensation in the lateral aspect of the leg below the level of the knee as well as to the foot is reduced. Deep sensations such as joint and position sense are also lost. The autonomic function is affected resulting in reduced circulation to the region. Sweating and temperature regulation may be poor in this region.

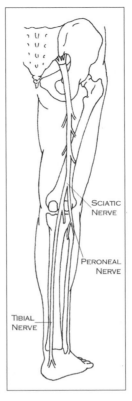

SCIATIC NERVE

PERONEAL NERVE

TIBIAL NERVE

If the injury is lower, flexion of the knee is present. But movement and sensations of the ankle are affected. If only the common peroneal is injured, dorsiflexion of the foot is impaired with loss of sensation in the anterior and lateral aspect of the leg and between the toes on the dorsum of the foot. Injury only to the tibial nerve results in impaired plantar flexion of the foot with difficulty in abducting and adducting the toes. The sensations are affected on the plantar surface as well as the lateral aspect of the foot.

Risk Factors:

See Cause.

Caution and Recommendations to Therapists:

Assess the motor and sensory function and keep a record of it. The extent of the loss can be kept on record using diagrams of outline of the legs and coloring

References

Turchaninov R, Cox CA. Medical massage. Scottsdale: Stress Less Publishing; 1998. p. 266-281.

Hall CM, Brody LT. Therapeutic exercise moving toward function. Philadelphia: Lippincott Williams & Wilkins; 1999.

areas where sensory and motor loss is present. An idea of the cause of the lesion can be obtained by a good history. Treatment should be modified according to the cause (eg. disc prolapse, piriformis spasm). For the muscles involved, the aim is to increase tone, reduce atrophy, prevent contractures and reduce edema. Pressure ulcers have to be watched for and prevented. Joint stiffness should be prevented or reduced. Position the limb neutrally and elevate it above the level of the heart to use the effect of gravity to reduce edema. The foot should be supported with pillows to maintain a neutral position ie. not excessively dorsiflexed or plantar flexed. The client can be positioned half prone, prone or lying on the side as the affected area is on the posterior and lateral aspect of the leg. Since the sensation is reduced, excessive pressure and force should not be used. Vibration, pinching and tapotement strokes can be used in the areas of sensory deficit.

Passively move all joints (do not forget the small joints of the toes) through as wide a range of motion as possible without using force. Use transverse friction around joints. A stimulatory massage helps to increase the tone of the muscles. Use broad strokes of effleurage and pétrissage to increase circulation and lymph drainage. Lymph drainage techniques can be used to reduce edema. Massage the stressed muscles of the pelvis, back and neck, which are overused to compensate for the lack of muscle control over the leg. Avoid massaging a wide area around pressure ulcers if present. Work in close conjunction with a Physiotherapist. See Appendix D for organizations and support groups.

Integumentary system

Scleroderma (Dermatosclerosis; Sclerema; Scleroma; Scleriasis; Hide bound disease; Systemic sclerosis)

A progressive, widespread disease of the connective tissue.

Notes

There is no cure for this condition. Immunosuppressants and corticosteroids are used to reduce symptoms. Physiotherapy may prevent contractures. For more details see Appendix C: Antiinflammatories - steroidal drugs; Immunosuppressants.

Cause:

The cause is not known. It may be due to the immunity of the body attacking tissues of self (autoimmune disease).

Signs and Symptoms:

This disease typically begins with vascular changes such as pallor, blue coloration or redness of the skin. Slowly, there is thickening of the skin through fibrosis. This fibrosis may fix the skin to the deeper tissues like the fascia covering tendons and muscle. The lesion may develop rapidly or as is more common gradually in a single or multiple area. It may be well localized or diffuse and ill defined, level, depressed or slightly elevated from the normal skin. The skin feels thick and leathery and cannot be pinched up in folds. The surface of the skin is usually smooth, but may be slightly scaly or nodular (see Appendix A: page 356). The shrinking and progressive thickening of the skin may greatly interfere with the function and nutrition of the parts beneath producing pain, edema and calcification. The muscles may atrophy as a result and the joints stiffen.

Pathology A to Z -

If the thickening is over the hands and fingers (*sclerodactylia*) the hands become stiff, immobile and useless. If over the chest, respiration may be compromised. If on the face, the natural folds disappear. Movements of the mouth and eyelids are inhibited and the person has a mask-like face. In some cases, the infiltration disappears gradually leaving a dry, wrinkled and parchment-like skin. This condition is systemic and can involve the central nervous system, lungs, esophagus, heart, duodenum and kidneys.

Risk Factors:

It is more common in women, African-Americans, in youth and the middle-aged.

Caution and Recommendations to Therapists:

It is not contagious. Local massage with oil or a mildly stimulating ointment is very beneficial. Friction strokes can reduce adhesions. Deeper strokes help increase circulation to the local area and improve nutrition and drainage. Passive and active movements of the joints help retain the range of movement. The individual may be on corticosteroids or immunosuppressants that lower the immunity. Ensure that they are not exposed to even mild forms of infection in the clinic as such infections can have serious consequences in these immuno-compromised individuals.See Appendix D for organizations and support groups.

References

Gilliland BC. Systemic sclerosis (Scleroderma). In: In: Isselbacher KJ et al, editors. Harrison's principles of internal medicine. 13th ed. New York: McGraw-Hill Inc; 1994. p. 1659.

Scoliosis

Musculoskeletal system

Bending of the vertebral column to one side with or without rotation of the bodies of the vertebrae.

Cause:

There is no known cause in general, but in some it may follow diseases like poliomyelitis, congenitally deformed vertebra, neurofibromatosis and cerebral palsy. Scoliosis may be compensatory to other deformities such as those of neck, arms, legs of uneven length, unilateral paralysis of muscles, injury to the spine and unilateral lung disease.

Signs and Symptoms:

Scoliosis may be present in the thoracic, thoracolumbar or lumbar region. It is noted by the deformity such as a high shoulder, prominent hip or protruding scapula.

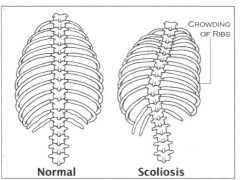

Normal   Scoliosis

Notes

Treatment aims to reduce progression and correct the deformity to an acceptable level. Scoliosis is classified as functional, postural, nonstructural or first degree scoliosis if it is due to muscular imbalance. This type can be corrected with exercises. Structural, second or third degree scoliosis refers to scoliosis caused by bony or connective tissue changes. This type is harder to correct. The type of treatment depends on the site and age of onset. Surgical treatment is done, if necessary, after adolescence. Surgery aims to fuse the joints of all the vertebrae within the primary curvature. Before surgery, orthotic braces (eg. Milwaukee brace) may be used.

Pain may be caused by the pressure on the ribs or the pelvis. The crowding of the intraabdominal structures may produce symptoms. There may be difficulty in breathing when the movement of the ribs is impaired by the deformity. Low back pain may be present due to the compensation made by muscles to maintain the posture. Of the two types of scoliosis, the postural type is a small curvature that corrects with bending. The structural type is one where the deformity is fixed.

Risk Factors:

Scoliosis is more frequent in adolescence and is more common in girls. In some there is a family history of scoliosis. Habitual asymmetric posture related to certain occupations can result in this condition.

Caution and Recommendations to Therapists:

Work in conjunction with the Physician and Physiotherapist. A thorough assessment is necessary to identify the extent of scoliosis, associated trigger points and spasm of muscles. The role of the Massage Therapist is to relax tense muscles, and increase blood flow to the fatigued muscles. The elongated and weakened muscles should be strengthened. The client should be positioned according to individual comfort and supported with pillows wherever necessary. In the postural type, the aim is to restore muscle tone and relax tense muscles while correcting the posture. Massage groups of muscles in the legs, lower back and gluteals that are put under excessive strain while the client maintains balance. Heat packs help alleviate low back pain. Deep muscle stripping, fascial work and joint mobilizations are other forms of therapy that should be used to stretch the shortened structures. Deep diaphragmatic breathing should also be employed to improve thoracic mobility.

Encourage client to do remedial exercises to maintain range of motion and to correct muscle imbalances. The frequency of massage should be varied according to the type of scoliosis. Initially, more frequent massages should be scheduled for postural/functional type of scoliosis, with the frequency reduced as the individual improves. For the structural type, massages are given once a week over a very long period. Physiotherapy is a major component of treating structural curves. Severe cases of structural scoliosis may require corrective surgery and/or braces. See Appendix D for organizations and support groups.

References

Turchaninov R, Cox CA. Medical massage. Scottsdale:Stress Less Publishing;1998. p370-375.

Hall CM, Brody LT. Therapeutic exercise moving toward function. Philadelphia: Lippincott Williams & Wilkins; 1999. p. 566-570.

Wine ZK. Russian medical massage: scoliosis. Massage 1994; 49(May/June): 32,34.

Nervous system

Seasonal Affective Disorder (SAD)

A periodic major depression which manifests at specific seasons.

Notes

It is treated with exposure to intense white light at a specified time of day for a specific duration. Antidepressants are also used. For more details see Appendix C: Antidepressants.

Cause:

It is thought to be due to a dysfunction of the natural biological rhythm. It has been associated with changes in hormonal secretions and certain neurotransmitters in the brain. Changes in sleep patterns have also been observed in people with depression.

Signs and Symptoms:

Episodes of depression occur in these individuals during the winter when the days are short and periods of darkness are longer. There is a marked reduction in the depression when the duration of light in the day becomes longer. The person exhibits easy fatigability, loss of interest in every day and pleasurable activities and insomnia. In severe depression, suicide may be attempted.

Risk Factors:

It is common in people living in the northern latitudes. There may be a family history of depression.

Caution and Recommendations to Therapists:

A general relaxation massage is recommended. Encourage the client to take the prescribed medications.

References

Judd LL, Britton KT, Braff DL. Mental disorders. In: Isselbacher KJ et al, editors. Harrison's principles of internal medicine. 13th ed. New York: McGraw-Hill Inc; 1994 p 2404.

Shin splints (Idiopathic compartment syndrome)

Inflammation of the proximal portion of any of the musculotendinous units originating from the lower part of the tibia.

Musculoskeletal system

Cause:

Repetitive stress of the muscles arising from the lower tibia may produce this condition. It may involve the group of muscle anterolateral to the tibia (tibialis anterior, extensor hallucis longus, and extensor digitorum longus) or that posteromedial to it.

Notes

In acute cases, the limb is rested for 2-3 days. Application of ice packs and elevation of the limb may help reduce swelling and inflammation. Activities that aggravate the condition should be avoided.

Signs and Symptoms:

The person complains of pain and tenderness lateral to the tibia if the anterolateral muscles are involved. The pain is increased on dorsiflexing the foot. The pain is localized to the posteromedial aspects of the lower tibial region, in the posteromedial type. In the later, the pain is increased on standing on the toes. There may be signs of inflammation viz. redness, swelling and warmth. The muscles surrounding the area may be in spasm with increased tone and trigger points. Weakness of the involved muscles may be seen in chronic cases. A common complication of shin splint is stress fractures.

Risk Factors:

Using shoes with hard heels, recurrent contact of heel on a hard surface as in running on hard, uneven or inclined surfaces, overzealous training can predispose to anterolateral shin splint. Ballet or other sports involving plantar flexion predispose to the posteromedial type.

Caution and Recommendations to Therapists:

In acute cases, the limb should be rested for 2-3 days. Apply ice packs, and elevate limb to reduce swelling and inflammation. Later, use friction massage to

References

Mercier LR. Practical Orthopedics. 4th edition. Mosby Year book Inc. St. Louis. Missouri 1995. P305.

increase blood flow and prevent adhesions. Gentle stretching also helps. Refer to Physiotherapist for strengthening exercises. Initially, short treatments lasting for half an hour are recommended at a frequency of two to three times per week.

Cardiovascular, Nervous systems

Shock

Profound and widespread reduction in the delivery of oxygen and nutrients to tissues.

Cause:

It is caused by any condition that affects the volume of blood pumped out of the heart per minute (cardiac output), and/or the resistance offered by the blood vessels to the flow of blood. Shock can be classified according to the cause as *cardiogenic shock* (due to abnormalities in the heart), *extracardiac obstructive shock* (conditions like fluid in the pericardium, pulmonary embolism, that affect outflow), *oligemic shock* (reduced blood volume as in hemorrhage, dehydration), *distributive shock* (conditions like infection in the blood, overdose of toxic products), and severe allergic reaction - *anaphylactic shock*, (sympathetic nervous system inactivity, endocrine disorders etc.).

Notes

The goal of treatment is to maintain the arterial pressure and maintain blood flow to organs such as the kidney, liver, lungs and central nervous system that are easily damaged by shock. Specific treatment is given according to the cause of shock. For example, if it is oligemic shock, blood or plasma expanders are rapidly infused. If due to myocardial abnormalities, the aim is to reduce ischemia and prevent further death of myocardial tissue. In septic shock, antimicrobial therapy is required in addition to other measures.

For more details see Appendix C: Blood/ plasma expanders; Antimicrobial - antibacterial agents.

Signs and Symptoms:

It is characterized by a lowered blood pressure, disorientation, palpitation, cold and clammy skin. Depending on the type of shock other symptoms may be present.

Risk Factors:

See Cause.

Caution and Recommendations to Therapists:

Shock is an emergency as it can produce irreversible damage to the brain if present for sometime. If you suspect shock in a client in your clinic call for medical help immediately. Loosen the clothes and allow client to be in a recumbent position with the leg end elevated until help arrives.

References

Parrillo JE. Shock. In: Isselbacher KJ et al, editors. Harrison's principles of internal medicine. 13th ed. New York: McGraw-Hill Inc; 1994. p. 187-192.

Respiratory system

Sinusitis

An inflammation of the paranasal sinuses.

Cause:

It is usually caused by a viral or bacterial infection. Sinusitis may also be a complication of common cold or allergy. The congestion of the nose results in blockage of the opening of the sinus into the nasal cavity and a build up of pressure in the sinus. There is a slow absorption of the air in the sinus and a

Notes

The treatment aims to promote adequate drainage of the sinuses. Nasal sprays that produce vasoconstriction may be used. Secretions may be loosened by the

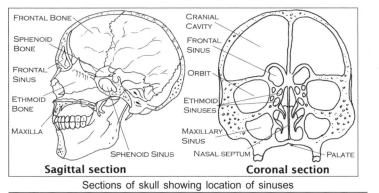

FRONTAL BONE		CRANIAL CAVITY
SPHENOID BONE		FRONTAL SINUS
FRONTAL SINUS		ORBIT
ETHMOID BONE		ETHMOID SINUSES
MAXILLA		MAXILLARY SINUS
SPHENOID SINUS	NASAL SEPTUM	PALATE

Sagittal section   **Coronal section**

Sections of skull showing location of sinuses

use of steam inhalation. If bacterial infection is suspected, antibiotics may be needed. In chronic cases, surgery may be done. For more details see Appendix C: Nose drops / Nasal decongestants; Antimicrobial - antibacterial agents.

partial vacuum is formed. All these processes are responsible for the characteristic symptoms.

Signs and Symptoms:

The symptoms are similar in acute and chronic sinusitis. There is nasal congestion followed by a mucous or purulent discharge from the nose. There is pain localized to specific areas depending on the sinus affected. If the maxillary sinus is affected there is pain over the cheeks and upper teeth. If ethmoid, over the eyes, if frontal, over the eyebrow and if sphenoid, the pain is felt behind the eye. The patient may have chronic cough due to the constant dripping of secretions in the back of the throat.

One of the complications of sinusitis is spread of infection into the cranium and /or eye.

Risk Factors:

Any condition that interferes with the drainage and movement of air in the sinuses can predispose to sinusitis. It is more common in individuals with deviated nasal septum, nasal polyps, diabetes, nasal intubation, immunosuppressed individuals and those using steroids over prolonged periods. Swimming in contaminated water also predisposes to this condition. Deep-sea diving and airplane travel, which is associated with fluctuating air pressure, may also precipitate sinusitis.

Caution and Recommendations to Therapists:

Local application of heat helps relieve pain. Encourage clients to complete the full course of antibiotics that have been prescribed. Steam inhalation also helps relieve the congestion. Accupressure and acupuncture are forms of treatment that have been found to be beneficial.

References

Maran AGD, editor. Logan Turner's diseases of the nose, throat and ear. 10th ed. London: Wright; 1988. p. 34-36, 42-50.

a Handbook for Massage Therapists

Sjögren's syndrome

A chronic, autoimmune disease with infiltration of lymphocytes into exocrine glands.

Notes

The treatment aims to alleviate symptoms as no cure exists. Frequent ingestion of fluids is advised. Eye drops may be given to help with tearing. Drugs such as antihypertensives, antidepressants and diuretics that exacerbate the condition should be avoided. For more details see Appendix C: Antihypertensives; Antidepressants; Diuretics.

Cause:

It is due to an autoimmune phenomenon where antibodies are developed against exocrine glands such as the salivary and lacrimal glands.

Signs and Symptoms:

Most patients present with dryness of the mouth and eyes. There is difficulty in swallowing food and to speak continually due to the dryness of the mouth. The incidence of dental caries is also higher. The parotid and other salivary glands may be enlarged. The patient complains of a sandy feeling in the eye, redness and itching due to dryness of the eye. If the exocrine glands in the respiratory or gastrointestinal tract are affected other symptoms may exist.

Risk Factors:

It is more common in middle-aged women. It may be associated with rheumatoid arthritis, systemic lupus erythematosus, scleroderma and fibromyalgia. Lymphomas are also common.

Caution and Recommendations to Therapists:

Other concomitant conditions have to be addressed if present. The Therapist may have to provide a glass of water beside the table during the session.

References

Moutsopoulos HM. Sjögren's syndrome. In: Isselbacher KJ et al, editors. Harrison's principles of internal medicine. 13th ed. New York: McGraw-Hill Inc; 1994. p. 1662-1664.

Sleep apnea

A condition where there is stoppage of breathing for 10 seconds or longer, 30 times or more during a 7 hour sleeping period.

Notes

Sleep apnea is treated in many ways according to the cause. While sleeping, nasal masks that literally push the air into the respiratory tract are sometimes used. Drugs are also used to stimulate the respiratory center.

Rarely, surgery is done to correct the nasal passage if the cause is due to abnormal nasal septum.

Cause:

The cause may be due to abnormalities in the respiratory center of the brain that controls the respiratory rate and depth (*central sleep apnea*) or due to obstruction to the airflow in the mouth or pharynx while sleeping (*obstructive sleep apnea*). In some individuals it may be due to both reasons (*mixed sleep apnea*).

Signs and Symptoms:

Noisy snoring, difficulty in falling asleep (insomnia), sleepiness during the day, abnormal movements during sleep are some of the symptoms. It may be associated with early morning headaches and psychological problems like sexual impotence and depression.

Risk Factors:

Encephalitis, poliomyelitis affecting the brain stem can predispose to central sleep apnea. Obstructive type is more common in middle-aged men and obese individuals. Alcohol and drugs that depress the central nervous system also predispose to obstructive sleep apnea.

Caution and Recommendations to Therapists:

Encourage clients to loose weight. Sleeping on the side instead of the back helps reduce obstructive type of apnea. Massage is not contraindicated in this condition. It helps relax these tired and depressed individuals.

References

Phillipson EA. Disorders of ventilation. In: Isselbacher KJ et al, editors. Harrison's principles of internal medicine. 13th ed. New York: McGraw-Hill Inc; 1994. p. 1236-1239.

Sleeping sickness (African trypanosomiasis)

Nervous system

An infection caused by the protozoal parasite Trypanosoma brucei that is transmitted by tsetse flies.

Cause:

The organism infects the tsetse flies when they take a blood meal from an infected mammal. The protozoa multiplies in the gut of the insect and migrates to the salivary gland to be subsequently injected into the body when it takes another blood meal. The organisms multiply in the body fluids.

Notes

The drugs used for treatment varies with the species that has affected the individual, the presence or absence of central nervous system disease, adverse reactions and drug resistance.

The disease can be prevented by taking measures to control the insects, wearing protective clothing, using insect repellents and actively treating those who are infected.

Signs and Symptoms:

There is inflammation at the site of the insect bite (*trypanosomal chancre*). As the parasites migrate in the bloodstream, high fever is seen. There is enlargement of the spleen (splenomegaly) and lymph nodes (lymphadenopathy).

Risk Factors:

It is common in the tropical rain forests of Central and East Africa. It is an occupational hazard for those working in the forests.

Caution and Recommendations to Therapists:

Ensure that your clinic is "insect proofed". Though an infectious disease it is not transmitted by direct contact. Avoid massage during the acute stage. Refer to Appendix B: Strategies for infection prevention and safe practice for some useful guidelines.

References

Morello JA, Mizer HE, Wilson ME, Granato PA. Microbiology in patient care. 6th ed. New York: McGraw-Hill; 1998. p. 500-501

Spina bifida (Meningocele; Myelomeningocele)

Nervous system

A defect in the fusion of the right and left half of one or more vertebrae during the development of the foetus resulting in malformation of the spine. There may or may not be protrusion of the spinal cord and meninges through the gap.

Cause:

Virus infection, exposure to radiation or other toxic environmental factors during the first three months of pregnancy - when the spinal cord and vertebrae develops, can produce malformation of the spine. Usually the defect is in the lower back - lumbosacral region.

Signs and Symptoms:

In spina bifida occulta - the commonest and least severe form, there is a depression, tuft of hair, birthmark or soft fatty tissue on the skin over the region. It may be asymptomatic or associated with weakness of the legs, urinary bladder or bowel dysfunction.

In the more severe defect, the menings and cerebrospinal fluid (CSF) protrude (*meningocele*) or there is protrusion of the spinal cord along with the meninges and CSF (*myelomeningocele*), producing a sac like appearance in the region. The severe forms are accompanied by weakness or paralysis of the legs. There may be associated hydrocephalus and mental retardation.

Risk Factors:

There is a genetic predisposition. Exposure to radiation, Rubella or other viral infections early in pregnancy also produces this condition.

Caution and Recommendations to Therapists:

In the less severe form avoid massage over the lumbosacral area. In the more severe form with neurological problems, the aim is to prevent contractures, pressure ulcers and reduce spasticity. Passive movements and range of motion exercises of joints prevent contractures of muscles. Use transverse friction strokes around joints. Do not use force to stretch muscles that are in spasm. These individuals are prone for decubitus (pressure) ulcers and edema in the dependent parts such as the legs or sacral region. The poor circulation in these areas makes the skin very fragile with a tendency to breakdown with minimal pressure. Avoid massaging areas with ulcers and bring it to the notice of the caregivers. Some clients may also have reduced sensations. Use mild to moderate pressure in these areas.

References

Adams JC, Hamblen DL. Outline of orthopaedics. 11 Ed. New York. Churchill Livingstone 1990. p. 133-136.

Nervous system

Spinal cord injury

Complete or partial damage to the spinal cord at any level resulting in loss of sensation, motor function and autonomic function.

Cause:

Trauma is the most common cause. The problems that result is not only due to the direct damage but also to the reaction of the body to the injury in the form of edema, bleeding, reduced blood supply and inflammation of the cord. Other causes include tumors.

Signs and Symptoms:

Within the first twenty-four hours the person looses all function below the level of injury - *spinal shock.* In spinal shock, sensations, motor activity as

Notes

Soon after injury, treatment is aimed to stabilize the medical condition, treat associated injuries and immobilize the client. Steroids may be used to reduce edema. The specific treatment of an individual with spinal cord injury is related to the level of lesion. The diagram of the dermatome (page 183) indicates regions where sensations may be lost according to the level of injury. Knowledge of the segmental innervation of muscles can

well as autonomic function is lost. In due course the functions resume depending on the extent and site of damage.

help determine the motor loss.

For more details see Appendix C: Antiinflammatories - steroidal drugs.

If the whole cord is cut, there is complete loss of sensations and motor function below the level of injury. If the injury is at the cervical region quadriplegia (paralysis of all four limbs) results. If above C4, the nerve supply to the diaphragm is affected and the person requires mechanical ventilation. If below the cervical region, paraplegia (paralysis of the lower limbs) results with or without involvement of the trunk muscles. Injury at the thoracic level affects the nerve supply to the intercostal muscles and impairs respiration making the person prone to respiratory infection.

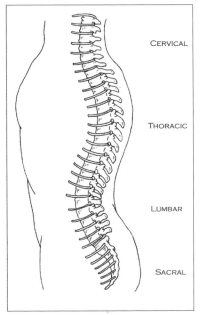

Vertebral column showing spinal nerves (cut)

The muscles are spastic (increased in tone) and the reflexes are exaggerated. The muscles have a tendency to get fixed in a flexed position. The lack of muscle tone makes the person prone to edema. Pressure ulcers are common due to lack of sensation and abnormal autonomic function. Bladder and bowel control is lost. The absence of stress on the bones supporting the paralyzed muscles results in osteoporosis. The absorption of calcium from the bone and excretion through the kidneys, along with the stagnation of urine in the bladder makes the person prone for stone formation in the kidneys and urinary tract infection. The absence of movement around the veins of the limbs makes them prone for deep vein thrombosis.

Lesions above the level of T6 can result in abnormal autonomic reflexes such as sudden increase in blood pressure, flushing, increased sweating and headache on even mild stimulation below the level of lesion. The lack of autonomic control affects the regulation of temperature and blood pressure. Erection may be possible by local tactile stimulation. Ejaculation and orgasm is possible in some patients. 1-5% of men with spinal cord injuries have sired children. A common problem encountered by patients with spinal cord injury is orthostatic hypotension. A few patients may experience intractable pain.

C 4 level. In these quadriplegic patients, the sternomastoids and trapezius and upper cervical muscles are spared. There is no voluntary function of the arms, trunk and lower limbs. Various functions may be achieved by using devices that capitalise on the movement of the head and mouth.

C 5 level: The deltoid and biceps are functional as C 5 is functioning. Support of the wrists and fingers are required. These patients may be able to use electrical wheelchairs.

C 6 level: The patient has use of shoulder musculature, elbow flexion and wrist extension and may be capable of dressing themselves, use wheelchairs and transfer themselves from bed to chair. Beginning at this level, patients should be able to drive an automobile with manual controls and other adapted equipment.

C 7 level: These patients have use of the triceps and the extrinsic finger flexors and extensors.

T 1 level: The patient has normal upper limbs and should be able to dress, feed and manage toileting needs.

T 6 level: The patient has upper intercostal and back musculature control.

T 12 level: Abdominal and back control is present. Orthoses may be used for standing and walking.

L 4 level: The patient has use of the hip flexors and knee extensors and can stand without orthoses and walk without external support. However, lack of ankle and gluteal power makes it difficult to walk without ankle-foot orthoses and crutches.

Risk Factors:

The most common cause is motor vehicle accidents.

Caution and Recommendations to Therapists:

Massage is indicated in the chronic phase. Work in conjunction with a Physiotherapist. Assessment of the client before massage is very important. Keep a record of the extent of the loss of function - both sensory and motor. The aim is to reduce spasticity, improve circulation, prevent edema and pressure ulcers, prevent contractures and maintain the range of motion in joints. Caution is required as the sensations are impaired and proper feedback may not be forthcoming. Also they are prone for deep vein thrombosis. Dislodgment of thrombus can cause further complications.

Position the client in a neutral position with the legs in line with the rest of body. A number of cushions may be required. Elevate the limbs with cushions if edema is present even before beginning treatment. Keep the client warm. Use lymphatic drainage techniques to help reduce edema. Watch for pressure ulcers and avoid areas of ulcers leaving a wide margin around it. Use gentle rhythmic and repetitive strokes in general. However, stimulatory massage to the extensor muscles can reduce the tone in the flexors, which are more hypertonic than extensors. Use tapotement and vibration strokes over chest wall to help drain the mucus. The head end can be lowered while massaging the chest as this uses the effect of gravity for drainage.

Give sufficient support when the position of the client is changed, as they are prone for postural hypotension. Involuntary spasms and movements are common in these clients so do not be alarmed. Passively move the joints through as wide a range of motion without using force. Transverse friction should be used around joints to prevent adhesions and contractures. Concentrate also on muscles that are excessively stressed by compensatory overuse. Massage is indicated on an ongoing basis. Schedule once or twice a week and modify the duration according to individuals. Special training may be required to treat individuals with spinal cord injury in order to understand the special challenges that are faced. Improve communications by seeking information on how to use words with dignity. See Appendix D for organizations and support groups.

Segmental innervation of muscles

Neck flexion, extension, rotation	C1,2,3,4
Shoulder flexion, abduction	C5,6
adduction, extension	C5,6,7,8
Elbow flexion	C5,6
extension	C7,8
Forearm pronation	C6,7
supination	C5,6,7
Wrist extension	C6,7
flexion	C6,7, T1
Hand extension of fingers	C6,7,8
Flexion of fingers	C7,8, T1
Fine digital motion	C8, T1
Back extension	C4-L1
Chest muscles for breathing	T2-T12
Diaphragm	C2,3,4
Abdominal muscles	T6-L1
Hip flexion	L2,3,4
abduction	L4,5, S1
adduction	L2,3,4
extension	L4,5, S1
rotation	L4,5, S1,2
Knee extension	L2,3,4
flexion	L4,5, S1
Ankle	L4,5, S1,2
Foot	L5, S1,2
Bladder	S2,3,4
Bowel	S2,3,4
Erection of penis	S2,3,4
Ejaculation	L1,2,3

References

Ropper AH, Martin JB. Diseases of the spinal cord. In: Isselbacher KJ et al, editors. Harrison's principles of internal medicine. 13th ed. New York: McGraw-Hill Inc; 1994. p. 2352-2355.

Sprain

A complete or incomplete tear in the ligament/s around a joint. There is no displacement of or instability to the joint.

Musculoskeletal system

Cause:

It follows a sudden, sharp twist to the joint that stretches the ligament and ruptures some or all of the fibres.

Signs and Symptoms:

Sprains are classified as mild, moderate or severe according to the extent of injury to the ligaments.

There is local pain (especially during joint movement), swelling, loss of mobility and discoloration of the skin over the joint due to the extravasation of blood into the surrounding tissues from the injured ligament. Sprains occur more commonly in the ankle, wrist and back. The patient usually gives a history of recent injury or prolonged overuse.

Risk Factors:

Occupations and sports that require use of ankles and wrists extensively have a high risk of causing sprain.

Caution and Recommendations to Therapists:

In acute cases, use ice pack intermittently to reduce pain and swelling. The joint should be elevated above the heart to use the effect of gravity to reduce edema. The joint is immobilized for a short while depending on the extent of the rupture. After the acute phase, controlled activity and rehabilitative exercises with optimal loading are of benefit. Movement of the joint within the extent of pain tolerance helps form stronger scar tissue that is laid out in the right direction. Passively move joints that are not affected. Massage adjacent muscles to increase circulation, reduce swelling and address trigger points. The aim of massage at the time of healing is to prevent adhesions. Deep transverse friction that move the ligaments over the bone are advocated. Deep moist heat helps soften scar tissue and increase circulation.

References

Hall CM, Brody LT. Therapeutic exercise moving toward function. Lippincott Williams & Wilkins. Philadelphia. 1999. Pp 165-173.

Mercier LR. Practical Orthopedics. 4th edition. Mosby Year book Inc. St. Louis. Missouri 1995. Pp 238-241.

Musculoskeletal system

Sprain - ankle (Anterior talofibular or calcaneocuboid ligament injury)

Partial or complete tear of one of the ligaments in the ankle.

Cause:

A forced stress on the ankle usually produces this condition. It is the most commonly sprained area in the body. Typically, it is seen in athletes who jump and land on the lateral border of the foot that has been plantar flexed or by excessive inversion of the foot as when a high heel gets caught on uneven ground.

Notes

Antiinflammatories and painkillers may be used in the acute stage. In severe cases, casts may be applied for a short period. Surgery is used as a last resort. For more details see Appendix C: Painkillers; Antiinflammatories - non steroidal drugs.

Signs and Symptoms:

It presents as pain over the ankle and/or pain referred distally or proximally. The severity of the pain does not correspond to the extent of injury. Mild or moderate injury produces more pain than a complete tear. There may be discoloration in the area due to the extravasation of blood. In acute cases, movement is painful and restricted due to effusion of fluid in the joint and muscle spasm. In chronic cases, passive foot movement is painless and hypermobility may be seen if there is complete rupture. In chronic, recurrent injuries, the sprain presents as sudden giving way of the ankle. This may be followed by swelling and pain for a few days.

Risk Factors:

It is common in active young individuals who are engaged in sports that involve jumping.

Caution and Recommendations to Therapists:

In acute cases, ice application and elevation of foot is recommended. To aid the healing process rest is advised. However, active movement should be encouraged to prevent stiffness and muscle atrophy. Passively move the joint in a direction that does not stress the ligament. Friction massage may be used in the subacute stage to prevent adhesions. It should be noted that although collagen fibres are laid down within the first few weeks it takes months for the collagen to mature, realign and regain original strength (see under Sprain for further details).

References

Hall CM, Brody LT. Therapeutic exercise moving toward function. Philadelphia: Lippincott Williams & Wilkins; 1999. p 165-173.

Mercier LR. Practical Orthopedics. 4th edition. St. Louis: Mosby Year book Inc; 1995. p. 238-241.

Sprain - knee

Musculoskeletal system

A complete or incomplete tear of the ligaments around the knee joint.

Cause:

It is usually caused by trauma to the knee. It is a common injury in football players while being tackled from the side. The sudden force from the side on the slightly flexed knee and planted foot produces forward movement of the femur and external rotation of the tibia resulting in tear in the medial collateral ligament and /or capsule and medial meniscus. The anterior cruciate ligament can be torn by forward forces on an extended or near extended thigh. The posterior cruciate ligament is stretched by a sudden backward movement of the tibia on the femur.

Notes

Antiinflammatories and painkillers may be used in the acute stage. In severe cases, casts may be applied for a short period. Surgery is used as a last resort. For more details see Appendix C: Painkillers; Antiinflammatories - non steroidal drugs.

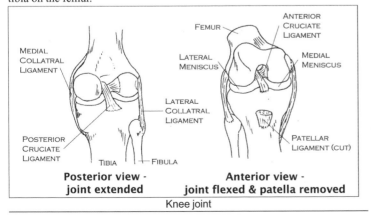

Posterior view - joint extended | Anterior view - joint flexed & patella removed

Knee joint

Signs and Symptoms:

The pain is localized to the site of the tear. There is joint swelling with synovial fluid or blood. The pain may be referred to the L3, L4 and S2 segment as nerves supplying the knee arise from here. Thus, pain may be felt in the lower lumbar region, front and back of thigh or back of calf. The pain is increased by moving the knee in directions that produce stress on the ligament. There is muscle guarding in the acute stage. The normal knee is capable of flexing 130-150 degrees, extending 0-3 degrees, and rotating internally or externally by 10 degrees.

In chronic sprains, the patient complains of giving way of the knee. There is also difficulty in performing specific activities like squatting, turning sharply or going down the stairs. There is associated atrophy of the quadriceps muscle and hypermobility of the joint.

Risk Factors:

Sprain of the knee is common in young active individuals.

Caution and Recommendations to Therapists:

Assess the joint to see if the sprain is mild - Grade I (very little loss of integrity of ligament, not hypermobile), moderate - Grade II (mild hypermobility) or severe - Grade III (marked hypermobility). In mild to moderate injury, use ice packs if acute. Compression and elevation is also used in this stage. In the subacute or chronic stage transverse friction massage is used - in a direction perpendicular to the line of ligament with the knee flexed at different degrees. This prevents adhesion to adjacent structures and also helps align the newly formed collagen fibres. For grade III sprains the limb is immobilized with cast. Massage muscles around cast to improve circulation. After removal of cast use transverse friction massage around the joint. Encourage client to do remedial exercises to maintain and improve range of motion. Always work in conjunction with a Physiotherapist (see under Sprains for more details). Half-hour schedules two to three times a week for the first few weeks are recommended.

References

Hall CM, Brody LT. Therapeutic exercise moving toward function. Philadelphia: Lippincott Williams & Wilkins; 1999. p. 165-173.

Mercier LR. Practical Orthopedics. 4th edition. St. Louis: Mosby Year book Inc; 1995. p. 238-241.

Musculoskeletal system

Still's disease (Juvenile rheumatoid arthritis)

An autoimmune disease that affects multiple systems in children, producing degenerative changes in connective tissue and inflammatory vascular lesions.

Notes

Treatment is similar to that of rheumatoid arthritis, with use of aspirin and other non-steroidal anti-inflammatory agents. Adequate rest, temporary splinting of inflamed joints and graduated exercises are other general forms of treatment. Surgery may be required to correct fixed deformities. For more details see Appendix C: Antiinflammatories - non

Cause:

It is due to the immune system of the body reacting to tissues of self as it would to foreign tissues.

Signs and Symptoms:

The symptoms are similar to that of rheumatoid arthritis in adults (see Arthritis - rheumatoid). The spleen and lymph nodes are also enlarged.

Risk Factors:

It affects children under 16 years of age and is more common in females. Viral or bacterial infections, emotional stress and trauma have been known to precipitate the disease.

Caution and Recommendations to Therapists:

Arthritis cannot be cured, but its relentless progress can be prevented. Stress reduction helps muscles to relax and reduce discomfort. In the early stages the aim should be to prevent contractures, deformity and to maintain joint range of movement. Hot packs help alleviate pain. Massage should not be given in the acute stages, but passive movements of the joints are encouraged. In the chronic stages, general massage helps reduce stress. Brisk but gentle effleurage and kneading can be used in the limbs. Friction strokes can be used around the joints to reduce the thickening in the periarticular tissues. But make sure that there is no pain.

In general, massage should be for a shorter duration. For clients with this condition, maximum benefit is obtained if the Massage Therapist works in conjunction with the Physician and Physiotherapist. Individualized therapeutic exercises are used to reduce pain, increase mobility and improve muscle performance. The exercises used should have minimal or no joint stress and shock. Water exercises are beneficial as, for example, waist level water reduces the body weight to 50% of that in land. The clients may be on painkillers and/ or anti-inflammatory drugs that suppress pain and symptoms. The suppressed pain sometimes may result in inadequate feedback from the clients. Care should be taken while massaging such clients as harm may be done to the joints inadvertently. Refer clients to local support groups (see Appendix D).

steroidal drugs; Antiinflammatories - steroidal drugs.

References

Field T, Fernandez-Reif S et al. Juvenile rheumatoid arthritis: Benefits from massage therapy. Journal of Pediatric Psychology 1997; 22: 607-617.

Stomatitis

Gastrointestinal system

An inflammation of the mucosa of the mouth.

Cause:

Stomatitis may be due to various factors. *Herpes stomatitis* is due to Herpes Simplex virus infection (see under Herpes Simplex). The cause of *Aphthous stomatitis* is unknown. *Allergic stomatitis* is due to hypersensitivity to food or lipstick. *Thrush* is another form of stomatitis caused by yeast infection.

Notes

Stomatitis heals spontaneously in 10-14 days. Antiseptic mouthwashes should not be used, as it is irritable to the inflamed area.

Signs and Symptoms:

In the type due to Herpes, the person also has systemic symptoms of fever, irritability, loss of appetite along with pain in the mouth. The submaxillary lymph nodes may be enlarged and painful. In the aphthous type, single or multiple shallow ulcers may be seen on the mucosa of the mouth, palate or lip. In thrush, patchy ulcers covered by a white cheesy material are seen in the mouth and pharynx.

Risk Factors:

Herpes Simplex infection in other areas may spread to the mouth. Stress, fatigue, anxiety, trauma, sunburn, hypersensitivity to drugs or food, or other systemic diseases can predispose to Aphthous stomatitis.

Caution and Recommendations to Therapists:

Stomatitis due to Herpes can spread to other areas in the person as well as to others on contact. Do not massage till completely treated. In other types, avoid massaging face and neck if the lymph nodes are enlarged and inflamed.

References

Lynch MA et al. Burket's oral medicine, diagnosis and treatment. 8th ed. Philadelphia: Lippincott; 1983.

Musculoskeletal system

Strain

A stretching injury to a muscle that results in partial or complete tear.

Cause:

Strains are usually caused by acute or chronic mechanical overloading.

Notes

Antiinflammatories and painkillers may be used in the acute phase. For more details see Appendix C: Antiinflammatories - non steroidal drugs; Painkillers.

Signs and Symptoms:

Pain, swelling and stiffness is seen in the affected area. Sometimes a snapping sound may be heard followed by rapid swelling soon after the injury. The muscle is tender and pain is increased on actively contracting or passively stretching the muscle. A few days later ecchymoses (small spots of bleeding under the skin) may be seen. If the strain is mild there is muscle spasm and tenderness over the region. There may be slight weakness of muscle. In moderate strain, along with more severe symptoms of mild strain, bruising may be seen. In severe strain, the function of muscle is lost, with excruciating pain if the muscle is not fully ruptured. If fully ruptured there may be no pain associated.

Strain is more common in the lower back and neck. In the hip the hamstrings, adductor longus, iliopsoas and rectus femoris are the most commonly strained muscles.

Risk Factors:

Overweight, strenuous exercises and poor posture are the commonest predisposing factors. Abnormal strength ratios of agonist and antagonist muscles as seen in weight trainers who concentrate on strengthening only one group of muscles, increases the risk of strain.

Caution and Recommendations to Therapists:

Use cold applications during the first 24-48 hours to reduce pain and swelling. The unaffected areas should be massaged to reduce muscle spasm and thereby lessen pain. Avoid massaging distal to the site of injury. Passively move all joints adjacent to the injury to maintain range of movement. Care should be taken not to stretch the injured muscle. In the subacute stage, techniques to reduce swelling should be employed. Later transverse friction massage is used

References

Hall CM, Brody LT. Therapeutic exercise moving toward function. Philadelphia: Lippincott Williams & Wilkins; 1999. p. 165-173.
Mercier LR. Practical Orthopedics. 4th edition. St. Louis: Mosby Year book Inc; 1995. p. 238-241.

to prevent formation of adhesions, and random alignment of the newly laid collagen fibres. Use gentle stretching manipulations. Refer to Physiotherapist for strengthening exercises. Initially, half hour treatments, once or twice a week is recommended. The frequency can be reduced according to the progress of the condition.

Stroke (Cerebrovascular accident; CVA)

Nervous system

A sudden reduction of blood supply to areas of the brain.

Cause:

The reduction in blood supply is due to either thrombosis/embolism which block the blood vessel, or hemorrhage. This results in reduced oxygen supply to the brain tissue. The hypoxia (reduced oxygen) causes congestion and edema of the brain. The latter produce the symptoms and signs associated with stroke. If the lack of oxygen supply lasts for a few minutes irreversible damage is done to the brain tissue.

Signs and Symptoms:

This varies with the artery that is affected and the duration of lack of blood supply and the ability of the surrounding arteries to compensate for the lack of blood supply to the area. If the left side of the brain is affected the symptoms are seen on the right side and vice versa. Some of the associated signs and symptoms seen are difficulty in speech, weakness of muscles in one side of the body with certain groups of muscles more affected than the others (*hemiplegia*), complete or partial loss of sight. There may also be accompanying loss or decrease in sensations. Poor coordination, abnormalities in gait are other signs that may be present. Disorientation, headache, convulsions, coma are other general symptoms. Autonomic problems like constipation may be present.

In patients who are in the recovery or rehabilitation phase of stroke the muscles are weak, spastic (rigid), with reflexes that are exaggerated. In these individuals, typically, the arm is held adducted with elbows partly flexed and pronated, and fingers flexed. The legs are extended with the foot plantar flexed. The facial muscles may or may not be affected with the cheeks lax and lip depressed on one side. The eyelids may droop on one side. Sensation may be altered and tremors of one of the limbs may be present. In patients with long-term paralysis, skin changes and contractures may also be seen. It may be accompanied by depression, lack of concentration and memory loss.

Risk Factors:

History of transient ischemic attacks, atherosclerosis, hypertension, postural hypotension, cerebral aneurysms, cardiac arrhythmias, diabetes mellitus, high cholesterol levels are high risk factors. A sedentary lifestyle, smoking, family history of cerebrovascular accidents and use of contraceptives are other predisposing factors.

Notes

Treatment varies with individuals. 90% of neurological recovery occurs in the first 3 months. The improvement in function depends on the environment in which the client is placed. Rehabilitation is begun when there is no progression of neurological deficits for 48 hours. The treatment aims to prevent complications such as intellectual regression, depression, development of contractures and dealing with bowel and bladder dysfunction. Range of motion exercises and stretching are an important part of the treatment. Regular aerobic and/or stretch exercises are helpful. Alternative therapies include yoga, tai chi, meditation and imagery.

Caution and Recommendations to Therapists:

The aim is to prevent joint stiffness and deformity, decrease spasticity, re-educate the perception of sensory stimuli and movement patterns, reduce skin changes and edema and address postural changes like scoliosis and kyphosis that may occur due to the weakness of muscles. Work in conjunction with a Physiotherapist and Occupational Therapist. Spend time to assess the sensory and motor functions and keep a good record of your findings in order to individualize treatment and track progress of the client.

For assessing motor function, test the range of motion possible in all joints. Note the level of spasticity. Spasticity is the resistance offered to a particular movement when the joint is passively moved. Careful assessment of the factors that precipitate a spasm in the client should be obtained. Stretching of muscles, pressure or irritation of the skin are some of the common stimuli for spasm. For assessment of sensory function, ask clients about decreased or loss of sensation in specific areas. These areas may be tested for perception to light touch - as with stroking with a feather, and for temperature and pain perception - by using warm and cold water in a small container. Also look for skin changes and pressure ulcers.

The pressure used during massage, and use of hydrotherapy should be modified according to the findings. Position the client with the spine and neck straight and the shoulder and pelvis aligned over each other. Cover the parts that are not being worked on making sure that the client is kept warm. All the affected joints should be moved passively through the full range of movement possible. Do not forcibly move spastic muscles. To help re-educate the limb ask the client to perform the same movement using the unaffected side. Stimulate the muscles antagonistic to the spastic muscles using tapotement. This can help reduce the spasticity eg. stimulating the triceps can reduce spasticity in the biceps muscle. The massage strokes should be slow and superficial, soothing and rhythmic. Excessive stimulation may increase the spasticity. Clonus - abnormal involuntary movements with alternate contraction and relaxation especially of the ankle joint is normal in these clients. This is seen if the ankle is dorsiflexed suddenly. Do not be alarmed if clonus is present.

Adjust pressure according to each client. The skin is fragile and easily damaged on the affected side. In addition, the sensation may be altered and the feedback from the client may be inadequate. Closely monitor the temperature of heating pads (if used) due to the reduced sensation in these clients. Massage the unaffected side - especially those areas that are overused. Encourage clients to use both affected and unaffected side. In the case of treating clients in the early stage -within a week or two, the muscles may be flaccid - with reduced tone. In such cases, use friction, effleurage and pétrissage as such strokes have been shown to increase muscle tone. The first few treatments should be short - not more than half an hour, once or twice a week. This should be slowly increased to durations of one hour.

The Therapist should be sensitive to issues such as bladder and bowel incontinence. Special training may be required by those who wish to deal with such individuals on a constant basis in order to understand the special challenges these individuals face. The clinic may have to be modified to make it accessible to clients on wheelchairs. Refer clients to local support groups. See Appendix D for resources.

References

Vickers A. Complementary therapy and disability: alternatives for people with disabling conditions. London: Chapman and Hall; 1993.

Wine ZK. Russian medical massage: massage treatments for strokes. Massage 1995; 55 May/June: 98-100,102.

Synovitis - acute

Musculoskeletal system

An acute inflammation of the lining membrane of joints.

Cause:

It usually follows any form of injury to the joint. Some inflammation of the synovial membrane is present in any type of arthritis.

Signs and Symptoms:

The joint shows sign of inflammation - redness, heat, swelling, pain and loss of function. The skin may be reddened if the inflammation has spread. The joint is swollen due to the movement of fluid into it. A dull and aching pain is present at rest. The pain increases on moving the joint. To minimize pain the patient keeps the limb in a position that relaxes the ligaments around the joint. Atrophy of the muscles around the joint may be seen in those with prolonged inflammation.

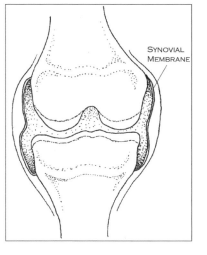

SYNOVIAL MEMBRANE

Notes

Antiinflammatories and painkillers may be used. For more details see Appendix C: Antiinflammatories - non steroidal drugs; Painkillers.

Risk Factors:

See Cause.

Caution and Recommendations to Therapists:

Care of the client should be directed towards preventing the spread of inflammation, relief of pain, reduction of swelling and assisting with the reabsorption of fluid and toxins thereby preventing adhesions. The aim should also be to prevent disuse atrophy of muscles and to help client regain joint range and function. The limb should be well supported with pillows.

During the first 24 hours, cold application gives relief. Cold packs or towels immersed in cold water and then wrung out can be applied over area. During the first few days mild heat helps reduce swelling and pain. In acute synovitis the client may be unable to tolerate much manipulation. Light squeezing movements

a Handbook for Massage Therapists

311

in an upward direction with each hand on the side of the limb may help. Gentle effleurage can be substituted according to the tolerance of the individual. Gentle finger kneading may be added over the joint to reduce the swelling and prevent adhesions.

To maintain circulation, the parts of the limb that can be reached without moving the affected joint should be massaged vigorously. When the inflammation has subsided and there is no pain, deep friction around the affected joint should be resorted to along with heat application. Passive movement also helps. Encourage client to exercise the joint at this stage.

References

Mercier LR, editor. Practical orthopedics. 4ᵗʰ ed. New York: Mosby-Year book Inc; 1995. p. 192-193.

Musculoskeletal system

Synovitis - chronic

A chronic inflammation of the lining membrane of joints.

Cause:

It can be caused by repeated acute synovitis, recurrent injuries or strains to the joint. Loose bodies like broken bones, bits of cartilage inside the joint or abnormal alignment of the articulating surfaces of the joint can also result in this chronic problem.

Notes

The treatment is similar to that of acute synovitis. Stretching and strengthening exercises play a more important role.

Signs and Symptoms:

Chronic synovitis is characterized by thickening of the synovial membrane and long-standing swelling of the joint. The muscles around the joint are atrophied and the joint tends to buckle due to the lax and stretched ligaments. There may be a dull, aching pain and stiffness of the joint.

Risk Factors:

See risk factors for Synovitis - acute.

References

Mercier LR, editor. Practical orthopedics. 4ᵗʰ ed. New York: Mosby-Year book Inc; 1995. p. 192-193.

Caution and Recommendations to Therapists:

Any form of heat is soothing. Use kneading and deep friction strokes over and around the joint. Passive movements of the joints also help break up adhesions.

Reproductive, Integumentary systems

Syphilis

A chronic, infectious, sexually transmitted disease.

Cause:

It is caused by the bacteria *Treponema pallidum*. It is transmitted by intimate physical contact. The bacteria enters the mucous membrane and spreads to the local lymph nodes and then to the blood stream producing systemic symptoms. It can spread to the fetus from infected mothers. Rarely, it may be transmitted by blood transfusion. The incubation period lasts for about 3 weeks.

Notes

Penicillin is the drug of choice for all stages of syphilis. For more details see Appendix C: Antimicrobial - antibacterial agents.

Pathology A to Z -

Signs and Symptoms:

Typically, it presents as painless, fluid-filled lesions in the genitalia and other regions of contact such as the mouth, tongue, nipples etc. These lesions (*chancres*) are firm to touch with raised edges. The local lymph nodes may be enlarged. The chancres may disappear within 3-6 weeks with or without treatment. If untreated, generalized lymph node enlargement and skin rashes occur within 8 weeks after the onset of chancres. These rashes are highly contagious.

The late stage of syphilis (very rare after the availability of antibiotics) which occurs 1-10 years after infection is noninfectious. But it is destructive and affects many systems.

Risk Factors:

The incidence is higher in urban regions, in drug users and those with AIDS.

Caution and Recommendations to Therapists:

Massage is contraindicated. Encourage clients with painless fluid filled lesions around the mouth, tongue etc. to seek medical help. Refer to Appendix B: Strategies for infection prevention and safe practice for some useful guidelines. Also see Appendix D for organizations and support groups.

References

Morello JA, Mizer HE, Wilson ME, Granato PA. Microbiology in patient care. 6th ed. New York: McGraw-Hill; 1998. p. 408-412.

Aral SO, king KH. Sexually transmitted diseases in the AIDS era. Sci Am. 1991; 264 (2): 62-91.

Systemic Lupus Erythematosus (SLE)

A chronic autoimmune inflammatory disease.

Cardiovascular, Musculoskeletal, Integumentary, Renal, Respiratory systems

Cause:

The cause is unknown. It is considered to be autoimmune, as there is production of autoantibodies and immune complexes that affect multiple systems.

Signs and Symptoms:

It is called "the great imitator" as the signs and symptoms resemble that of many other diseases. The onset may be acute or chronic and there is exacerbation and remission of the disease. Most patients present with joint pain. Chronic inflammation of the joint makes the ligaments, tendons and capsule lax and susceptible to deformities. In the acute form of SLE, a butterfly-shaped rash is seen over the nose and cheek. Glomerulonephritis (inflammation in the kidney), pulmonary effusion (fluid collection in the lungs), pericarditis (inflammation of the membrane surrounding the heart) are some of the other manifestations. The patient may also have central nervous system effects such as psychosis, depression, confusion and dementia. Lymph node enlargement may be seen in some. See Appendix A: pages 357 & 358.

Risk Factors:

It is more common in females especially in the childbearing age group. Estrogens favor the development of the disease while androgens protect. African-

Notes

There is no cure for SLE. Treatment aims to control acute, severe flares and to suppress symptoms. Non-steroidal anti-inflammatory drugs and steroids are used to suppress symptoms. Immunity may be suppressed by using cytotoxic agents. For more details see Appendix C: Antiinflammatories - non steroidal drugs; Antiinflammatories - steroidal drugs; Painkillers; Immunosuppressants.

Americans and Asians are at less risk. There is a genetic predisposition. SLE can be triggered by ultra-violet light, chemicals such as hair dyes, drugs, some types of food and infectious agents.

Caution and Recommendations to Therapists:

Clients may be on corticosteroids and anti-inflammatory drugs. Some may also be on other drugs that suppress immunity. Care should be taken to minimize exposure of such clients to any form of infection. A whole body relaxation massage is indicated. Avoid areas that are acutely inflamed. Special care of joints such as passive movements and friction to reduce adhesions are required for those with chronic arthritis. Application of warm packs may be beneficial. See Appendix D for organizations and support groups.

References

Ginzler E, Schorn AK. Outcome and prognosis in systemic lupus erythematosus. Rheum Dis Clin North Am. 1988; 14:67.

Hahn BH. Systemic lupus erythematosus. In: Isselbacher KJ et al, editors. Harrison's principles of internal medicine. 13th ed. New York: McGraw-Hill Inc; 1994. p. 1643-1648.

Musculoskeletal system

Temporomandibular joint dysfunction syndrome (Mandibular pain dysfunction syndrome; Arthrosis temporomandibularis; Temporomandibular joint arthrosis; Myofascial pain syndrome; Costen's disease)

A collection of symptoms and signs produced by temporomandibular joint disorders.

Cause:

It is caused by inappropriate alignment of the joint and/or laxity of the supporting ligaments and muscle. There may be degenerative changes in the joint.

Signs and Symptoms:

This syndrome is characterized by unilateral or bilateral muscle tenderness and reduced motion. There is a dull aching pain around the joint, often radiating to the ear, face, neck or shoulder. The syndrome may start off as clicking sounds in the joint. There may be protrusion of the jaw or hypermobility on opening the jaw accompanied by pain. Slowly it progresses to decreased mobility of the jaw. Locking of the jaw may occur. If the problem is unilateral, the jaw may deviate to the side affected with resultant hypermobility and subluxation (loss of alignment) of the other jaw. The criteria used for diagnosis include: a) muscle pain and tenderness in one or more muscles of mastication, b) clicking or popping noises in the temporomandibular joint, and c) restricted mandibular range (<35 mm).

Risk Factors:

It is more common between 20-40 years of age and is more frequently seen in women. Gum chewing, nail biting, mouth breathing, prolonged use of pacifiers and bottles, biting off large chunks of hard food, habitual protrusion of jaws, stress translated into tension of muscles of neck and back and clenching of jaw,

Notes

Being a controversial disease, multiple treatment options exist and one or more options may be used concurrently. Treatment includes physical exercises, anesthetic sprays, use of painkillers, anti-inflammatory drugs and steroids, adjustment of bites, intraoral appliances and surgery.

The goal of short-term treatment is to reduce pain and spasm, increase range of motion and decrease adhesions. Long term treatment aims to restore joint mechanics and muscle strength. Education of the client is an important component.

For more details see Appendix C: Antiinflammatories - non steroidal drugs; Painkillers.

predispose to this condition. Injury/ trauma, whiplash injuries, improper braces are other risk factors. In some people a genetic predisposition has been identified. Rarely, rheumatoid arthritis may affect this joint.

Caution and Recommendations to Therapists:

It is important to assess and palpate the specific muscles both intra and extra orally. Ensure that latex gloves are worn while palpating intra orally. The masseters, temporalis muscle and pterygoids both medial and lateral should be palpated for spasm, tenderness and trigger points. The range and symmetry of movement of the jaw should also be tested. The aim of treatment is to reduce the pain and spasm of muscles and to relax and strengthen the muscles involved. The cause has to be identified in order to produce long term improvement.

In the acute stage, hot packs can be used to relieve muscle pain and spasm. Ice packs can be used if inflammation of the joint is present. The muscles of the neck, occiput and shoulders have to be thoroughly massaged to reduce spasm and trigger points. Later soft tissue mobilization techniques are employed.

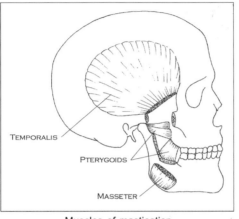

Muscles of mastication

Deep friction massage is given to the capsule of the joint. Gentle stroking or kneading at the insertion of the temporalis and medial and lateral pterygoids intra-orally may also be used. Myofascial release techniques help relax the muscles of mastication such as the masseter, temporalis, supra and infra hyoid muscles. Mobilization techniques like caudal traction, protrusion, medial-lateral glide can be used. The client has to be educated to relax the muscles. This can be done by asking the client to clench the jaw firmly and concentrate on the sense and feeling of tightness of jaw. Then he/she is asked to relax and let the jaw fall open. Alternately, the jaw is opened against resistance provided by the Therapist, followed by total relaxation. Other movements to the right and left are also performed with and without resistance and then allowed to relax. The client can also be advised on maintaining proper posture and breathing techniques. Passive and active stretches are other forms of treatment used.

Consult Dentist and Physiotherapist for specific treatment techniques. Ensure that the client does not harbor any infective disease that can be transmitted by secretions, at the time of treatment. Always use disposable latex gloves while manipulating intra orally. Remember to wash hands after removal of gloves.

References

Turchaninov R, Cox CA. Medical massage. Scottsdale: Stress Less publishing Inc; 1998. p. 360-365.

Goodheart G. Applied kinesiology in dysfunction of the temporomandibular joint. Dental Clin North Am 1983: 27(3):613-630.

Tendinitis - Achilles

Inflammation of the Achilles tendon (tendo calcaneus).

Notes

To avoid and prevent continued trauma and irritation, supportive devices such as splint or braces may be used. Sometimes steroid injections are given at the site. For more details see Appendix C: Antiinflammatories - non steroidal drugs; Antiinflammatories - steroidal drugs; Painkillers.

Cause:

It is caused by overuse of the gastrocnemius and soleus muscles.

Signs and Symptoms:

There is gradual onset of pain behind the ankle, that increases on inverting, everting or dorsiflexing the foot. The pain is made worse when wearing low-heeled shoes and is improved when wearing higher heels. The pain may be in areas proximal to the insertion of the tendon to the calcaneus ie. in the region with the poorest blood supply.

The pain may also be associated with inflammation of the infratendinous and supratendinous bursa. There may be swelling of the tendon. Crepitations (abnormal crackling sounds) may be heard on moving the ankle in the case of inflammation of the connective tissue around the Achilles.

Risk Factors:

High impact sports such as basketball, running, volleyball predispose to this condition.

Caution and Recommendations to Therapists:

In the acute state, the part should be rested. Ice, compression and elevation of the limb are used to minimize swelling. Passive and active exercise of surrounding joints should be encouraged to maintain range of motion. With time, exercises to strengthen muscles have to be introduced. Deep transverse friction massage is used to reduce adhesions. Transverse friction massage is an important component of treatment in chronic tendinitis. It mobilizes scar tissue that is forming or which has already developed and also increases blood flow to the area thus speeding up healing. Deep moist heat should be used to soften scars and adhesions before friction massage. Without lubricant, use pad of index finger, middle finger or thumb over the tendon and apply light pressure. Move the skin over the site forward and backward, two to three times per second for 1-2 minutes, in a direction that is perpendicular to the direction of fibres in the tendon. Even if tenderness is felt initially, it should disappear or reduce. If tenderness increases, stop treatment.

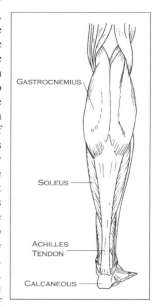

GASTROCNEMIUS

SOLEUS

ACHILLES TENDON

CALCANEOUS

Skin blisters may develop if improper techniques (which increase friction between skin and the massaging finger) are used. To reduce friction, gather and support the skin over the tendon with the thumb and fingers of the opposite hand. Do not do friction massage over skin of clients with already poor blood circulation. Such a condition is seen in clients on long-term corticosteroids or with peripheral vascular disease

References

Adams JC, Hamblen DL. Outline of orthopaedics. 11 Ed. New York: Churchill Livingstone; 1990.

Hall CM, Brody LT. Therapeutic exercise moving toward function. New York: Lippincott Williams & Wilkins; 1999.

Fu F. Sports injuries. Baltimore: Williams & Wilkins; 1994, 195.

Tendinitis - bicipital

Musculoskeletal system

Inflammation of the tendon of the biceps near its insertion.

Cause:

It is commonly caused by acute trauma to the elbow or recurrent overuse. Other musculoskeletal disorders such as rheumatic diseases, congenital defects, postural misalignment or hypermobility may also cause this.

Signs and Symptoms:

There is a gradual onset of pain in the front of the elbow radiating down the forearm. Painful twinges are also felt when the elbow is flexed or supinated. Biceps tendinitis can be recognized by the pain produced on extending the elbow with the shoulder extended.

Risk Factors:

Activities that involve recurrent flexion of the elbow or supination of the forearm predispose to this condition.

Caution and Recommendations to Therapists:

In acute cases, ice application and restriction of movement is beneficial. However, joints should be moved gently to minimize loss of extensibility of the muscle and tendon and to prevent stiffening. Such a treatment should be continued for 3-4 days. In chronic cases, strong repetitive movements should be restricted as long as pain persists. Heat therapy can help reduce pain. Start with gentle effleurage and kneading strokes and later, use deep transverse friction. Transverse friction promotes proper orientation of the fibres along line of stress without causing additional trauma to the healing tendon. Later, add stretches to the line of treatment by extending elbow with the forearm pronated. Exercises to strengthen the atrophied muscles should be added last. Clients on anti-inflammatory therapy will have a higher threshold for pain and there are chances of overtreating the client inadvertently.

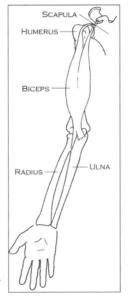

SCAPULA
HUMERUS
BICEPS
RADIUS — ULNA

Notes

To avoid and prevent continued trauma and irritation, supportive devices such as splint or braces may be used. Sometimes steroid injections are given at the site. For more details see Appendix C: Antiinflammatories - non steroidal drugs; Antiinflammatories - steroidal drugs; Painkillers.

References

Adams JC, Hamblen DL. Outline of orthopaedics. 11 Ed. New York: Churchill Livingstone; 1990.

Hall CM, Brody LT. Therapeutic exercise moving toward function. New York: Lippincott Williams & Wilkins; 1999.

Fu F. Sports injuries. Baltimore: Williams & Wilkins; 1994, 195.

Tendinitis - elbow (Tennis elbow; Epitrochlear bursitis; Golfer's elbow)

Inflammation of the origin/insertion of muscles and tendons around the elbow.

Cause:

It is due to overstrain of muscles while playing tennis or other activities that involve forceful grasp, extension of wrist against resistance, or repeated rotation of the forearm. *Lateral tennis elbow* involves the origin of the extensor carpi radialis brevis, or the common aponeurosis of the extensors at the lateral epicondyle. *Medial epicondylitis* or *golfers elbow* involves the inflammation of the flexor tendons as they arise from the medial epicondyle. Posterior tennis elbow is rare and involves the inflammation of the triceps tendon.

Signs and Symptoms:

There is a gradual onset of pain in the elbow. The pain radiates to the back of the arm and wrist on grasping objects. Tenderness may be present over the lateral or medial epicondyle, or head of radius. Increased temperature, swelling and reduced range of motion may be seen during the acute phase. The grip may also be weaker.

Risk Factors:

Occupations that involve overstrain of the muscles that originate/insert at the elbow increase the risk.

Notes

To avoid and prevent continued trauma and irritation, supportive devices such as splint or braces may be used. Sometimes steroid injections are given at the site. For more details see Appendix C: Antiinflammatories - non steroidal drugs; Antiinflammatories - steroidal drugs; Painkillers.

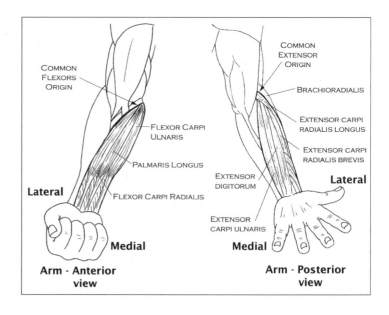

Caution and Recommendations to Therapists:

Assessment is done with the elbow extended and supported between the Therapist's elbow and side, and with the clients forearm cradled on the forearm and hand. In lateral tennis elbow, pain or restricted movement is noted on wrist flexion, ulnar deviation with the forearm pronated and flexed. In medial tennis elbow, pain is felt when the wrist and fingers are fully extended and the forearm supinated. In acute cases, ice application along with restriction of movement helps. However, the joints should be moved gently to minimize loss of extensibility of the muscle and tendon. Such a treatment should be continued for 3-4 days. Start with gentle effleurage and kneading strokes during the acute stage.

In chronic cases, strong repetitive movement should be restricted as long as pain persists. Heat therapy helps reduce pain. Passively move all joints to prevent stiffening. Use deep transverse friction over the tendon. Transverse friction promotes proper orientation of the fibres along line of stress without causing additional trauma to the healing tendon tissue. To access the tendon, the wrist is positioned fully flexed, with the elbow in semi-flexion, and the arm abducted and internally rotated. Follow the friction with ice massage. Add stretches to the line of treatment. The muscles can be stretched by extending the elbow with the forearm pronated, wrist ulnar deviated and the wrist and fingers flexed. Exercises to strengthen the atrophied muscles should be added last.

Clients on anti-inflammatory therapy will have a higher threshold for pain and there are chances of overtreating the client inadvertently. Half hour treatments daily or three times a week followed by twice a week for one week and once a week for another two weeks are recommended. Advice the client to refrain from activities that may cause tendinitis for 2-6 weeks or until healing has occurred.

References

Adams JC, Hamblen DL. Outline of orthopaedics. 11 Ed. New York: Churchill Livingstone; 1990.

Hall CM, Brody LT. Therapeutic exercise moving toward function. New York: Lippincott Williams & Wilkins; 1999.

Fu F. Sports injuries. Baltimore: Williams & Wilkins; 1994, 195.

Tendinitis - patellar (Jumper's knee)

Musculoskeletal system

Inflammation of the patellar or quadriceps tendon as it attaches to the tibial tuberosity and the patella.

Cause:

Overuse of the quadriceps muscle can cause this.

Signs and Symptoms:

There is pain over the knee along with swelling and joint tenderness. The pain increases on extension of the knee.

Risk Factors:

The incidence is higher in occupations that involve repetitive extension of the

Notes

To avoid and prevent continued trauma and irritation, supportive devices such as splint or braces may be used. Sometimes steroid injections are given at the site. For more details see Appendix C: Antiinflammatories - non steroidal drugs; Antiinflammatories - steroidal drugs; Painkillers.

leg. Sports activities like basketball or volleyball that require repetitive jumping can predispose to this.

Caution and Recommendations to Therapists:

Ice massage reduces inflammation in the acute stage. Friction massage to the tendon is helpful once the inflammation has subsided. Stretching of the muscle and ice application should be given following friction. The spasm and trigger points in the proximal and antagonist muscles should be addressed as well. The range of motion of the knee joint should be maintained by passive movements.

References

Adams JC, Hamblen DL. Outline of orthopaedics. 11 Ed. New York: Churchill Livingstone; 1990.

Hall CM, Brody LT. Therapeutic exercise moving toward function. New York: Lippincott Williams & Wilkins; 1999.

Fu F. Sports injuries. Baltimore: Williams & Wilkins; 1994, 195.

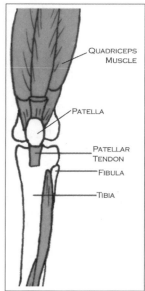

Knee - Anterior view

Musculoskeletal system

Tendinitis - popliteal/semimembranosus

Inflammation of the popliteal or semimembranosus tendon.

Cause:

It is caused by overuse of the muscles by repetitive flexion of the knee.

Signs and Symptoms:

Pain is felt over the lateral surface of the knee especially over the attachment of the muscle to the lateral surface of the femoral condyle.

Risk Factors:

It is more common in long distance runners.

Caution and Recommendations to Therapists:

Advice the client to rest. Use ice massage for the first 72 hours. Follow up by stretches and passive movements. Friction around the joint is beneficial. Use deep strokes to soften and stretch adhesions and scar tissue after the inflammation has subsided.

Notes

To avoid and prevent continued trauma and irritation, supportive devices such as splint or braces may be used. Sometimes steroid injections are given at the site. For more details see Appendix C: Antiinflammatories - non steroidal drugs; Antiinflammatories - steroidal drugs; Painkillers.

References

Adams JC, Hamblen DL. Outline of orthopaedics. 11 Ed New York: Churchill Livingstone; 1990.

Hall CM, Brody LT. Therapeutic exercise moving toward function. New York: Lippincott Williams & Wilkins; 1999.

Fu F. Sports injuries. Baltimore: Williams & Wilkins; 1994, 195.

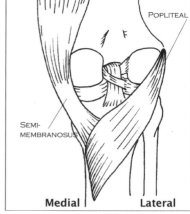

Tendinitis - supraspinatus, infraspinatus

(Shoulder impingement syndrome)

Musculoskeletal system

Painful inflammation of the supraspinatus/infraspinatus tendon at the muscle-tendon attachment to the humerus.

Cause:

The supraspinatus tendon, being attached to the greater tuberosity of the humerus is prone to compression between the acromion of the scapula and the humerus when the arm is abducted and the humeral head slips under the acromion. Prolonged overuse causes thickening of the tendon and bony spur formation which increase the chances of compression. In addition, compared to other muscles of the rotator cuff, the supra and infraspinatus are less vascular and more prone to degenerative changes. Tendinitis is commonly caused by acute trauma to the shoulder or recurrent overuse. Other musculoskeletal disorders such as rheumatic diseases, congenital defects, postural misalignment or hypermobility can also result cause this.

Signs and Symptoms:

The patient has restricted abduction of shoulder due to the compression of the inflamed and swollen tendon against the acromion. There is localized pain that presents as a sharp twinge on abducting the arm between 50 and 130 degree arc. The pain is often severe at night and is felt in the lateral aspect of the arm extending from the acromion to the insertion of the deltoid. There may be swelling due to fluid accumulation. A crepitus (crackling sound) may be felt over the site of the tendon.

Risk Factors:

It is more common in young active individuals. Activities such as tennis, swimming, racquetball, and baseball, which involve repeated elevation of arm to or above the level of the shoulder predispose to this condition.

Caution and Recommendations to Therapists:

If the inflammation is acute, ice can be applied to reduce swelling and pain. Transverse friction massage is an important component of treatment in chronic

Notes

Use of anti-inflammatory drugs and ultrasound to resolve inflammatory exudates, increase blood flow and reduce pain are the options used to treat the problem. For more details see Appendix C: Antiinflammatories - non steroidal drugs; Antiinflammatories - steroidal drugs; Painkillers.

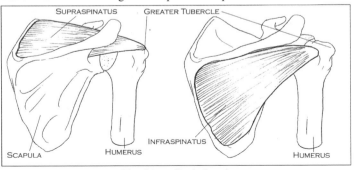

Shoulder - Posterior view

tendinitis. It mobilizes scar tissue that is forming or which has already developed and also increases blood flow to the area thus speeding up healing. Deep moist heat should be used to soften scars and adhesions before friction massage.

For transverse friction massage to the shoulder, the client should be seated, the shoulder exposed completely, and the elbow supported to reduce muscle tension. To access the supraspinatus tendon, the limb should be placed in adduction, and internal rotation, by asking the client to flex the elbow and keep the forearm close to the small of the back. The insertion can be felt near the acromion, on the highest impression of the greater tubercle of the humerus.

To access the infraspinatus tendon, the arm should be flexed, adducted and laterally rotated. Such a position may be obtained by asking the client to lie prone, with the body resting on the elbow of the laterally rotated limb. Without lubricant, use pad of index finger, middle finger or thumb over the tendon, which is between the acromion and the greater tuberosity of humerus, and apply light pressure. Move the skin over the site forward and backward, two to three times per second for 1-2 minutes, in a direction that is perpendicular to the direction of fibres in the tendon (ie. for the supraspinatus tendon, move in an antero-posterior direction). Even if tenderness is felt initially, it should disappear or reduce. If tenderness increases, stop treatment.

Skin blisters may develop if improper techniques (which increase friction between skin and the massaging finger) are used. To reduce friction, gather and support the skin over the shoulder with the thumb and fingers of the opposite hand. Do not do friction massage over skin of clients with already poor blood circulation. Such a condition is seen in clients on long-term corticosteroids or with peripheral vascular disease. Passive movement of the arm within the limits of pain should also be employed. Work in close conjunction with the Physiotherapist. Encourage client to do remedial strengthening exercises. Increase duration of treatment from 5-6 minutes in the first treatment to a maximum of 12-15 minutes. Usually a maximum of 6-10 sessions over 2-3 weeks are required for resolution.

It is common for increased soreness to be felt after the first or second session. Ensure that the treatment is given over the lesion and not in the site of the pain. The latter may be referred to a different site. Therapists should take care not to overstress the distal interphalangeal joints while massaging. This can be avoided by supporting the massaging finger as well as by alternating different fingers for treatment.

References

Lowe W. Shoulder Impingement syndrome. Journal of soft tissue manipulation 1998; 6(1): 14,16,18.

Hall CM, Brody LT. Therapeutic exercise moving toward function. New York: Lippincott Williams & Wilkins; 1999. p. 175-184.

Fu F. Sports injuries. Baltimore: Williams & Wilkins; 1994, 195.

Musculoskeletal system	**Tenosynovitis** (Stenosing tenovaginitis; Hoffman's disease)
	Inflammation of the synovial sheath of muscles.

Cause:

Synovial sheaths are synovial fluid-filled sacs that are seen around certain tendons. It functions as a cushion that reduces friction between tendons and between bone and tendon.

It is caused by overwork of muscle, stretching or wrenching of a tendon or spread of inflammation from surrounding tissues. In injuries that break the skin and expose the tissue to the exterior, bacterial infection may cause this.

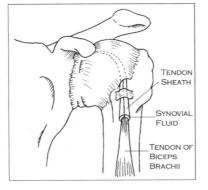

TENDON SHEATH

SYNOVIAL FLUID

TENDON OF BICEPS BRACHII

Notes

Anti-inflammatory drugs may be given. Corticosteroids or a local anesthetic is injected into the sheath to reduce pain and inflammation. Occasionally, surgical incision of the sheath is performed. Ultrasound, friction massage are other treatment options. The treatment aims to maintain and increase mobility of the tendons within the sheath and to help resolve the chronic inflammatory process.

For more details see Appendix C: Antiinflammatories - non steroidal drugs; Antiinflammatories - steroidal drugs; Painkillers; Anaesthetics.

Signs and Symptoms:

There is swelling in the affected sheath with tenderness and pain on using the muscles. Crepitus (crackling sounds) may be produced by the friction between the roughened sheath of the tendon.

Risk Factors:

Overwork of individual muscles predisposes to this condition.

Caution and Recommendations to Therapists:

The aim is to smooth the roughened walls of the sheath and tendon and to free the tissues from adhesions. Deep transverse frictions should be used across the affected tendon. Keep the tendon stretched while massaging. Hot packs may help relieve pain. Regular massage over three months may be required. Half hourly treatment twice weekly is recommended.

References

Adams JC, Hamblen DL. Outline of orthopaedics. 11 Ed. Ney York: Churchill Livingstone; 1990.

Hall CM, Brody LT. Therapeutic exercise moving toward function. New York: Lippincott Williams & Wilkins; 1999.

Fu F. Sports injuries. Baltimore: Williams & Wilkins; 1994, 195.

Tenosynovitis - bacterial

Musculoskeletal system

An inflammation in the synovial sheath of muscle, due to infection.

Cause:

(See Tenosynovitis for description of synovial sheath). Injuries that break skin and allow the entry of bacteria into the area cause this. The effects are particularly severe if it affects the thumb or fingers as it can spread all along the common synovial sheath up to the wrist. The flexor pollicis longus tendon has a long sheath from 2 inches proximal to the wrist to its insertion. The flexor sheath of the little finger is common with the sheath of the flexor profundus and sublimis. The sheaths of the middle fingers are unconnected with the common sheath.

Signs and Symptoms:

Pain, swelling and redness is seen along the length of the affected sheath. General symptoms such as fever are also seen. If pus has formed it may break through and spread to the surrounding tissues. It heals by fibrosis causing adhesions between adjacent structures and compromising the mobility. There

Notes

Anti-inflammatory drugs may be given. Corticosteroids or a local anesthetic is injected into the sheath to reduce pain and inflammation. Antibiotics are used in addition to control the infection. Occasionally, surgical incision of the sheath is performed. Ultrasound, friction massage are other treatment options. The treatment aims to maintain and increase mobility of the tendons within the sheath and to help resolve the chronic inflammatory process.

For more details see Appendix C: Antiinflammatories - steroidal drugs; Anaesthetics; Antimicrobial - antibacterial agents.

may be generalized symptoms of fever, fatigue and loss of appetite.

Risk Factors:

Any injury close to the sheath increases the risk.

Caution and Recommendations to Therapists:

In the acute stages refer to Physician. The client may require surgery to release the pus. Antibiotic treatment is also required. Do not massage until the infection has been treated completely. In the chronic stage, deep effleurage, finger kneading and deep friction are required to release adhesions. Joints are often kept immobilized by the client due to the pain and this leads to stiffness of joints. Passive movement help mobilize the stiff joints. Use olive oil while massaging to soften the tissues. Improvement is very slow in this condition.

References

Adams JC, Hamblen DL. Outline of orthopaedics. 11 Ed. New York: Churchill Livingstone; 1990.

Hall CM, Brody LT. Therapeutic exercise moving toward function. New York: Lippincott Williams & Wilkins; 1999.

Fu F. Sports injuries. Baltimore: Williams & Wilkins; 1994, 195.

Tenovaginitis - De Quervain's

Musculoskeletal system

Inflammation and swelling of the synovial lining of the common sheath of the abductor pollicis longus and extensor pollicis brevis as the tendons pass over the distal end of the radius.

Notes

Anti-inflammatory drugs may be given. Corticosteroids or a local anesthetic is injected into the sheath to reduce pain and inflammation. Occasionally, surgical incision of the sheath is performed. Ultrasound, friction massage are other treatment options.

The treatment aims to maintain and increase mobility of the tendons within the sheath and to help resolve the chronic inflammatory process. For more details see Appendix C: Antiinflammatories - non steroidal drugs; Antiinflammatories - steroidal drugs; Painkillers; Anaesthetics.

Cause:

It is usually caused by trauma to the area.(See Tenosynovitis for description of synovial sheath).

Signs and Symptoms:

There is a slow onset of pain over the radius that may radiate to the thumb or proximally to the forearm. This pain is more on abducting or extending thumb as in performing wringing or grasping movements. There is tenderness over the tendon sheath as it passes over the styloid process of the radius. A spindle shaped thickening 2-3 inches long is felt over the distal end of the radius.

Risk Factors:

Occupations involving repeated abduction and extension of thumb can predispose to this condition.

Caution and Recommendations to Therapists:

Assess by stretching the sheath. Pain is present on deviating the wrist towards the ulna while keeping the thumb flexed. When acute, use ice to reduce pain and swelling. When the inflammation has subsided, deep transverse friction is used at the rate of 3-5 times per week for one to two weeks. Transverse friction helps to resolve the inflammatory process and increase the mobility of the tendon within the sheath. Regular massage over a period of three months may be required. Half-hourly massage, twice weekly is recommended. The client should be advised not to overly exert the hand during the period of therapy.

References

Adams JC, Hamblen DL. Outline of orthopaedics. 11 Ed. New York: Churchill Livingstone; 1990.

Hall CM, Brody LT. Therapeutic exercise moving toward function. New York: Lippincott Williams & Wilkins; 1999.

Fu F. Sports injuries. Baltimore: Williams & Wilkins; 1994, 195.

Tetanus

A bacterial neurological disorder characterized by increased muscle tone and spasms.

Cause:

It is caused by the toxin tetanospasmin released by the bacteria *Clostridium tetani*. The organism and its spores are found worldwide in soil, animal and sometimes human feces. The spores can survive for years and are resistant to various disinfectants and even boiling water for 20 minutes. However, the organisms are killed by antibiotics.

The organism enters through a contaminated wound and produces the toxin. Since it does not require oxygen for survival, it thrives in dead tissue, wounds contaminated with foreign bodies and active infection. The toxin released by the organism enters the motor neuron in the area and migrates through the axon, across synapses to reach the spinal cord and brain stem where it blocks the release of certain neurotransmitters that normally inhibit the impulses in the motor neuron. As a result, the motor neuron fires more than usual causing rigidity in the muscles. The toxin also affects the sympathetic system increasing its activity. Sometimes tetanus affects only the nerves supplying the affected muscle (local tetanus). In others it may enter the blood stream and have a generalized effect. It takes 7-10 days for the symptoms to present after the injury.

Signs and Symptoms:

It is characterized by an increase in muscle tone and spasm of muscles. Initially, the person notices spasm of the masseters (*trismus* or *lockjaw*). Soon there is pain and stiffness in the neck, shoulder and back muscles. As the toxin affects more regions, the abdomen and proximal limb muscles become stiff. The spasms of the facial muscles appear as if the individual is grimacing or sneering - *risus sardonicus*. The contraction of the back muscles may produce an abnormal curvature of the back. In severe cases, the muscles may be thrown into violent spasm with the slightest stimulus threatening the entry of air into the lungs.

The increased activity of the sympathetic system presents as an exaggerated fight or flight response with palpitation, sweating and increased blood pressure.

Complications of tetanus include fractures and muscle rupture (due to the violent spasms), pneumonia, inflammation of veins, decubitus ulcers and muscle death.

Risk Factors:

Tetanus can occur in individuals who are not immunized or are partially immunized and in those immunized individuals who have not had the required booster doses. The disease is common in areas where soil is cultivated, in rural areas, in regions with a warmer climate and in summer months. In countries where immunization is not given major importance, tetanus may be seen in newborns.

Notes

Hospitalization is required for tetanus and the patient is kept in an environment where stimulation is minimized. The goal of treatment is to eliminate the source of toxin, neutralize unbound toxin, prevent muscle spasms and provide support until recovery. Wounds are cleaned thoroughly. Antibiotics are given to eradicate the bacteria.

Tetanus toxoid - antibodies that neutralize the toxin are given immediately to act against free toxins. Drugs are given to reduce and control muscle spasms. The course of tetanus lasts for 4-6 weeks. Muscle pain and spasms can last for many months.

Tetanus can be prevented by active immunization. The primary series for adults consists of three doses, the first and second being given 4-8 weeks apart with the third dose being given 6-12 months later. A booster dose is required every 10 years.

For more details see Appendix C: Immunization; Antimicrobial - antibacterial agents.

Tetanus can occur in inadequately cleaned wounds. It may also complicate ulcers, abscesses and gangrene.

Caution and Recommendations to Therapists:

Tetanus is a serious illness that requires hospitalization. However, tetanus is entirely preventable by proper immunization. Encourage clients to get immunized against tetanus. The Therapist should keep a record of her/his own vaccine schedule. Ensure that the clinic has a first aid kit and clean all wounds thoroughly with disinfectant and hydrogen per oxide. Refer to Appendix B: Strategies for infection prevention and safe practice for some useful guidelines. Also see Appendix D for organizations and support groups.

References

Morello JA, Mizer HE, Wilson ME, Granato PA. Microbiology in patient care. 6th ed. New York: McGraw-Hill; 1998. p. 516-517.

Thoracic outlet syndrome (First rib syndrome; Scalenus syndrome)

Cardiovascular, Musculoskeletal, Nervous systems

It includes conditions that produce symptoms of pressure on structures that exit from the thorax.

Cause:

This syndrome is caused by entrapment or pressure on structures like nerve plexuses, arteries and veins that pass through the thoracic outlet to enter the limbs. Cervical ribs, ribs that are not aligned, spasm of neck muscles (scalenes) or other muscles like pectoralis minor lying close to the structures passing through the thoracic outlet can result in this syndrome. *Scalene Anterior Syndrome*, is a term given to conditions that put pressure on the brachial plexus as it passes between the scalene anterior and medius. This may occur due to scaring and adhesions after whiplash injury. *Pectoralis syndrome* is caused by pressure on the brachial plexus and blood vessels as they pass between the pectoralis minor and coracoid process of the scapula. *Costoclavicular syndrome* is a term given to conditions that put pressure on the nerves and vessels as they pass between the clavicle and the first rib.

(Also see Nerve entrapment syndrome).

Signs and Symptoms:

Edema or heaviness of the arms, numbness, tingling or weakness of the upper limb are some of the symptoms.

Risk Factors:

It could be familial if a cervical rib is present in other members of the family. Kyphosis and bad posture may also predispose to this condition. Pressure in the armpit as in the use of crutches can damage the nerves going to the limb. Whiplash injury or similar trauma that produces spasm of the neck muscles are other predisposing factors.

Notes

Treatment depends on the nature and severity of the problem. It has to be ensured that the cause of the problem is due to mechanical encroachment of the space between the clavicle and the first rib. Exercises may be done to strengthen the muscles in the neck, improve posture thus opening the outlet. When the symptoms are mild, painkillers are given. In severe cases, the brachial plexus is explored surgically and the scalenus anterior and scalenus medius divided or the first rib divided. For more details see Appendix C: Painkillers.

Caution and Recommendations to Therapists:

Assess the range of motion of neck and upper limbs. The pulse may weaken and symptoms may be precipitated or reduced on changing the position of the limb. This indicates the presence of this syndrome. Massage helps reduce stress, relax muscles and thereby relieves symptoms of this syndrome especially if the cause is spasm of muscles. Position the client as comfortably as possible, using supporting pillows and towels if postural defects are present. Keep the upper limb elevated above the level of the heart with pillows throughout the treatment if edema is present.

Initially with the client supine, massage the chest, shoulder and neck using broad strokes of effleurage and pétrissage. Then concentrate on the muscles of the neck and shoulder, passively moving the neck through the full range of movement. Massage the sternocleidomastoid, trapezius, levator scapulae, pectoralis major and minor and scalene muscles, using special techniques for trigger points and for releasing adhesions. Massage all these muscles from origin to insertion.

Use lymphatic drainage techniques on the limb to reduce edema. Deep moist heat can be used to reduce pain and to soften the connective tissue. Fascial stretches, muscle stripping, and exercises are other techniques used. Finish treatment with a whole body relaxing massage. Encourage client to sleep in a supine position with just one soft pillow under the head. Initial treatment schedules of twice a week for three weeks have been recommended.

References

Hall CM, Brody LT. Therapeutic exercise moving toward function. Philadelphia: Lippincott Williams & Wilkins. 1999. p. 617-625.

Phaigh R. Tests for thoracic outlet syndrome. Massage Therapy Journal 1995; 34(2): 26-27.

Tinea versicolor

Integumentary system

A fungal infection of the skin.

Cause:

A fungi *Malassezia furfur* causes this condition.

Signs and Symptoms:

The fungus commonly affects the back and upper chest with lesions that appear scaly and multicolored - from yellow, pink to brown. The patches appear lighter in color as compared to the normal skin as the fungi do not allow the affected area of skin to tan. The patient may not take notice of the lesions, as they are painless. Often treatment is sought only for cosmetic reasons. The disease is rarely contagious. See Appendix A: page 358.

Risk Factors:

It is more common in those with lowered immunity or diabetes.

Caution and Recommendations to Therapists:

Do not massage clients with lesions. Boil and steam press bedding, towels and clothes if contact has been made. Advice client to get treated. Refer to Appendix B: Strategies for infection prevention and safe practice for some useful guidelines. Also see Appendix D for organizations and support groups.

Notes

Topical antifungal creams have to be used for cure. For more details see Appendix C: Antimicrobial - antifungal agents.

References

Ray TI. Candidiasis and other yeast infections. In: Sams WM, Lynch PJ. Editors. Principles and practice of Dermatology. 2nd ed. New York: Churchill Livingstone; 1996. p. 145-147.

Tonsillitis

An inflammation of the tonsils. The tonsils are rounded masses of lymphoid tissue located in the pharynx. It is one of the lymphatic organs.

Notes

Antibiotics are given for 10-14 days. Increased fluid intake and warm salt water gargling are beneficial. If the infection is chronic with a potential for abscess formation, surgery may be done to remove the tonsils (*tonsilectomy*). For more details see Appendix C: Antimicrobial - antibacterial agents.

Cause:

The inflammation is due to a bacterial infection. It is more commonly produced by *Beta haemolytic streptococci*. The disease spreads by direct contact with respiratory secretions or saliva. The incubation period is 1-3 days. Rarely, it may be caused by a virus or other bacteria.

Signs and Symptoms:

The person presents with sore throat, difficulty in swallowing, fever and painful lymph node enlargement. Joint and muscle pain, headache and chills are other symptoms. The symptoms last for 3-7 days. In chronic tonsillitis there is recurrent sore throat with a pustular discharge from the tonsils. Chronic tonsillitis can lead to abscess formation.

Risk Factors:

It is more common in children between the ages of 5-10.

Caution and Recommendations to Therapists:

Encourage client to complete the full course of the prescribed antibiotic treatment that should be for 10-14 days. Increased fluid intake, warm salt water gargling are other forms of treatment used. Do not massage until two days after start of treatment with antibiotics. A Therapist with tonsillitis should be excluded from work for at least

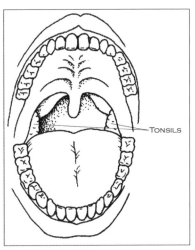

TONSILS

two days after the start of antibiotic treatment. This is to avoid spreading the infection to clients and others in the work place. Refer to Appendix B: Strategies for infection prevention and safe practice for some useful guidelines.

References

Maran AGD, editor. Logan Turner's diseases of the nose, throat and ear. 10th ed. London: Wright; 1988. p. 84-85.

Tooth decay (Dental caries)

A slow disintegration of the surface of the tooth.

Cause:

The formation of plaques/coating on the surface of the teeth by dead cells, food, bacteria etc. alter the acidity of the environment around the tooth. This results in the demineralisation and disintegration of the tooth.

Signs and Symptoms:

It starts as a blackening of the tooth. If left untreated the tooth is corroded further with resultant tingling and pain. It may be super-infected and become a tooth abscess.

Risk Factors:

Unhealthy hygiene of the mouth predisposes to this condition.

Caution and Recommendations to Therapists:

Pain may be referred to other areas of the face depending on the tooth affected. Hydrotherapy may help reduce pain and swelling. If there is an infection, the lymph nodes in the neck may be enlarged. Avoid massaging over enlarged lymph nodes.

Notes

Treatment of caries involves removal of the infected and dead tissue, sealing of the dentine that is exposed and restoration of the lost tooth structure with silver amalgam, gold, plastic or porcelain. Patient education on oral hygiene is an important component.

References

Genco et al. Contemporary Periodontics. St. Louis: Mosby; 1989

Torticollis (Wry neck)

A malposition of the head and neck due to the shortening of the muscles of the neck such as sternocleidomastoids.

Musculoskeletal system

Cause:

It may be congenital or acquired. The congenital form is due to fibrosis or shortening of one of the sternocleidomastoid muscle. It may be due to malpositioning of the fetus inside the uterus, or injury to the neck muscles by forceps delivery. The acquired form, which is rare, could be due to spasm of the muscle on exposure to cold or compression of the nerve supplying the muscle. Whiplash injury can result in injury to and inflammation of the muscle. Healing by fibrosis can cause shortening of the muscle and lead to wry-neck.

Signs and Symptoms:

There is shortening of the sternocleidomastoid or hardening of other muscles such as the scalenes, trapezius and splenius. The head is fixed in a bent position with the face tilted. Usually the muscle feels hard but there is no pain. There is scoliosis in the cervical region. In the congenital form there may be associated deformity of the face with the eye and mouth on the affected side drawn down. The nose may be deviated. (The changes in the face disappear once the position of the head is corrected). Pain may be present due to the development of trigger points in the sternocleidomastoid muscle. This pain may be referred to other areas like the ear, cheek and sternum. Autonomic symptoms like watering of the eye, dizziness and ringing in the ear may be present.

Risk Factors:

The congenital form is more common in girls. Occupations that require prolonged tilting of the head can predispose to this condition.

Caution and Recommendations to Therapists:

The aim is to relax the neck, stretch the contracted muscle, improve the range of

Notes

It is important to diagnose and treat the congenital form using daily stretching. Treatment started within the first month and continued for at least a year, results in complete and permanent correction in 90% of the children. Recurrent and resistant torticollis may be treated by surgery where the sternocleidomastoid is divided and the surrounding tissue loosened.

motion and release trigger points. Massage in the seated position may be best for these clients. Lying on the side or supine positions are also well tolerated. Deep moist heat can be used to reduce spasm and soften the connective tissue. Use firm but light strokes with the tips of the fingers. The strokes should be directed along the length of the muscle. Fascial stretching techniques can be used for the contracted muscles.

Passive movements of the head with the head over the edge of the table, but well supported with hands help stretch the muscle. The head and shoulder areas should be thoroughly massaged. Care should be taken to avoid pressure over the carotid artery that lies superficially in the neck. In people with narrowed arteries or with inadequate blood flow to the brain, manipulation of the neck may produce dizziness. Avoid turning the head to one side in these individuals. Work in close conjunction with the Physiotherapist. Encourage client to do remedial exercises to stretch the sternocleidomastoid and scalene muscles. Initially, massage should be scheduled twice a week for a month, and the frequency altered according to improvement. See Appendix D for organizations and support groups.

References

Adams JC, Hamblen DL. Outline of orthopaedics. 11 Ed. New York: Churchill Livingstone; 1990. p. 145.

Toxemia of Pregnancy (Eclampsia; Preeclampsia; Pregnancy-induced hypertension)

Reproductive system

A condition where there is increased blood pressure, protein loss in the urine and severe edema produced usually after twenty weeks of pregnancy.

Cause:

The cause is not known. It has been thought to be due to the changes in the responsiveness of the blood vessels to circulating hormones. Prostaglandins have been implicated. Abnormalities in coagulation, dietary deficiencies/excesses and genetic predisposition are other theories associated with the etiology of preeclampsia.

Signs and Symptoms:

The blood pressure in a normal pregnancy decreases during the first trimester being at its lowest during the second trimester.

In a person with this condition, the systolic blood pressure is more than 140 millimeters of Mercury (mmHg) or has increased by 30 mmHg or more as compared to previous levels, and the diastolic pressure is above 90 mmHg or has increased by 15 mmHg or more than levels before 20th week of pregnancy. There is a gain in weight of more than 3 lb per week indicating retention of fluid and edema. The person also passes less than 400 ml. of urine a day (normal about 1000 ml). Other associated general symptoms include headache, irritability, heartburn and blurring of vision. The growth of the fetus is also retarded. In the more severe condition - *eclampsia*, the person has convulsions, with premature labor or stillbirth. Liver failure may occur in the mother.

Notes

The condition is serious because of the complications such as kidney failure, liver failure and persistent hypertension. It is treated with careful monitoring, high protein and low salt diet, nutritional supplementation with adequate calcium, magnesium and zinc, bed rest, sedatives, anti-convulsants, antithrombin agents and anti-hypertensives. Due to the threat to the mother, some advocate early induction of labor. Early diagnosis and prompt treatment is required.

For more details see Appendix C: Antiepileptics/Anticonvulsants; Anticoagulants; Antihypertensives.

Risk Factors:

It is more common in pregnant adolescents or those over the age of 35.

Caution and Recommendations to Therapists:

Refer pregnant clients to Obstetrician if a sudden increase in weight or edema is noted. Discourage all pregnant clients from smoking or drinking alcohol. Consult Obstetrician before massaging a client with preeclampsia. Massage with its psychological relaxing effects can be therapeutic. The effect of massage on the autonomic nervous system can help lower the elevated blood pressure. The client may be massaged seated or turned to the left side. A gentle, relaxing massage of shorter duration is recommended. Do not try to reduce the edema as the underlying cause of edema in this case is due to kidney and liver and not improper drainage of interstitial fluid.

References

Alvarez RR. Preeclampsia, eclampsia, and other hypertensive disorders of pregnancy. In: Aladjem S, editors. Obstetrical practice. London: CV Mosby Co; 1980. p. 576-611.

Trachoma

Nervous system

An infection that causes chronic inflammation of the conjunctiva.

Cause:

It is a chlamydial infection produced by the organism *C. trachomatis*. The organism is transmitted from eye to eye via hands, flies, towels and contaminated surfaces. It may also be transmitted by contact of infected genital secretions with the conjunctiva.

Notes

It is treated with antibiotic ointments such as tetracycline and erythromycin. Surgery may be needed to correct complications. Trachoma can be prevented to some extent by taking measures to control flies and improve personal hygiene. For more details see Appendix C: Antimicrobial - antibacterial agents; Eye drops.

Signs and Symptoms:

Initially, small follicles are seen in the conjunctiva. Inflammation in the cornea may result in clouding and formation of new blood vessels. With time, scars begin to form in the conjunctiva deforming the eyelids. The eyelashes that are turned inwards irritate the cornea and lead to corneal ulcers and blindness. If the lacrimal glands are affected, tearing is reduced leading to dryness and bacterial infection.

Risk Factors:

It is endemic in north Africa, sub-Saharan Africa, Middle East and parts of Asia. The incidence is higher in the southeastern parts of the United States.

Caution and Recommendations to Therapists:

Massage is contraindicated until the person is not contagious. Refer to Appendix B: Strategies for infection prevention and safe practice for some useful guidelines. Also see Appendix D for organizations and support groups.

References

Miller SH. Parsons' diseases of the eye. 18th edition. New York: Churchill Livingstone; 1990.p. 135-138.

Morello JA, Mizer HE, Wilson ME, Granato PA. Microbiology in patient care. 6th ed. New York: McGraw-Hill; 1998. p. 428-429.

Transient Ischemic Attack (TIA)

A sudden onset of neurological abnormalities that lasts for less than 24 hours and clears soon after.

Notes

A high risk of stroke is present in individuals with TIA. Hence the goal of treatment is to prevent a stroke. These patients are treated with aspirin and anticoagulants. For more details see Appendix C: Anticoagulants.

Cause:

It is caused by temporary clogging of arterial branches in the brain by small emboli released from thrombi or spasms of arteries that lasts for a short duration.

Signs and Symptoms:

The symptoms are the same as for stroke except that it lasts from a few hours to a day and the person is completely normal again. The symptoms include, speech abnormality, loss of vision, weakness of one side of the body, gait abnormalities, dizziness etc. The symptoms depend on the site of the brain affected.

Risk Factors:

There is a higher incidence over the age of 50. It is more common in Afro-Americans and in men.

Caution and Recommendations to Therapists:

These clients are prone to bleeding if on anticoagulant therapy. Avoid using excessive pressure, as bleeding may occur under the skin. Since this condition predisposes to stroke, the Therapist should refer client to the treating Physician immediately or call for help if s/he complains of tingling, numbness, acute onset of loss of motor function during a session. See Appendix D for organizations and support groups.

References

Isselbacher KJ et al: Harrison's principles of internal medicine. 13th ed. New York: McGraw-Hill Inc; 1994. p. 2240.

Trigeminal neuralgia (Tic douloureux)

A painful condition produced by irritation of the trigeminal nerve (5th cranial nerve).

Notes

Painkillers are given as the first line of treatment. If it fails, surgery may be done to destroy the sensory ganglion. It results in partial numbness of the face. For more details see Appendix C: Painkillers.

Cause:

The cause is not known. It may be a reflex phenomenon at the sensory nerve level or at the level of the brain. It may also be due to pressure on or reduced blood supply to the nerve.

Signs and Symptoms:

It is characterized by excruciating, intermittent pain confined to one or both sides along the distribution of the trigeminal nerve - ie. on the face. The pain may be triggered by any touch or movement such as chewing, eating, swallowing, shaving etc. In some people even a draft of air, exposure to heat or cold may trigger an attack. Trigger zones may be at the tip of the nose, cheeks or gums. The pain may be of burning or jabbing type lasting for a few minutes.

Pathology A to Z -

There may be a dull ache in the region between attacks. Many people are symptom-free between attacks. There is no loss of sensation.

Risk Factors:

Scarring, pressure on the 5th cranial nerve can predispose to this. It is more common over the age of 40 with a higher incidence in women than men. It may occur in individuals with multiple sclerosis or shingles.

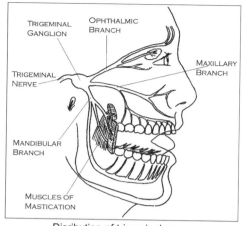

Disribution of trigeminal nerve

Caution and Recommendations to Therapists:

Get a good history of the signs and symptoms and treatment and get clearance from a Physician. Make a note of possible triggers to an attack. The individual may not allow you to touch the side of face where attacks occur. In such cases, avoid the local area and do a general relaxation massage. If the client finds massage beneficial, initially use effleurage and friction over the skull with the client in a seated position. Use effleurage for about two minutes then stroke gently and continuously starting from the middle of the face towards the temple and periphery. Start in the least sensitive area and move towards sensitive areas. Do not overwork specific areas as it may irritate the nerve and cause more pain. Do not repeat the strokes more than thrice in one area. The duration of the massage should be for 10 minutes with almost half the time spent on the skull. Schedule a total of 10-15 treatments at a frequency of one treatment every day or every other day.

See Appendix D for organizations and support groups.

References

Turchaninov R, Cox CA. Medical massage. Scottsdale: Stress Less publishing Inc; 1998. p. 226-228.

Tropical pulmonary eosinophilia

Respiratory system

A syndrome seen in individuals infected with lymphatic filarial species.

Causes:

The rapid clearance of the the microfilariae from the blood into the lungs by the immune system result in allergic and inflammatory reactions and symptoms of the disease.

Signs and Symptoms:

The person lives in an area where filariasis is endemic. It presents as cough and

Notes

The condition is treated with the drug diethylcarbamazine. For more details see Appendix C: Antihelminthic agents.

wheezing usually more at night. It is accompanied with weight loss, fever and lymphadenopathy. The eosinophil count in the blood is high - hence the term eosinophilia. The reaction in the lungs is due to allergic and inflammatory response to the microfilariae. If not treated, the inflammation resolves by fibrosis leading to further pulmonary complications.

Risk Factors:

It is more common in countries such as India, Pakistan, Sri Lanka, Brazil and Southeast Asia. The incidence is higher in men.

Caution and Recommendations to Therapists:

Though due to response to microfilaria, this condition is not infectious and is not transmitted from person to person. Relaxation massage with focus on the respiratory muscles is beneficial. Refer to Appendix B: Strategies for infection prevention and safe practice for some useful guidelines.

References

Ottesen EA, Nutman TB. Tropical pulmonary eosinophilia. Annu Rev Med 1992; 43:417.

Musculoskeletal system

Tuberculosis - bone (Pott's disease)

Tuberculous infection of bone, usually the spine.

Cause:

It is caused by an infection of the spine by *Mycobacterium tuberculosis*. The infection is usually spread from another part of the body such as the lungs or lymph nodes.

Notes

Also see Tuberculosis - lung. Plaster jacket or reinforced corset may be required to support the back and relieve pain. Abscesses may have to be drained surgically. Sometimes surgery may be done to remove dead bone. For more details see Appendix C: Antimicrobial - antitubercular agents.

Signs and Symptoms:

There is bone destruction and abscess formation. The lower thoracic vertebrae are most frequently affected. The vertebrae collapse under the weight of the body with deformity of the spine. The patient feels pain at the site of the infection. Referred pain may be felt along the dermatome if there is pressure on the roots of the nerve. The spasm of the back muscles immobilizes the affected spine and produces rigidity in the area. The gait and posture is altered in order to support the affected vertebrae. Angular deformities of the spine can be seen. Complications include abscess formation, compression of nerves and spinal cord by the collapsed vertebrae and spread to other areas.

Risk Factors:

Tuberculosis is more common in people of poor hygiene, living in overcrowded homes. (See Tuberculosis - lung). Bone TB is seen more frequently in children.

Caution and Recommendations to Therapists:

Acute cases are treated by immobilization and anti-tuberculous drugs. Consult the Physician and ensure that the client is not infective. Encourage client to take the full course of treatment. If the client is not infectious, massage may be given to the unaffected areas. Refer to Appendix B: Strategies for infection prevention

References

Schatz A. Tuberculosis and Massage. Massage. 1994: 50 (July/August): 32,34,35.

Morello JA, Mizer HE, Wilson ME, Granato PA. Microbiology in patient care. 6th ed. New York: McGraw-Hill; 1998. p. 260-267.

Daugherty JS, Hytton MD, Simone PM. Prevention and control of tuberculosis in the 1990s. Nurs Clinics North Am 1993; 29(3): 599-611.

TB. A global emergency. 1993. World Health 46(4): entire issue.

Tuberculosis - lung (Phthisis; Consumption; TB)

An acute or chronic bacterial infection that primarily affects the lungs. It may affect any system in the body.

Respiratory, Gastrointestinal, Renal, Nervous, Musculoskeletal, Lymphatic systems

Cause:

The infection is caused by the bacteria *Mycobacterium tuberculosis*. The bacteria are transmitted by airborne droplets that are produced by infected individuals when they cough, sneeze or talk. The droplets can remain suspended in the air or be transported over long distances. It may also be spread by ingestion eg. milk from a tuberculous cow - leading to tuberculosis of the gastrointestinal tract. The incubation period is 4-12 weeks. The bacteria cause a reaction in the lungs when they are inhaled. The macrophages ward off the infection by forming fibrous tubercles around the infected site, which may later become calcified. Here the bacteria can lie dormant over years and get reactivated when the individuals are susceptible. The tissue reaction may progress to formation of cavities and fibrosis in the lungs.

Signs and Symptoms:

Initially, the individual is asymptomatic. Respiratory tuberculosis presents as chronic cough and blood in sputum. Low-grade fever, weight loss and fatigue are other general symptoms.

Risk Factors:

People living in crowded, poorly ventilated buildings and those malnourished are at higher risk. Uncontrolled diabetes, AIDS, Hodgkin's disease, silicosis, individuals on corticosteroids/immunosuppressants and substance abusers are prone. It is more common in infants and the elderly.

Caution and Recommendations to Therapists:

In general, tuberculosis is not infectious from 2-4 weeks after start of adequate treatment with antitubercular drugs. Do not massage unless sure that the client is no longer infective. Consult Physician regarding infectivity of individuals. Be cautious while treating clients with history of prolonged cough (more than 3 weeks), weight loss, fatigue and low-grade fever. Refer such clients to a Physician before you treat. Massage Therapists should periodically get screened for tuberculosis by skin tests. Keep track of the epidemiology of tuberculosis in your area. If exposed to tuberculosis inadvertently, consult Physician immediately and watch for results of skin testing and take preventive treatment. Ensure that the local exhaust and general ventilation of the clinic is functioning properly.

Refer to Appendix B: Strategies for infection prevention and safe practice for some useful guidelines. Also see Appendix D for organizations and support groups.

Notes

Tuberculin Skin testing or *Mantoux test* is done to screen individuals. A positive test only indicates that the person has been exposed to tuberculosis. It does not indicate that the individual is infectious.

Not all those with TB are infectious ie. able to spread the disease. Only 10% of individuals progress to active disease. Individuals are infectious only when the disease is active. The majority of individuals enter a latent phase from which there is a lifelong risk of reactivation. If a person has active tuberculosis, work should not be resumed unless cleared by Physician ie. until three consecutive sputum smears are negative for tuberculous bacilli and clinical improvement is seen. TB is treated with multiple drugs for at least 6-9 months. For more details see Appendix C: Antimicrobial - antitubercular agents.

References

Schatz A. Tuberculosis and Massage. Massage 1994: 50 (July/August): 32,34,35.

Morello JA, Mizer HE, Wilson ME, Granato PA. Microbiology in patient care. 6th ed. New York: McGraw-Hill; 1998. p. 260-267.

Daugherty JS, Hytton MD, Simone PM. Prevention and control of tuberculosis in the 1990s. Nurs Clinics North Am 1993; 29(3): 599-611.

TB. A global emergency. 1993. World Health 46(4): entire issue.

Tularemia (Rabbit fever; Deer fly fever)

An infection caused by the bacillus Francisella tularensis.

Cause:

The bacillus *F. tularensis* is found in animals such as rabbits, squirrels, muskrats, beavers, deer, cattle, sheep, fish and amphibians etc. is transmitted to humans by direct skin contact or via insects. Rarely, infection can be caused by ingestion or inhalation of the bacterium. Ticks and deer flies can transmit the bacterium. The bacterium is found in the feces of the insects.

Signs and Symptoms:

Once the bacterium enters the skin it multiplies there and within 2-5 days there is an inflammatory reaction at the site with formation of an itchy, red, painful papule. The papule enlarges and ulcerates. Spread of bacteria to the local lymph nodes results in lymphadenopathy. Spread to liver, spleen and other lymph nodes produce similar reactions in these organs. Symptoms of pneumonia are seen if the bacterium infects the lungs. Fever with chills, body pain and lethargy are other associated symptoms. Pharyngitis, conjunctivitis, nausea and vomiting occur if the pharynx, conjunctiva and gastrointestinal tracts are infected.

Risk Factors:

It is found only in the northern hemisphere. Hunters, game wardens, trappers and others who may come in contact with wild animals are more at risk.

Caution and Recommendations to Therapists:

Ensure that the clinic is "insect proofed". Refer to Appendix B: Strategies for infection prevention and safe practice for some useful guidelines. Also see Appendix D for organizations and support groups.

Notes

It is treated with antibiotics. Tularemia can be prevented by avoiding exposure to the bacteria and by vaccinating high-risk individuals. Gloves should be used to handle wild life carcasses.

In areas where ticks are present, insect repellents should be used. For more details see Appendix C: Antimicrobial - antibacterial agents; Immunization.

References

Morello JA, Mizer HE, Wilson ME, Granato PA. Microbiology in patient care. 6th ed. New York: McGraw-Hill; 1998. p. 450-453.

Typhoid fever (Enteric fever)

An acute bacterial infection that affects many systems.

Cause:

It is usually caused by the bacteria *Salmonella typhi*. Other species *Salmonella paratyphi A, paratyphi B* may also cause the disease. Most often it spreads from a carrier who may harbor the bacteria for over 50 years. Contamination of water or food by a human carrier is the most common form of spread of disease. Carriers may harbor the bacteria in their gall bladder from where it enters the intestines through the bile and is excreted in the feces.

On being ingested, the organisms enter the small intestines. They can multiply inside macrophages and monocytes that engulf them. Soon the organism enters the gall bladder and other areas. The incubation period is variable and depends

Notes

Specific antimicrobials such as chloramphenicol are used to treat typhoid. Salicylates should be avoided to reduce the danger of intestinal bleeding. Prompt surgery is done to manage complication such as intestinal bleeding and perforation.

It is very difficult to eradicate the carrier state. Prolonged antimicrobial treatment is given. Precautions have to be taken by carriers while handling food. The incidence of typhoid can be reduced

on the immunity of the host and the number of organisms ingested and may extend from 3-60 days.

Signs and Symptoms:

It presents as prolonged high fever associated with headache, apathy and chills. If untreated the fever may last for 4-8 weeks. Ulcers in the intestine may cause indigestion, bleeding and sometimes perforation. The chance of perforation is highest in the third or fourth week after symptoms. There may be tenderness and swelling of the liver and spleen. Often abdominal pain is present. Sometimes, rashes may be seen over the chest and abdomen in the first week of infection. Complications of typhoid can occur in almost all systems.

Risk Factors:

Those travelling to endemic areas such as Mexico, Pakistan, India, Chile and Peru are at higher risk. Also, the incidence is higher in individuals with a lowered immunity such as those with AIDS, the elderly etc.

Caution and Recommendations to Therapists:

Ensure that the clients with a history of typhoid are not carriers. In those clients recovering from typhoid it is important to avoid the abdominal area during massage as it takes sometime for the intestinal ulcers to heal, and the swelling of the liver and spleen to subside. Encourage clients to get vaccinated before travelling to areas that are endemic for typhoid. Refer to Appendix B: Strategies for infection prevention and safe practice for some useful guidelines.

markedly by improving sewage disposal and water supplies. Travelers going to endemic areas can be immunized. For more details see Appendix C: Antimicrobial - antibacterial agents; Immunization.

References

Morello JA, Mizer HE, Wilson ME, Granato PA. Microbiology in patient care. 6th ed. New York: McGraw-Hill; 1998. p. 348-359.

Typhus fever

Integumentary system

Infectious disorders caused by rickettsiae.

Cause:

Notes

It is treated with antibiotics. Measures to eliminate rodents and insects can be used to prevent the condition. For more details see Appendix C: Antimicrobial - antibacterial agents.

There are many types of typhus fever. *Endemic (murine) typhus fever* is caused by the organism *R. typhi* and is transmitted by fleas present in small rodents. The organism is transmitted into humans by inoculation of infected flea feces into broken skin. *Epidemic typhus fever* is transmitted by body lice found in humans and animals such as flying squirrels. The inoculation of the louse feces into broken skin is responsible for the disease in humans. The organism causing this disease is *R. canada* and *R. prowazekii*.

Brill-Zinsser disease (Recrudescent typhus) is another form of typhus fever that recurs many years after the original attack. *Scrub typhus* caused by the organism *R. tsutsugamushi* is transmitted by mites found in wild rodents. Humans are infected by mite bites.

Signs and Symptoms:

Typically the condition presents as fever lasting for many days. Body ache, headache, nausea and vomiting are other symptoms. A cutaneous rash is seen a few days after the fever. Initially the rash is confined to the axilla and inner surface of the arm. Later, the rash becomes generalized and may be pea-sized and discrete. The rash disappears after about 8 days. There may be dry cough and mild hemoptysis (blood in sputum). If the nervous system is affected, delirium, and coma may ensue.

The severity and progress of the illness vary with the type of typhus fever. For example in epidemic typhus, circulatory disturbances such as hypotension, tachycardia and cyanosis are seen.

Risk Factors:

See Cause.

References

Morello JA, Mizer HE, Wilson ME, Granato PA. Microbiology in patient care. 6th ed. New York: McGraw-Hill; 1998. p. 487-488.

Caution and Recommendations to Therapists:

Ensure that the clinic is "insect proofed". Refer to Appendix B: Strategies for infection prevention and safe practice for some useful guidelines.

Renal system

Urinary tract infection

An infection of one or more structures of the urinary tract.

Cause:

It is caused by bacteria when the local defenses in the bladder are broken down.

Notes

It is treated with specific antibiotics after determining the sensitivity of the organism. For more details see Appendix C: Antimicrobial - antibacterial agents.

Signs and Symptoms:

Frequency of urination, burning sensation on passing urine are the common symptoms. The urine may be blood stained and cloudy. Fever, low back pain and tenderness over the suprapubic area are other symptoms. Inflammation of the urethra is known as *urethritis*. *Pyelonephritis* denotes infection of the kidney.

Risk Factors:

It is more common in women due to the shortness of the urethra. Any kind of obstruction in the urinary tract predisposes to this infection. Catheterization, pregnancy, loss of bladder control as in spinal cord injuries, renal stones, birth defects of the urinary tract make a person more susceptible to infection.

References

Paulson D. The urinary system. In: Sabiston DC (ed.): Textbook of Surgery 14th ed. Philadelphia: WB Saunders Company; 1991. p. 1438-1439.

Caution and Recommendations to Therapists:

Do not massage during the acute phase. Encourage the client to take the full course of antibiotics. Avoid massaging the abdominal area until all pain has subsided.

Cardiovascular system

Varicose ulcers (Stasis ulcers)

Chronic ulcers in the leg.

Cause:

It is seen in individuals with varicose veins. The sluggish flow of blood in the legs makes the skin prone to injury. Healing is also delayed and this results in ulceration.

Signs and Symptoms:

Typically there is a slow onset of ulcers in the medial aspect of the leg in a person who has varicose veins. There is edema and congestion of blood vessels. The ulcer may follow a mild injury to the leg with varicose veins, which later gets infected. Healing is sluggish due to the poor circulation in the limb. The skin around the ulcer may be hardened, edematous and discolored. The hardening is due to slow healing by fibrosis, which further compromises the blood flow to the area. If there is superinfection the patient will have fever, and signs of inflammation - redness, heat, swelling and pain. There may be pus discharge from the ulcer and the ulcer may appear yellow or white. See Appendix A: page 359.

Risk Factors:

See Varicose veins.

Caution and Recommendations to Therapists:

These clients are prone for thrombosis. After clearance from the Physician, the Therapist should aim to reduce edema and prevent venous and lymphatic stasis. The client should be massaged with the leg raised above the level of the heart. To reduce edema and congestion, deep and slow effleurage and kneading movements should be used starting from the thigh and continuing down the limb. To soften the hardening around the ulcer and to improve circulation, deep friction around the ulcer should be employed.

Notes

Treatment of varicose veins facilitates the healing of ulcers. Proper cleaning of wound and use of antibiotics will prevent superinfection. For more details see Appendix C: Antimicrobial - antibacterial agents.

References

Flye WM. Venous disorders. In: Sabiston DC, editor. Textbook of Surgery 14th ed. Philadelphia: WB Saunders Company; 1991. p. 1490-1495.

Varicose veins
Cardiovascular system

Abnormally dilated and tortuous veins of the lower limbs or other areas.

Cause:

The veins in the limbs are of two types - superficial and deep. The superficial veins (the long and short saphenous veins in the lower legs) drain blood from the skin and subcutaneous areas, which in turn flow into the deeper veins via communicating veins. Valves, as well as the pumping action of the surrounding skeletal muscles, prevent back flow. In patients with varicose veins, prolonged dilatation and stretching of the vessel wall make the valves incompetent and result in backflow and stagnation of blood in the veins of the lower limbs.

Varicose veins may be primary or secondary. When the varicosity is due to the superficial veins the cause is said to be primary. Secondary varicose veins result from defects in the deep veins. The latter may be due to infection of the veins - *thrombophlebitis*.

Notes

Varicose veins are treated with elastic bandages or stockings and exercise programs, in mild cases. In chronic or severe cases surgery is done where the vein may be stripped (removed), ligated (tied off) or destroyed with a sclerosing agent. For more details see Appendix C: Sclerosing agents.

Varicosities can also occur in other areas like the esophagus, rectum. (See Esophageal varices and Hemorrhoids.) In the esophagus, veins are dilated when the blood is shunted from the abdomen to the thorax through alternative routes when the architecture of the liver is distorted as in cirrhosis.

Signs and Symptoms:

The patient complains of pain or ache in the lower legs, especially on using them. S/he may also complain of progressive heaviness of the leg on prolonged standing. Some edema may be present.

Tortuous veins may be visible. In those patients with chronic varicose veins, ulcers may be seen. Superficial injuries take a longer time to heal in these patients. See Appendix A: page 359.

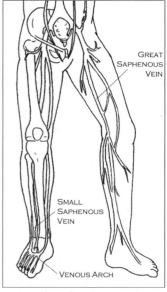

Location of saphenous vein

Risk Factors:

Varicose veins are more common in people whose occupation requires prolonged standing. The hormones, estrogen and progesterone relax the smooth muscles of the veins thus making women more prone for venous insufficiency. The risk is even higher during pregnancy. Varicose veins may be familial, as it has been shown that the number and competency of the valves in the veins differs from person to person. Obesity predisposes to varicose veins.

Caution and Recommendations to Therapists:

In those with MILD varicosity, light, local massage helps move blood and lymph towards the heart. If possible keep the leg elevated for 15 to 30 minutes before massage and throughout the treatment period to use the effects of gravity on venous drainage. The aim is to help blood flow in the collateral circulation.

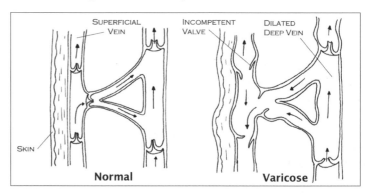

Use strokes such as effleurage, kneading, squeezing and picking up. Massage the proximal areas before moving to the distal areas. This helps decongest the proximal blood vessels that eventually drain blood from the distal vessels.

If the short saphenous vein is affected, massage first the thigh then the anterior tibial group and finally the calf. Avoid massage directly over the dilated vein. Gentle passive movements of the joints are also helpful. If the client is on supporting bandages or stocking, remove the bandage after the positioning of the client and reapply before the client gets off the table. DO NOT MASSAGE OVER SEVERE VARICOSITIES.

In those clients with twisted and hard veins, with ulceration and edema, local massage is contraindicated as prolonged stasis in the veins tend to promote thrombi formation. Massage can dislodge the thrombus if present. The emboli thus formed can in turn block arteries in the lungs, heart or brain and result in pulmonary edema, myocardial infarction, or stroke respectively. A simple test (*Homan's sign*) to eliminate the possibility of thrombosis in the deep vein is to dorsiflex the foot with the knee extended. If the client complains of pain in the calf it may indicate presence of deep vein thrombus.

Another complication of severe varicose veins is rupture of the weak walls with even the slightest of injuries. If such an emergency occurs call a Physician. Apply firm pressure pads above and below the injury with the client lying with the leg well raised. Always consult the attending Physician if the varicosity is chronic. Advice client to keep leg elevated above heart level whenever possible. For those clients who have had surgery, massage helps relieve the general fatigue in the legs. Use deep transverse friction strokes over the incision scars to prevent adhesions.

References

Flye WM. Venous disorders. In: Sabiston DC, editor. Textbook of Surgery 14th ed. Philadelphia: WB Saunders Company; 1991. p. 1490-1495.

Venous thrombosis

Cardiovascular system

Presence of thrombus in a vein.

Cause:

A thrombus is a blood clot attached to the walls of a blood vessel.

Clotting is a natural phenomenon that prevents loss of blood by clogging abnormal or potential openings in the vessel wall. Factors that promote clotting in the blood vessel such as stagnation of blood, injury to the vessel wall and alteration in the coagulability of blood promote thrombus formation.

Venous thrombosis can form in superficial or deep veins and is more common in the veins of the lower limbs. The major complication of thrombosis is the formation of emboli and resultant pulmonary edema, myocardial infarction or stroke.

Signs and Symptoms:

Since a thrombus is accompanied by inflammation in the vessel wall - *thrombophlebitis*, the patient may present with pain, swelling, and muscle

Notes

Since there is a risk of pulmonary embolism, deep vein thrombosis has to be prevented and treated promptly. Deep vein thrombosis is treated with strict bed rest and prolonged anticoagulant therapy. The affected limb is elevated above the level of the heart to reduce edema and tenderness. Thrombolytic drugs may be used in addition. For more details see Appendix C: Anticoagulants.

tenderness in and around the local area. The arterial pulse in the leg may be reduced or absent and the leg may appear pale. Fever and general malaise may also be present. In individuals with deep vein thrombosis, pain in the calf is felt if the ankle is dorsiflexed with the knee extended (*Homan's sign*).

Risk Factors:

Prolonged bed rest and immobilization, absence of blood factors which prevent clotting, or increased levels of factors like fibrinogen that promote clotting predispose to the formation of venous thrombosis. Increased levels of clotting factors are seen in those using oral contraceptives as well as during, and soon after pregnancy. Infections, trauma, surgery and catheterization also promote thrombi formation.

Caution and Recommendations to Therapists:

References

Alexander D. Deep vein thrombosis. Journal of Soft Tissue Manipulation. 1995; 3(1): 2,16.

Kravitz E, Karino T. Pathophysiology if deep vein thrombosis. In Leclerc JR, editor. Thromboembolic disorders. Philadelphia: Lea & Febiger; 1991. p. 54-64.

Local massage is contraindicated in venous thrombosis. Apart from increasing the pain and inflammation, the thrombus can be dislodged resulting in major complications including death. In a client under treatment for venous thrombosis, massage should be done only in consultation with the Physician. Since treatment for thrombosis includes drugs that inhibit clotting, such clients have bleeding tendencies and deep massage can result in small bleeds (petechiae, ecchymosis) under the skin.

Integumentary system

Vitiligo

White irregular patches on the skin.

Cause:

Notes

It is considered as a cosmetic disorder by many. However, the disease has psychological implications and in many cultures individuals are socially ostracized.

Many therapeutic approaches exist. Techniques to increase pigmentation are employed to treat this condition. Creams and exposure to sunlight/ultraviolet light and corticosteroids may be used. Use of cosmetic camouflage, sunscreens are other approaches. Surgical treatment includes skin grafting, melanocyte transplantation and micropigmentation. For those with extensive lesions, depigmentation is an option.

For more details see Appendix C: Antiinflammatories - non steroidal drugs; Sunscreen.

References

Grimes PE. Diseases of hypopigmentation. In: Sams WM, Lynch PJ, editors. Principles and practice of Dermatology. 2nd ed. New York: Churchill Livingstone; 1996. p. 843-850.

The cause is unknown. There is loss of pigment cells in the area. Genetic, immunologic, viral and biochemical mechanisms, among others, have been implicated.

Signs and Symptoms:

Hypopigmented patches are seen on the skin. The patches may be symmetrical and bilateral, and are more common around the eyes, mouth, and body folds. There may not be any inflammation. See Appendix A: page 359.

Risk Factors:

The incidence is higher between 10 and 30 years of age. There may be a family history. It may be associated with other diseases like thyroid disease, Addison's disease, diabetes mellitus etc. Stress, severe sunburn, surgery or pregnancy may precipitate vitiligo.

Caution and Recommendations to Therapists:

Infection by tinea versicolor (which is infectious) should be ruled out. Apart from the cosmetic effects, vitiligo is a harmless condition. A high degree of sensitivity to the emotional needs of the client is required in the part of the Therapist.

Volkmann's ischaemic contracture

Contracture seen in the hand following death of muscle tissue in the forearm and replacement by fibrous tissue.

Cause:

It usually follows when the blood flow to the muscles in the forearm is compromised for six hours or longer. This may be due to injury of the arm near the elbow with resultant spasm/injury to the brachial artery. The edema that follows in the rigid osteofascial compartment affect blood supply to the muscle. The degenerated muscle is replaced by fibrous scar tissue that gradually shortens producing the typical deformity. Usually the flexor digitorum profundus and flexor pollicis longus are more affected.

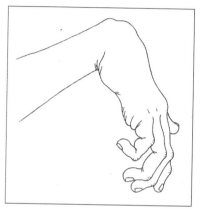

Notes

The most important aspect is prevention. The cause is identified and dealt with immediately. Established contractures may require reconstructive operations such as muscle release, nerve grafts and tendon transfers to minimize the disability.

Signs and Symptoms:

In the early stage, there is pain that is aggravated on extending the fingers passively. Soon there is flexion of the interphalangeal joints of the fingers. The fingers can be partially extended when the wrist is flexed.

Risk Factors:

The injury most frequently complicated by this condition is supracondylar fracture of the humerus. Pressure by haemorrhage and tight plasters or bandages can also result in this condition.

Caution and Recommendations to Therapists:

If a client who has just had a plaster cast applied complains of weakness and pain on movement of the limb in the cast or if the fingers are white or blue, or passive extension of the fingers is painful and restricted, advice the client to seek medical help immediately.

Application of heat to soften the connective tissue followed by friction massage and stretching may be helpful in established cases. Focus on the flexor group of muscles of the forearm especially the flexor digitorum profundus and flexor pollicis longus. Passively move all joints. Stimulatory massage should be used for the extensors that are elongated and weak. Do not apply excessive pressure if there are areas with sensory deficit. Once established, the limb cannot be restored to normal.

References

Adams JC, Hamblen DL. Outline of orthopaedics. 11 Ed. New York: Churchill Livingstone; 1990. p. 243-246

Vulvitis

An inflammation of the female external genitalia - vulva. The vulva includes the structures - labia majora, labia minora, mons pubis, clitoris and adjacent areas.

Notes

Vulvitis is treated according to the cause. General measures include keeping the area dry and clean, and decrease itching by application of cortisol cream. For more details see Appendix C: Antiinflammatories - steroidal drugs.

References

Berek JS. Novak's gynecology. 12th ed. Philadelphia: Williams & Wilkins; 1996. p. 282, 379.

Cause:

It is commonly caused by yeast (candida albicans) infection. It may also be transmitted sexually in which case it may be of viral origin. Other causes may be a reaction to chemicals such as laundry products, soaps, sprays etc. In older women, symptoms may be due to atrophy of the tissue with age.

Signs and Symptoms:

Severe itching is the most common symptom.

Risk Factors:

It is common in those with diabetes mellitus.

Caution and Recommendations to Therapists:

Have clients wear underclothes during treatment.

The female external genitalia

Warts (Verruca vulgaris)

A viral infection of cutaneous or mucosal surfaces producing a fleshy growth.

Notes

There is no reliable cure for warts. Traditionally, treatment has been to destroy the warts. Since up to two-thirds of the warts resolve by themselves within two years, treatment depends on the age, general health and level of motivation of the client.

Topical salicylic acid preparations, liquid nitrogen cryotherapy, curettage and light electrodesiccation, injection of destructive agents into the wart and lasers are some of the options used to destroy the lesion. Those with genital warts should be educated to use condoms or practice abstinence until fully treated.

For more details see Appendix C: Antimicrobial - antiviral agents; Curettage; Cryotherapy.

Cause:

Warts are caused by the *human papilloma virus*. The papilloma virus is transmitted by contact with an affected individual or sloughed infected epidermal cells. The virus probably enters through breaks in the skin. Flat warts of the beard in men and of the legs in women may be spread by shaving. After it is acquired it may spread by autoinoculation. The type of wart, the amount of virus it contains and the susceptibility of the host determines how contagious the condition is. The incubation period is 2-3 months.

Signs and Symptoms:

Warts are classified according to their appearance, location and the strain of virus that produces the lesion. *Flat warts* or *verrucae planae* are barely raised skin-colored papules usually found in the hands or face of children. *Plantar warts* are seen on the soles of the feet and may appear as small depressions, as

Pathology A to Z -

large thin plaques or as deep plaques. *Genital warts* or *condyloma acuminata* are seen in the skin of the genitalia or mucous membranes of the vagina, rectum or urethra. Warts are painless, fleshy, multiple growths seen on the surface of skin. In the dry skin, they appear as pink growths of different consistency, sizes and shapes - soft, cauliflower-like, or flat and granular, or small, pointed and firm. See Appendix A: pages 359 & 360.

Risk Factors:

Direct contact with an infected person puts one at risk. Smoking, immunosuppression, other sexually transmitted diseases and oral contraceptives increase the risk of contracting the disease. As well, these factors place an infected person at a higher risk for malignant changes.

Caution and Recommendations to Therapists:

Observe strict hygienic procedures while massaging all clients. Avoid massaging individuals with warts and advice medical treatment, as it is a precancerous condition. Refer to Appendix B: Strategies for infection prevention and safe practice for some useful guidelines. Also see Appendix D for organizations and support groups.

References

Morello JA, Mizer HE, Wilson ME, Granato PA. Microbiology in patient care. 6th ed. New York: McGraw-Hill; 1998. p. 425-426.

Stone MS, Lynch PJ. Viral Warts. In: Sams WM, Lynch PJ, editors. Principles and practice of Dermatology. 2nd ed. New York: Churchill Livingstone; 1996. p. 127-135.

Whiplash (Acceleration deceleration injury)

A condition produced by damage to muscles, ligaments, intervertebral disks and nerve tissues of the cervical region by sudden hyperextension and/or flexion of neck.

Musculoskeletal system

Cause:

The most common cause is automobile accidents - especially the type where an immobile car is struck from behind. The inertia of the head in relation to the body results in hyperextension of the neck. Whiplash can also result from contact sports such as football, or high velocity sports such as skiing. There may be micro or complete tearing of the sternocleidomastoid muscle, longus coli muscle and the anterior longitudinal ligament of the vertebral column. The cervical intervertebral disk may be prolapsed or torn away from the vertebral body.

Signs and Symptoms:

Symptoms start immediately in severe injury. In mild cases, the symptoms may start after 12-24 hours. There is pain in the anterior and posterior regions of the neck. The cervical muscles may be rigid to touch due to the spasm. There is pain, swelling, stiffness, spasm and soreness of the sternocleidomastoid. The skin may be warm and red indicating inflammation.

Different groups of muscles are affected depending on the type of injury. In an extension injury, the sternocleidomastoid, scalenes, infrahyoid, suprahyoid, levator scapulae, longus coli, suboccipitals and rhomboids are likely to be injured.

Notes

The prognosis of the injury is related to the direction of the initial impact. In general, prognosis is worst for those involved in accidents where the impact was from the rear (symptoms persist up to or beyond a year after accident). It is a little better in impacts from the side (symptoms last for a few months). The best prognosis is for those involved in head-on collisions (symptoms last a few weeks). The extent of injury is less in flexion injuries as the movement of the neck is limited by the chin in front and the shoulder in the side. Extension injuries are worse as the backward movement is not limited unless a high headrest is present.

As with other sprains, whiplash can be considered as an acceleration extension sprain of the neck, treatment includes splinting and use of analgesics. Splinting may be provided by a removable plastic cervical collar. If the injury is severe, the client has to lie in bed for a week or more to take the weight off the neck. Intermittent cervical traction may be needed if neck

pain and arm pain persist. For more
details see Appendix C:
Antiinflammatories - non steroidal drugs;
Painkillers.

In a flexion type of injury, the trapezius, splenius capitus and semispinalis capitus - ie. muscles behind the neck are likely to be injured.

An injury from the side is likely to affect the sternocleidomastoid, suboccipitals, levator scapulae, splenius capitus and splenius cervicis. Muscles of the upper and lower limbs may be injured in association with those of the neck. The pectoralis major and minor may be injured by the seatbelt.

Disturbances of the vestibular apparatus of the inner ear may result in dizziness, nausea, vomiting, headache and gait disturbances. Disturbance of the cochlea of the inner ear may result in *tinnitus* (ringing in the ear) and *nystagmus* (rapid eye movement). Injury to the nerves exiting from the cervical region may produce numbness in the arms. Blurring of vision and dizziness may be due to injury to the cervical sympathetic nerves. There may be difficulty in swallowing due to hemorrhage in the wall of the oral pharynx and esophagus.

Whiplash may also present as restlessness, mood changes and insomnia if concussion to the brain has occurred in addition.

Risk Factors:

The risk is increased if driving without proper seatbelt and padded headrests.

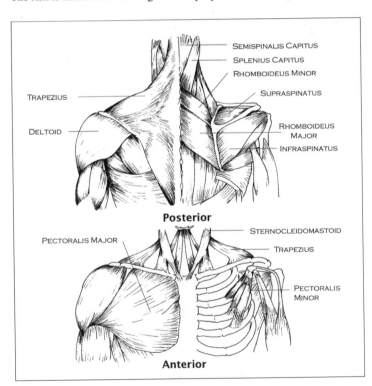

Some muscles of the neck and shoulder

Caution and Recommendations to Therapists:

Consult Physician about the extent of the injury. Assessment should be done very cautiously in the acute phase. Assess the active range of movement of the cervical spine and shoulder girdle. The acute phase is assessed by the physical findings and not by the duration of the symptoms. This phase may last up to 2-3 weeks. The client may be treated seated or lying to the side. Use hot compresses to neck to relieve pain and spasm in acute cases. Cold compresses may be used to reduce edema. If tolerated by the client, passively move the neck within limits of pain to maintain range of motion. Lymphatic drainage techniques may be used in the shoulder and neck regions.

The subacute phase, is when the pain and swelling of the muscle has subsided. There is no tenderness of muscle. However, pain may be referred to the interscapular region, upper limbs, head and shoulders. Thoroughly massage the back and shoulders using broad strokes. There may be tender points in the sternocleidomastoid, suboccipital, multifidus and other neck muscles. The aim of treatment in this phase is to increase the flexibility of the neck. Stretching exercises should be used.

Stretch the sternocleidomastoid by rotation and lateral flexion. Massage the sternocleidomastoid from origin to insertion using gentle friction strokes. For this to be effective, the client should be in a supine position with the Therapist sitting at the head. Grasp the sternocleidomastoid between thumb and fingers and roll and massage the muscle between the fingers. Gently stretch the muscle by running the hand from the head toward the sternum with the head held slightly flexed in the opposite direction of the muscle being stretched. Stretch to the suboccipital muscle can be produced by mild traction to the occiput. The scalenus muscle can be stretched by rotating the head towards the side of muscle to be stretched and laterally flexing away from the side to be stretched. Isometric exercises can be used to strengthen the multifidus. With the client lying prone and head over the table, support head with hand and slowly allow the client to take the weight of the head and maintain the position at different degrees of extension. Do not overstretch as it may damage the delicate facet joints of the vertebra.

In the chronic phase, the healing is complete but the muscles may be shortened by fibrosis with limitation of the range of motion. The posture may be altered with the head thrust forward. Deep, aching pain may be present. Deep moist heat can be used to reduce pain. Passively move joints, taking care not to overstretch. Use friction massage over the sternocleidomastoid and other neck muscles. Vigorous rotation and stretching should be avoided. Remember that in the case of whiplash it is better to undertreat than overtreat. Initially, treatment scheduled for half-hour duration at a frequency of two to three times a week for two weeks is recommended. The frequency may be reduced to one or two times a week for another two weeks and then rescheduled after assessment.

Since lawsuits may be involved in whiplash injury, keep accurate records of assessment and treatment and do not allow access of any other individual to the records.

References

Mercier LR, editor. Practical orthopedics. 4th ed. New York: Mosby-Year book Inc; 1995. p. 41.

Deans GT et al. Neck sprain: a major cause of disability following car accidents. Injury 1987; 18:10.

Pennie BH, Agambar LJ. Whiplash injuries. J Bone Joint Surg (Br) 1990;72:277.

Yaws (Pian; Framboesia; Bubas)

A chronic infectious disease caused by the organism Treponema pallidum.

Cause:

It is spread by direct contact of skin with infected lesions or by insects.

Signs and Symptoms:

It presents as single papules at the site of inoculation. The lesion becomes larger and red and its surface erodes to be covered by a yellow crust. This lesion is known as '*mother yaw*'. The fluid that oozes out is infective. There may be enlargement of local lymph nodes. The secretions can infect other areas of the skin. The lesion may take 6 months to heal. Healing may occur with scarring and pigmentary changes.

Lesions may be seen in the bones as well and destruction of the nose, maxilla, palate and pharynx may occur.

Risk Factors:

It is more common in warm, humid climates and is common between the regions between the Tropic of Cancer and Capricorn. Children are more prone.

Caution and Recommendations to Therapists:

Do not massage an individual with this condition until all lesions have healed. Encourage client to take the full course of antibiotics. Friction massage can be used over old healed scars to reduce adhesions. Refer to Appendix B: Strategies for infection prevention and safe practice for some useful guidelines. Also see Appendix D for organizations and support groups.

Notes

It is treated with penecillin injections. For more details see Appendix C: Antimicrobial - antibacterial agents.

References

Perine PL. Endemic treponematoses. In: Isselbacher KJ et al, editors. Harrison's principles of internal medicine. 13th ed. New York: McGraw-Hill Inc; 1994. p. 737-738.

Zollinger-Ellison syndrome (Gastrinoma)

A syndrome of ulcers in the upper gastrointestinal tract, increase in acid secretion and tumors of the pancreas.

Cause:

The tumors also known as *gastrinomas* secrete the hormone gastrin that stimulates acid secretion in the stomach. They may also secrete other hormones such as glucagon, melanocyte-stimulating hormone etc.

Signs and Symptoms:

The symptoms are similar to those of peptic ulcers. But these ulcers do not respond very well to medical and surgical treatment. The ulcers may be multiple and are present in the stomach and first part of the duodenum. Diarrhea may be present. This is a result of excessive secretion of acid and the reduction in pH in the jejunum. The activity of the enzymes in the intestines is affected by the pH changes and digestion of food is impaired.

Risk Factors:

There is a genetic predisposition. It presents itself more commonly between the ages of 30-60 years.

Caution and Recommendations to Therapists:

Avoid abdominal massage.

Notes

The treatment has to be individualized as the severity varies. Drugs are given to reduce acid secretion. Using sophisticated methods, the location of the gastrinoma/s can be identified and the tumor/s surgically removed. Limited success has been obtained by using chemotherapy. For more details see Appendix C: Antacids; Cancer chemotherapy.

References

Kaplan LM. Endocrine tumors of the gastrointestinal tract and pancreas. In: Isselbacher KJ et al, editors. Harrison's principles of internal medicine. 13th ed. New York: McGraw-Hill Inc; 1994. p. 1539-1540.

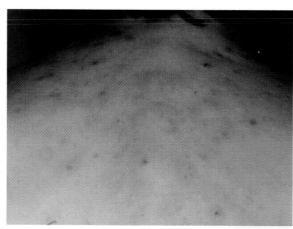

Acne conglobata
- inflammation of sebaceous glands on the back

Acne vulgaris
- inflammation of sebaceous glands on the face with papules, pustules and comedones (whiteheads/black heads)

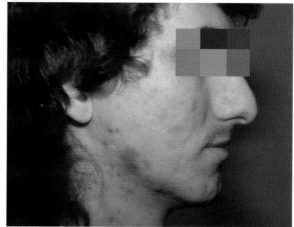

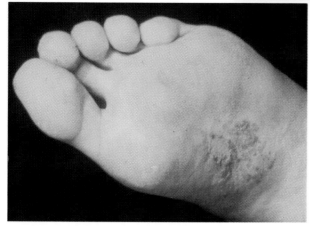

Athlete's foot
- fungal infection on the sole of foot with scaling, fissuring and multiple vesicles

Appendix A

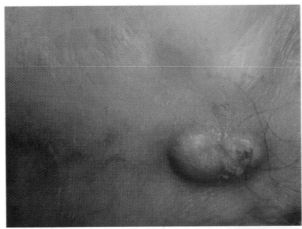

Carbuncle
- localized collection of pus with inflammation

Contact dermatitis
- inflammation of the eyelids due to cosmetics

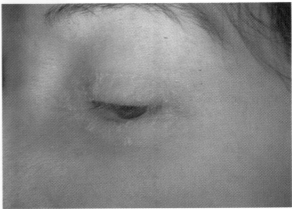

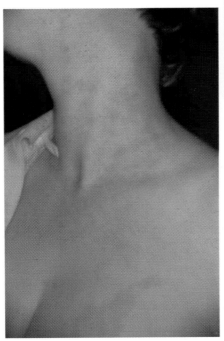

Contact dermatitis
- inflammation of the skin due to necklace

Pathology A to Z

Erythema multiforme
- round, red, edematous lesions in the hand;
immune reaction in the skin following
exposure to a drug

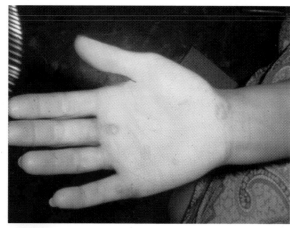

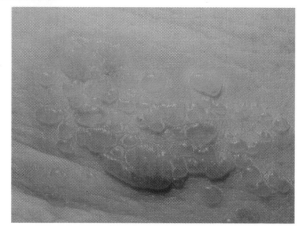

Gangrene - dry
- dry, scaly skin with blackened dead
tissue

Herpes zoster
- fluid-filled crops of vesicles along the
distribution of a sensory nerve

Appendix A

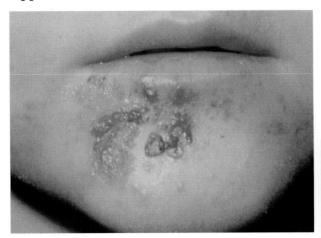

Impetigo contagiosa
- multiple, pustular, weeping vesicles covered by honey-colored crusts on an erythematous base

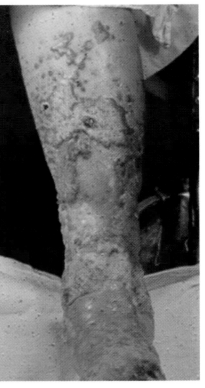

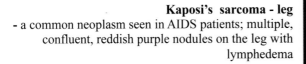

Kaposi's sarcoma - leg
- a common neoplasm seen in AIDS patients; multiple, confluent, reddish purple nodules on the leg with lymphedema

Kaposi's sarcoma - foot
- common neoplasm seen in AIDS patients; early lesions - small, discrete, raised, reddish purple nodules on the skin

Pathology A to Z

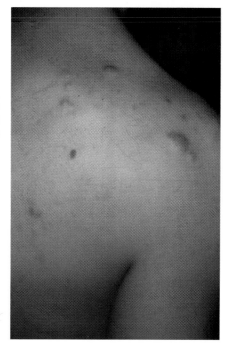

Keloid
- firm, flesh-colored to reddish nodules of scar tissue; these lesions resulting from acne

Lichen planus - lip
- small, papular, white, glistening lesions in the mucous membrane

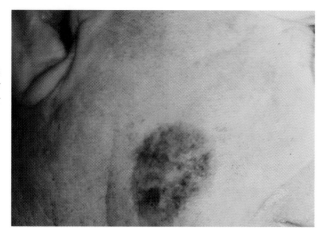

Malignant melanoma
- a pigmented lesion with an irregular border

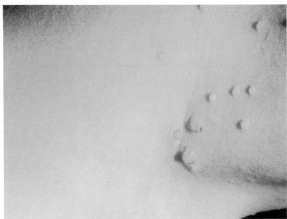

Molluscum contagiosum
- pearl-like, dimpled crops of lesions

Paronychia
- inflammation and pus formation around the nails

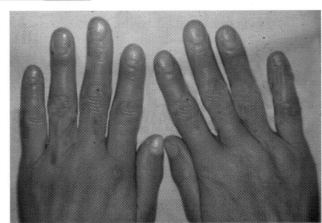

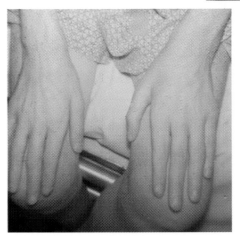

Pellagra
- symmetric, bilateral changes in skin; skin appears darkened and scaly; note muscle wasting in hands

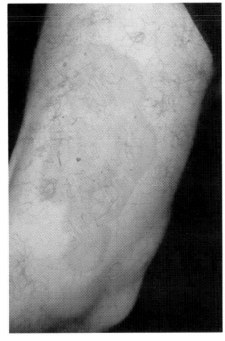

Psoriasis - arm
- well-defined red patches with thick, silvery, adherent scales

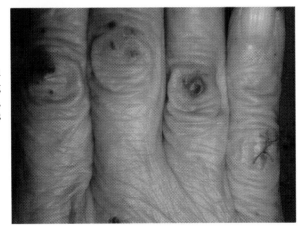

Psoriasis - palm
- symmetric, erythematous, papules and plaques with silvery scales

Purpura
- tiny purplish spots indicating bleeding under the skin; seen in bleeding disorders, platelet deficiency and collagen disorders

Appendix A

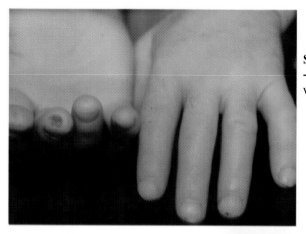

Scleroderma - hand
- pale, edematous skin with absence of wrinkles

Scleroderma - trunk
- pale, edematous skin with absence of wrinkles

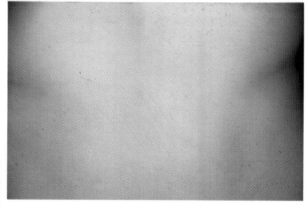

Seborrheic dermatitis
- central, facial erythema with overlying greasy, yellowish scales

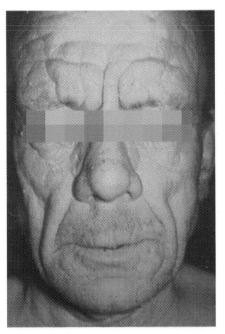

Solar damaged skin
- wrinkled, blotchy, roughened, irregular and "weather-beaten" appearance due to chronic exposure to the sun

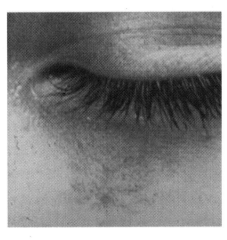

Spider nevi
- superficial, spider-like dilated blood vessels; common in liver disease

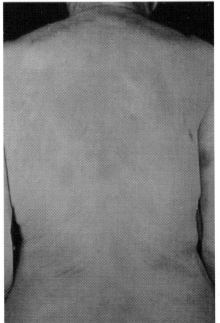

Systemic Lupus Erythematosus - body
- erythematous, raised, scaly lesions over the back

Appendix A

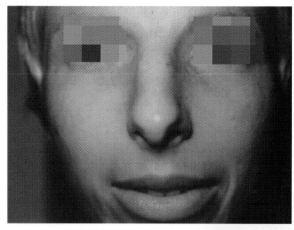

Systemic Lupus Erythematosus - face
- typical butterfly-shaped rash over bridge of nose and cheeks

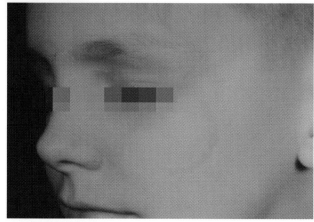

Tinea corporis
- typical, raised and red outline of the lesion with clearing in the central region

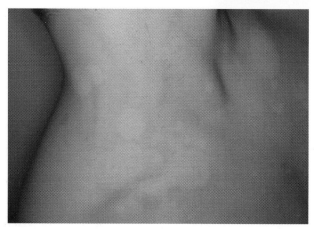

Tinea versicolor
- pale, tan, hypopigmented patches on the neck, shoulder and chest

Pathology A to Z

Varicose ulcers
- ulcers on the medial aspect of legs surrounded by hardened, edematous and discolored skin

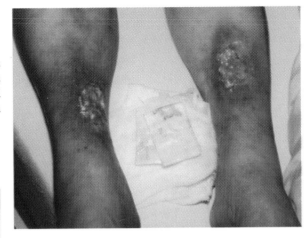

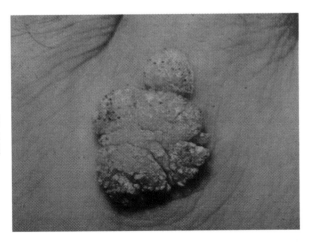

Vitiligo
- striking cutaneous depigmentation, as a result of loss of melanocytes

Warts - hand
- discrete, cauliflower-like, fleshy growth on the dorsum of hand

Appendix A

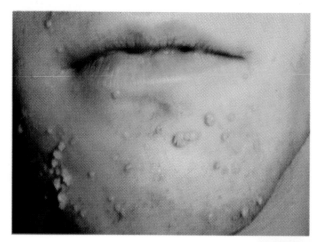

Warts - face
- irregular and branched crops of lesions on the face

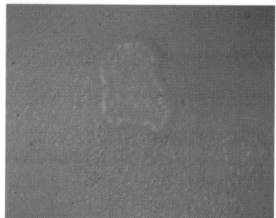

Warts - arm
- discrete, pink, slightly raised growths

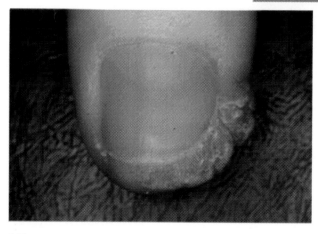

Warts - nail
- fleshy growth in and around the nail (periungual warts)

Pathology A to Z

Strategies
for infection prevention and safe practice

The most important strategy is good, well-balanced nutrition, a healthy, active lifestyle and a positive outlook in life.

Among the various causes of diseases, infection gains importance as it can be transmitted from person to person in the clinic and preventive measures can be taken easily. Some knowledge of infectious agents and how infection spreads can go a long way in preventing morbidity and mortality due to many major illnesses.

Infectious agents

Infectious agents are classified according to their structure. Arranged in order of structural complexity, they include Viruses, Rickettsiae, Chlamydiae, Bacteria, Fungi, Algae, Protozoa, Metazoa and Insecta.

Viruses are the smallest of these agents. They contain DNA (deoxyribonucleic acid) or RNA (ribonucleic acid) strands enclosed in a protein coat and require a living cell for replication and survival. They are actually particles and it is difficult to classify them as living creatures. On entering a host cell, the virus directs the nucleus of the cell to function differently and enable viral replication. New viral particles are formed in the host cell and these particles are liberated into the extracellular fluid to infect more cells.

Rickettsiae, Chlamydiae and **Bacteria** are simple cells that are very small – about 1 micron in size with the DNA material enclosed in a cell membrane. They lack a nuclear membrane. These organisms need specific environments for survival. The rickettsiae and chlamydiae, like viruses, depend on host cells for survival to a large extent. Some bacteria are aerobic organisms requiring oxygen for energy. Others are anaerobic organisms that can survive without oxygen. The bacteria are also of different shapes and sizes and are named accordingly eg. rod-shaped - *bacilli*, rounded - *cocci*.

Algae, Protozoa and **Fungi** are microorganisms that have membrane-bound organelles and proper nucleus. Algae are organisms that produce oxygen as a product of photosynthesis. Protozoa are the largest unicellular organisms that may contain flagella. They have a more complex life cycle. Fungi are microorganisms that grow as a mass of branching, interlacing filaments and include molds. Yeasts, also forms of fungi, do not have a branched appearance.

Metazoa and **Insecta** are multicellular parasites that affect man. Metazoa include worms and flukes and Insecta includes the parasites like ticks, fleas and Sarcoptes scabiei (produces scabies).

The ability of the infectious agent to cause disease is called **pathogenicity**. Organisms that cause disease readily are said to be **virulent**. Organisms that cause disease only when the immunity is low in a host are said to be **opportunistic pathogens**. Knowledge of the characteristics of the various organisms helps man to coin strategies to keep infections at bay.

Pathways of entry of infection

The various routes of entry of organisms are protected by the body by defense mechanisms. These mechanisms are breached in some way when infection occurs. Once inside the body, the infection may spread directly, via blood or lymphatics. An important way of containing and preventing infections is to protect these pathways and maintain the barriers.

Infection can be transmitted by:

Contact: Infection may be acquired through the skin *by direct contact* (eg. herpes simplex, ringworm,

Appendix B

impetigo) from person to person such as kissing, touching, sexual intercourse, fecal and oral contact; *by infection when the skin is disrupted* (eg. tetanus) or it may be *by injection into the skin by vectors carrying infectious agents* (eg. malarial parasites being injected by mosquitoes). Infections may also be acquired by *injection by humans.* This includes transfusion of infected blood and blood products and contaminated needles. Some infections are spread by *direct penetration of the skin by the infectious agent* (eg. hookworm larvae).

Infection may also be transmitted by *indirect contact* with infected body fluids via towels, shared utensils, bedding etc.

Droplet mechanisms: Sneezing, coughing, talking, singing etc. can disseminate infective particles into the air. Viruses and bacteria can be carried by dust particles and small droplets in air currents.

Vehicle: Infection can also be transmitted by substances that maintain the life of the agent until it is ingested or inoculated into the susceptible host eg. Water, blood, serum, food, feces.

Vector: Infection can be transmitted by vectors eg. insects that transmit agents by biting the susceptible host or by depositing the agent on skin or food eg. Mosquito, ticks, flies, rats.

Protective barriers

Skin

The keratinized epithelium, sweat, sebum etc are some of the protective barriers present in skin. When the continuity of skin is breached by maceration, burns or reduced blood supply, the barrier is no longer effective and there is an increased incidence of infection.

Respiratory tract

Entry of pathogens through the respiratory tract is prevented by the presence of mucus and cilia. The cilia move the mucus towards the mouth. Defense cells, antibody secretions and lymphoid tissue (tonsils) in the mouth and pharynx also protect the tract to a large extent. Depression of the cough reflex by drugs, interference with ciliary transport as in alcoholism or cold, loss of ciliated cells due to smoking and bronchial obstruction due to various causes can all contribute to

the weakening of the barrier and higher incidence of infection. Inhalation of droplets carrying infectious agents is the usual mechanism of transmission.

Gastrointestinal tract

This tract is protected by lysosomes, antibodies present in various secretions and the pH of secretions that are not conducive to growth and multiplication of microorganisms. The mucosal lining and the growth of natural intestinal flora in the colon serve as a protective barrier too. Entry of infectious agents through the gastrointestinal tract is via infected food and drinks, including fecal contamination.

Genitourinary tract

This tract is normally sterile. But risk of infection is increased by obstruction to urinary flow, catheterization, and alteration in normal flora by prolonged use of broad-spectrum antibiotics etc. In women, entry of infection through this tract is more common because of the shortness of the urethra.

Vaccines available and schedules

One of the important methods of preventing infectious diseases in humans is to develop active immunity. This usually occurs when a person is infected by a specific organism. Immunization can be artificially induced by using vaccines.

Many infectious diseases can be and have been controlled by the introduction of mass immunization programs. Smallpox has been completely eliminated. Some of the vaccines available are against tetanus, diphtheria, yellow fever, pertussis, poliomyelitis, measles, mumps, rubella, influenza, chicken pox, cholera, plague, typhus and typhoid fever. Some of the vaccines are used only in selective populations who are at high risk of being exposed to the infectious agent. Specific vaccines may be necessary for people traveling internationally. Current information on vaccines necessary can be accessed at: http://www.cdc.gov or at a local Public Health Service.

It is important to remember that vaccines do not necessarily produce lifelong protection and booster doses are necessary.

Pathology A to Z

Rarely, in some individuals, severe reaction may be produced to the vaccine or its components. Due to these rare occurrences being highlighted, many mothers do not immunize their children at all. It is important to identify those who are prone to develop these rare side effects and in the case of children, the parents have to make an informed choice about immunization in these cases.

It has to be kept in mind that if a large population of individuals who have not been immunized against a particular infection exist in one area, the whole population becomes very vulnerable to that infection. In such situations, an epidemic of that particular disease can wipe out the entire population. Presently, such a situation has not risen as those who have been immunized are shielding individuals who have not been immunized from contracting these deadly diseases.

Recommended immunization schedule for children

Age	Vaccine administered
2 months	HB, DTP. IPV, Hib
4 months	HB, DTP. IPV, Hib
6 months	HB, DTP. IPV, Hib
12 to 15 months	DTP, Hib, MMR, Varicella
4 to 6 years	DTP, OPV, MMR
14 to 16 years	TD (repeat every 10 years)

HB: hepatitis B; DTP: diptheria-tetanus-pertussis; IPV – trivalent inactivated polio; OPV – trivalent oral polio; Hib: haemophilus influenzae type b conjugate; MMR: measles-mumps-rubella; Varicella: live, attenuated varicella virus; TD – tetanus-diphtheria.

Vaccines for active immunization of normal civilian adults

Vaccines	Schedule and target group
Combined diphtheria and tetanus toxoid	Each 10 years; all adults
Inactivated influenza vaccine for current year	Yearly in autumn. All adults from age 65
Live measles vaccine	One dose. All adults without history of infection or immunization
Live mumps vaccine	One dose. All adults without history of previous infection or immunization
Live rubella vaccine	One dose. All females

Skin tests

Sometimes skin tests are used to detect the status of an individual in relation to a particular disorder. The skin test may indicate if a person has been exposed to the specific disease earlier or is currently having the disease. However, the reaction of the individual to the test will depend on their immune status. There may be no reactions if the person is immunocompromised.

One of the tests used is for tuberculosis. The protein antigen of the tubercle bacilli is injected under the skin and inflammatory reaction observed. Standardized doses and techniques are used for the test and the preferred test is known as the **Mantoux test.** The reading is taken in 48 hours (no later than 72 hours). A positive reaction (reddened, slightly raised area of induration at least 10mm in diameter) indicates past infection that may or may not be active. No reaction is present in those who have never been infected, those immunocompromised or those with advanced stage of tuberculosis, or those in very early stages of infection.

Skin tests may be used to detect present or past exposure to many types of fungal infections.

Strategies for safe practice

Remember that blood, and other secretions/excretions of the body are potentially infectious material.

Knowing that infection can spread **through the skin**, we can:

- be careful about whom we have intimate contact with and take precautions accordingly.

Appendix B

- Another simple method is hand washing. Handwashing is the single most effective way of preventing infection.

- When the skin is disrupted we can clean the wound carefully and apply suitable dressing.

- Prevent mosquito and other insect bites by using mosquito nets, repellents, using techniques to reduce propagation of these insects in the vicinity.

- We can use only disposable needles when injections are necessary.

- Hospitals can ensure that blood donors are screened properly to prevent spread of disease through transfusion products.

- By being knowledgeable about agents that can penetrate directly into the body, we can take necessary precautions. For example, the hookworm larvae enters the body when a person walks barefoot in contaminated soil. Its entry can be prevented by wearing footwear!

- Knowing that some infective organisms can live in utensils, bedding, linen etc. used by an infected person, the spread can be stopped by proper cleaning and disposal of secretions.

Knowing that infection can spread **through the gut** we can:

- Ensure that what we put into our mouth is safe. By drinking safe water, washing vegetables and fruits under water, eating fresh or well-cooked food and washing hands, many of the infections can be prevented.

Knowing that infection can spread **through the urinary and reproductive tracts**, we can:

- Keep these areas clean and dry. The use of condoms can prevent many sexually transmitted diseases.

Care of self in the clinic:

- Avoid eating, drinking, smoking and applying lip balm or contact lenses in the clinic area.

- Do not allow pets in area (except seeing eye dogs), as they may be carriers of vectors. Also, some clients may be allergic to the hair/fur.

- Request clients to take a shower before coming in for massage.

- Do not treat clients who are immunocompromised – such as clients with AIDS, on immunosuppressive drugs, on long-term corticosteroid treatment or on chemotherapy if you have any infection even if mild, as it can lead to serious or fatal infection in such susceptible individuals.

- Smoking is the cause of many diseases. Its long-term effect especially on the respiratory system makes an individual susceptible to infection. If a smoker, avoid smoking in the clinic, in the presence or absence of clients as smoke lingers in the air.

- Ensure that you are not under the influence of alcohol or drugs while working with a client.

- Use various strategies to prevent body and breath odor.

- Do not use perfume, as some clients may be sensitive to specific smells.

- Neatly tie hair back, if long, as it may fall on the client.

- Wear clothes that are modest. It may be advisable to use uniforms during the session. Ensure that the clothes used absorb perspiration as massage does increase metabolism.

- Do not wear jewelry, especially in parts that come in contact with the client, as they can be a potential source of transmitting infective organisms.

- Adopt a suitable exercise routine to keep fit.

- Learn and use proper techniques to avoid detrimental effects on your body, especially the hands. Stretch and strengthen muscles that you use during massage.

- Have a proper medical evaluation and reevaluations at regular intervals.

- If you have a communicable infection yourself, ensure that you stay away from clients during the communicable period.

- Get vaccinated. Vaccines are available against many disorders such as Hepatitis B virus, influenza, measles, mumps, rubella, poliomyelitis, diphtheria, and tetanus among others.

- Be informed about endemic disorders in your area and epidemics, if any.

Care of Clinic

Care of the room/s:

- Ensure that the local exhaust is working and the general ventilation is adequate in the clinic. The ventilation should be regularly monitored.This is important especially when you are dealing with a client with communicable infection or allergy.
- Disinfect clinic regularly, including doorknobs, and keep written record of the frequency of disinfection. 70-90% ethyl or isopropyl alcohol is adequate. Follow the product label for dilution while using germicidal detergent solutions. Some examples of other disinfectants are: bleach –10% solution; Quaternary Ammonium compounds (Quats); Phenol – 10% solution. Immersing items under water and boiling the water for about 20 minutes is another form of disinfection.
- Carpets are harder to clean than other floors, consider alternate floor style in massage area.
- To clean up spills of body fluids (which might occur inadvertently on rare occasions) use 10% bleach on and around area and mop dry without splashing. Be sure to soak and clean mop with disinfectant. Put the soiled material in a labeled, double plastic bag and dispose off carefully. Remember to wear disposable gloves.
- A first aid kit should be maintained in the clinic and the contents checked and replenished regularly.
- Doors and windows of the clinic should be tight fitting to prevent insects, rodents and other vectors from entering.
- All rooms should have heating capabilities with proper lighting.
- Sewage and other liquid waste should be disposed off in proper sewage system.
- The drinking water available should be safe, with disposable cups provided.
- The smoke detector should be working and a fire extinguisher should be available in the premises.

Care of equipment/accessories

- Use towels to cover ice/hot packs or other objects that are reused and come in direct contact with clients.
- Periodically clean ice/ice machines.
- The massage table including the face cradle should be cleaned as frequently as possible – preferably before every client. 70-90% alcohol or 10% bleach solution can be used.
- Oil and other lubricants should be stored in proper containers and dispensed into smaller ones while using them. Care should be taken not to contaminate the lubricants by dipping the fingers directly into the larger containers. Periodically clean the outside of the containers. Unused lubricants that have come in direct contact with the therapist or client should be discarded.

Care of linen

Linen used in the clinic includes towels, sheets,uniforms, pillowcases and other material that comes in contact with the client.

- Clean linen should be stored in closed cabinets.
- Dirty linen should be stored in closed containers until laundered. Don't wait too long to launder especially oil-stained material.
- Wash linen using detergent and hot water. Add one cup of household bleach to every load of laundry. Dry using the hot cycle. Ensure that the linen is rinsed well to avoid skin reactions in allergic individuals.

Client Education

- Keep brochures, articles on health for clients to take home
- Keep health magazines and pamphlets at vantage points for use by clients while waiting in the clinic.
- Refer client to support groups/associations and other resources. (See Appendix D)

Self Education

- Be well informed about infectious diseases so that you can recognize them in your client and avoid further harm to the client, yourself or others visiting the clinic.

Appendix B

- Keep reference books, medical dictionary and other resource materials in the clinic for easy and ready reference about rare disorders.
- Read the health sections of newspapers to be aware of local endemics and epidemics.

- Join local, national and international massage organizations and subscribe to journals to be current with progress made in the field and other health related issue.

Some infections caused by:

Virus AIDS, Chicken pox, Common cold, Conjunctivitis, Encephalitis, German measles, Hepatitis, Herpes simplex, Herpes Zoster, Infectious mononucleosis, Influenza, Laryngitis, Measles, Meningitis, Mumps, Molluscum contagiosum, Poliomyelitis, Rabies, Sinusitis, Stomatitis, Vulvitis, Warts

Bacteria Abscess, Anthrax, Arthritis -infective, Botulism, Brucellosis, Carbunculosis, Cellulitis, Cholera, Conjunctivitis, Cystitis, Diarrhea, Dysentery, Encephalitis, Furunculosis, Gonorrhea, Impetigo, Laryngitis, Leprosy, Lyme disease, Meningitis, Osteomyelitis, Peptic ulcer, Plague, Pneumonia, Q fever, Relapsing fever, Sinusitis, Syphilis, Tenosynovitis, Tetanus, Tonsillitis, Trachoma, Tuberculosis, Tularemia, Urinary tract infection, Yaws

Fungi Encephalitis, Candidiasis, Fungal infections, Ring worm, Tinea versicolor

Protozoa Giardiasis, Dysentery

Parasites Chagas' disease, Helminthic infections (Abdominal Angiostrongyliasis, Anisakiasis, Ascariasis, Capillariasis, Dracunculiasis, Enterobiasis, Hookworm, Larva migrans, Loiasis, Schistosomiasis, Strongyloidiasis, Taeniasis, Trichinosis, Trichuriasis, Malaria, Pediculosis, Scabies

Rickettsiae Typhus fever

Some diseases transmitted by:

Droplet/airborne mechanisms

Anthrax, Brucellosis, Chicken pox, Common cold, Infectious mononucleosis, Influenza, Laryngitis, Leprosy, Measles, Mumps, Poliomyelitis, Tuberculosis (lung), Tularemia, Pneumonia, Fungal infections, Meningitis, Sinusitis

Ingestion

Anthrax, Brucellosis, Encephalitis, Infectious mononucleosis, Influenza, Mumps, Poliomyelitis, Tuberculosis, Tularemia.

Contact – direct or indirect

Abscess, AIDS, Anthrax, Brucellosis, Candidiasis, Carbunculosis, Cellulitis, Chicken pox, Common Cold, Conjunctivitis, Diarrhoea, Dysentery, Furunculosis, Giardiasis, Helminthic infections (Enterobiasis, Hookworm, Larva migrans, Strongyloidiasis), Hepatitis, Herpes simplex, Impetigo, Influenza, Molluscum contagiosum, Pediculosis (lice), Poliomyelitis, Q fever, Relapsing fever, Ringworm, Scabies, Syphilis, Tenosynovitis – bacterial, Tetanus, Tinea versicolor, Trachoma, Tularemia, Warts, Yaws

Vehicle

Water/food borne

Botulism, Brucellosis, Cholera, Diarrhoea, Dysentery, Folliculitis, Giardiasis, Helminthic infections (Abdominal Angiostrongyliasis, Anisakiasis, Ascariasis, Capillariasis, Dracunculiasis, Enterobiasis, Larva migrans, Schistosomiasis, Taeniasis, Trichinosis, Trichuriasis), Hepatitis, Q fever, Tuberculosis, Typhoid fever.

Blood/serum
AIDS, Chagas' disease, Hepatitis, Infectious mononucleosis, Malaria

Vector

Black flies - Helminthic infection - Onchocerciasis
Deer flies - Helminthic infection - Loiasis
Fleas - Plague, Typhus fever
House Flies - Cholera, Dysentery, Trachoma
Insect bites (in general) - Anthrax, Impetigo, Tularemia, Yaws
Lice - Relapsing fever, Typhus fever
Mites - Scabies, Typhus fever

Mosquito - Encephalitis, Helminthic infection - Filariasis, Malaria
Rodents/other animals - Anthrax, Ebola virus infection, Rabies, Plague, Typhus fever
Ticks - Encephalitis, Lyme disease, Q fever, Relapsing fever
Reduviid bugs
Chagas' disease

Sexually transmitted diseases (STD)

AIDS, Conjunctivitis, Gonorrhea, Hepatitis, Herpes, Simplex, Pediculosis (Lice), Pelvic inflammatory disease, Syphilis, Vulvitis

Needle /Surgery/ Equipment

AIDS, Creutzfeldt-Jakob disease, Endometritis, Folliculitis, Hepatitis Meningitis, Osteomyelitis, Prostatitis

Across placenta/birth

AIDS, Conjunctivitis, Gonorrhea, Hepatitis

Appendix B

Commonly used drugs/therapies/ investigations and procedures

Contents

Appendix C

Introduction:

Along with their beneficial effects, drugs are linked with the risk of adverse effects. Aside from the illness/death produced, the adverse effects of drugs complicate diagnosis as they can involve almost all organs and systems of the body. The incidence of adverse effects is increased in the elderly as the number of drugs taken by them at a given time is more than others. Over-the-counter drugs - nonprescription drugs are common causes of side effects as, frequently, the right dosage is not taken.

In general, the most frequent type of adverse effect is from an exaggeration of the actual, required action of the drug. Other side effects are due to the toxic effect of the drug on organs and systems unrelated to the predicted action. These may be direct toxic effects on tissues, triggering of abnormal immune responses by the body or changes in the metabolic processes of the body especially in those people with genetic enzyme defects.

The exaggeration of the actual action may be due to increased levels of the drug at the site of action. This risk is increased if the drug is not metabolized at the expected rate - as in liver dysfunction, or excreted at a slower rate as in kidney disease. Also, other drugs taken simultaneously may interfere with the breakdown and excretion of a drug.

The magnitude of drug-induced disease is large. It has been estimated that 2-5% of patients admitted in hospitals are due to drug induced disease. Ninety percent of the reactions are produced by a small group of widely used drugs as those given below. The description given here deal with some common agents and their common side-effects, to give the massage therapist an overview - though a superficial one. Also, the given examples of drugs is not an exhaustive list.

Adrenergic drugs

Adrenergic drugs are those that mimic the activity of the sympathetic nervous system. The sympathetic nervous system is responsible for producing the effects of 'fight and flight' reaction. When this system is stimulated, the pupils dilate, the heart rate and force of contraction increases; the bronchi dilate; and the respiratory rate increases. The motility of the gut decreases – ie. muscles of the intestines relax while the sphincters close; and the intestinal secretions decrease. The blood flow to the skin decreases and the general metabolic rate increases.

The neurotransmitter involved is noradrenaline and the receptors stimulated vary from organ to organ. The effects produced by the adrenergic or sympathomimetic drugs depend on the receptors that they affect. For example, some organs (blood vessels etc) have alpha-receptors, while others (bronchi, peripheral blood vessels, heart etc have beta-receptors). There are sub types of these receptors too.

Adrenergic drugs are used in allergic states, to treat asthma, heart failure, hypotension, as nasal decongestants etc.

Examples

Epinephrine, isoproterenol, ephedrine; phenylephrine hydrochloride

Common side effects

The side effects include *arrhythmias, fear, dizziness, anxiety, anginal pain* and an *increase in blood pressure, dryness of mouth, constipation, tremors etc. Headache, flushing of the face* and *sweating* may be seen. All these side effects are symptoms that resemble excessive stimulation of the sympathetic nervous system. With the advent of drugs that affect specific receptors, the side effects are much less.

Anaesthetics

Anaesthetics are drugs that are used to ' put the body to sleep'. These drugs are of different types. They are used to produce *general anaesthesia* – where the whole body is affected; *regional anaesthesia* – where only part of the body is affected; or *local anaesthesia* where a small region is affected. Anaesthesia can be said to have four components – amnesia – where a person forgets an experience; analgesia – where the stress response to surgery is removed; hypnosis or sedation – sleep, and muscle relaxation – where the muscle fails to respond to motor nerve stimulation. Different anaesthetics have varying effects on each of these components. Depending on the type of anaesthesia required, one or more anaesthetics are used.

Anaesthetics generally work by blocking the transmission of impulses in nerves or by affecting the neurotransmitters. They may be administered as inhalations or injections.

Examples

General anaesthetics - Nitrous oxide, enflurane, isoflurane; regional and local anaesthetics – lidocaine (Xylocaine), procaine (Novocain); muscle relaxants – curare, succinylcholine

Common side effects

The side effects of general anaesthetics vary with the drug used. *Respiratory depression, nephrotoxicity* and *cardiac depression* are some. Regional and local anaesthetics can produce toxic reactions like *tremor, irritability, convulsions, increased blood pressure* etc, if large concentrations enter the blood. *Allergic reactions* may occur as well.

Analgesics

Analgesics are drugs that provide pain relief. The drugs may produce relief by affecting the free nerve endings located peripherally, preventing them from transmitting impulses to the brain, or by having an effect on the central nervous system and thereby inhibiting the perception of pain or the reaction to pain. The reaction to pain may be in the form of: autonomic response – increase in blood pressure, sweating etc; skeletal muscle response – increased tension in muscles; or the psychic response – suffering of pain.

Drugs that act peripherally generally reduce the production of prostaglandins and stimulation of the nerve fibers in inflamed tissue.

Examples

Non-opiates – aspirin-like drugs – naproxen, indomethacin, ibuprofen

Opiates – morphine, codeine, meperidine, hydromorphone, and methadone

Common side effects

The non-opiate drugs such as aspirin can produce *gastric irritation*. They may increase the *tendency to bleed* as the platelet activity is affected. They may also produce ringing in the ear (*tinnitus*).

The opiate drugs can produce *sedation, confusion,*

headache, floating feeling etc. They may predispose to *addiction. Hypotension* and *tachycardia* may be produced. The respiratory system may be depressed. *Constipation, urinary retention, dry eyes* and *blurring of vision* are other effects.

It is important for the therapist to find out the type of analgesics the patient is using, and when it was last taken. Apart from the side effects, the analgesic effect may prevent the person from giving proper feedback to the therapist.

Antacids

Antacids are one of the agents used to treat peptic ulcers. Peptic ulcers are seen in areas of the gastrointestinal tract that are directly exposed to acid and pepsin. Drugs used to treat peptic ulcers act by either neutralizing the acid or by reducing the production of acid. Antacids are agents that neutralize the acid. They are also used to treat acid indigestion, reflux esophagitis, and to prevent stress ulcers.

Examples

Aluminium hydroxide gel (Amphojel), magnesium hydroxide gel combined with aluminium hydroxide.

Common side effects

Prolonged and excessive use of antacids such as aluminium hydroxide can lead to lower levels of phosphate in the body (the antacid binds to phosphate preventing intestinal absorption) with resultant *loss of appetite, malaise* and *muscle weakness*. Some antacids that contain sodium – like over-the-counter drugs (Soda Mint, Instant Metamucil) are absorbed easily into the system and can result in *electrolyte imbalances*. Aluminium and calcium products tend to produce *constipation* while magnesium products tend to produce *diarrhoea*. There may be a tendency to form *stones in the kidney*, especially in those with kidney dysfunction.

Antiarrhythmic drugs

Antiarrhythmic drugs act at different levels of the conducting system of the heart. Some of them reduce the responsiveness of the cardiac tissue to stimulus while others slow down the rate of conduction of impulses. Depending on their action, specific drugs are prescribed for the different types of arrhythmias.

Appendix C

Quinidine, lidocaine, flecainide, propranolol, verapamil

Common side effects

The side effects vary with the primary mode of action. One of the common side effects is complete *blockage of conduction* across the heart chambers. Other side effects include *nausea*, *vomiting* and *diarrhea*. Some of the drugs act by blocking adrenergic receptors (receptors that respond to sympathetic stimulation). As a result, side effects could include *vasodilation* and *hypotension*. Some individuals may develop an *allergic reaction* to the drug.

Antiasthmatics

Although elimination of the causative agent from the environment is the most successful means for treating asthma, drugs are often needed to prevent or reduce the severity of an attack. The mode of action of the drugs used vary. In general, they relax the smooth muscles of the bronchus and reduce the congestion and inflammation. Some drugs prevent the release of histamine and other molecules from mast cells.

Since relaxation of the bronchial smooth muscles is brought about by the sympathetic nervous system, the drugs resemble the neurotransmitters released by the sympathetic nerves viz adrenaline. The drugs may also be in the form of antagonists to the neurotransmitters released by the parasympathetic nerves viz acetylcholine as the parasympathetic system has the opposite action of the sympathetic. Steroids help reduce symptoms through their antiinflammatory and other effects. Thus a single or a combination of drugs can be used in asthma. To increase the local effect and reduce the adverse reactions, many of these drugs are taken as inhalations.

Examples

Adrenergic stimulants - epinephrine, isoproterenol, isoetharine, rimiterol, hexoprenaline, salbutamol, albuterol, terbutaline, fenoterol; methyl xanthines - theophylline; mast cell stabilizing agents - cromolyn sodium, nedocromil sodium; anticholinergics - atropine, ipratropium bromide

Common side effects

One of the common side effects of the adrenergic stimulants is *cardiac arrhythmias*. The side effects resemble that of excessive sympathetic stimulation ie *fight or flight reaction*. The methyl xanthines may cause *nervousness, vomiting, anorexia* and *headache*.

Anticholinergic drugs

Anticholinergic drugs are those that inhibit the action of acetylcholine (ACh). Acetylcholine is the neurotransmitter primarily secreted by the parasympathetic nerves. Hence a drug that inhibits ACh would have an effect opposite to that of parasympathetic nerves or similar to that of sympathetic nerves. They may be used in conditions such as postural hypotension, to dilate the pupils, to reduce the motility of the gut, to reduce secretions and to reduce spasms in Parkinsonism.

Examples

Atropine, scopolamine, cyclopentolate

Common side effects

Some of the common side effects are *dryness of mouth, blurred vision, constipation, difficulty in urination, palpitation* etc (all symptoms similar to sympathetic stimulation).

Anticoagulants

Anticoagulants are given to those who have a tendency to develop or have developed thrombi in the blood vessels. For example, it is used in those with deep vein thrombosis and heart disease.

Examples

heparin, warfarin, urokinase, streptokinase

Common side effects

The most common side effect is the *tendency to bleed*. Anticoagulants increase the chances of bleeding especially in those who are predisposed - eg in those with active bleeding, bleeding tendency, uncontrolled hypertension, pregnancy and during/after surgery.

As a Therapist, special care should be taken not to use excessive pressure as bleeding may occur under the skin. In some cases, the bleeding can be fatal.

Antidepressants

Antidepressants are drugs given to treat mood disorders where depression is present. It has been shown that reduction in the level of norepinephrine and/or serotonin - the neurotransmitters in some areas of the brain, can result in depression. The antidepressants primarily produce changes at the synaptic level, to increase the levels of these neurotransmitters. Antidepressants are primarily of two types - tricyclic antidepressants and monoamine oxidase inhibitors.

Examples

Desipramine hydrochloride; doxepin hydrochloride, imipramine hydrochloride; phenazine sulfate

Common side effects

The effects are similar to inhibition of parasympathetic system (anticholinergic effects). This includes *orthostatic hypotension, constipation, dry mouth, blurred vision, dizziness, sedation* and *drowsiness*.

The therapist has to watch for hypotension and dizziness when a person on these drugs gets off the table. Due to the sedative effects, feedback from the client may be inadequate.

Antidiabetics

Diabetes is treated in many ways. The goal of the treatment is to maintain the glucose levels as close to normal at all times and thereby prevent/ reduce complications. Diabetes can produce complications in almost all systems of the body. Mild diabetes is treated by changes in lifestyle and dietary habits. Diabetes that cannot be controlled conservatively, has to be treated with oral antidiabetic drugs or insulin. Since insulin is a protein and can be digested in the intestines, it has to be given in the form of injections.

Examples

sulfonylurea (glyburide, glipizide, tolazamide, acetohexamide), biguanide (metformin), insulin

Common side effects

Hypoglycemia is the most common side effect. Hypoglycemia may manifest as sweating, palpitation, anxiety, giddiness and coma. Since prolonged hypoglycemia can produce irreversible brain damage, glucose has to be administered to the diabetic client as soon as possible. Sometimes giddiness and coma may be due to *hyperglycemia*. This can occur if the dosage and frequency of administration of the antidiabetic agent is wrong. The therapist should ensure that all diabetics have their drugs handy when they come for massage. A contact address should also be recorded in case of emergencies.

Other toxic reactions include *skin rash* and *jaundice*. In the case of clients on insulin, *sterile abscesses* may form at the site of injection. Common sites of injection are the anterior abdominal wall, anterior thigh, buttocks, posterior arm. Special care should be taken while massaging injection sites as it is important for these areas to be clean. Also, massage over an injection site can speed up the absorption of insulin and cause a sudden drop in glucose levels in the blood.

Insulin allergy is another adverse effect. Itching, swelling and redness of the injection site may be seen. In those clients who inject insulin at the same site, *lipohypertrophy* (increased fat accumulation) may be seen. *Lipoatrophy* may be seen in injection sites if impure insulin is injected.

Antidiarrheal drugs

Antidiarrheal drugs are those given to reduce the frequency of stools and to solidify the stools. It may also be given to reduce the discomfort that accompanies diarrhea. These drugs may act locally as adsorbents, astringents and intestinal flora modifiers or they may act systemically as anticholinergic drugs that reduce the motility and spasm.

Adsorbents bind to gas, toxins and irritants. They also adsorb normal nutrients and enzymes from the bowel. Diarrhea that often follows antibiotic treatment is due to the effect of the antibiotics on the normal bacteria present in the gut. These bacteria help to break down and digest food. Intestinal flora modifiers help the growth of normal flora. Systemically active antidiarrheals are opium products or belladonna. Opiates reduce motility and result in longer retention of the feces in the intestines. This results in more absorption of water and electrolytes and solidification of the feces. Infective diarrheas are treated with antibiotics.

Appendix C

Adsorbents – kaolin, activated charcoal, bismuth salts

Intestinal flora modifiers – Lactinex (lactobacillus acidophilus), Bacid

Opiates – paregoric tincture (contains morphine), Parelixir (contains opium and pectin), meperidine (Demerol); diphenoxylate hydrochloride (Lomotil)

Belladonna – atropine, hyoscine

Common side effects

Adsorbents tend to cause more *fluid* and *electrolyte loss*. They may cause *bowel obstruction*. The systemic antidiarrheals – especially the opiates can be *addictive*. The anticholinergics can result in *dryness of mouth, blurred vision* etc.

Antiepileptics/Anticonvulsants

These drugs act by reducing the seizures by suppressing the part of the brain that is the focus of abnormal nerve impulse discharge or by preventing the spread of the impulses.

Examples

Phenytoin, carbamazepine, ethosuximide, valproic acid

Common side effects

Phenytoin has an effect on the cerebellum (controls gait and coordination) and the vestibular apparatus (responsible for perception of orientation of body in space). Side effects include *ataxia, double vision, dizziness, drowsiness* etc. *Coarsening of facial features, hypertrophy of gums* and *growth of facial hair* (in women) are other side effects. The drug may have an effect on blood cells presenting with *anemia* and *leucopenia. Hypotension* is another side effect. *Nausea, vomiting* and *loss of appetite* may occur in some.

Antihelminthic agents

Specific drugs are used according to the type of parasitic infection. The mode of action varies from drug to drug. Generally, they have a direct toxic effect on the parasite causing immobilization and death.

Examples

Mebendazole (Vermox), pyrantel palmate, metronidazole

Common side effects

Nausea, loss of appetite, and *vomiting* are some common side effects. *Allergic skin rashes* may be seen in some individuals.

Antihistamines

These drugs are given to reduce itching and to control inflammation. They antagonise the secretion and action of histamine which is responsible for the itching, swelling and redness particularly prominent in allergic conditions.

Example

diphenhyrdamine, chlorpheneramine, tripelenamine hydroxyzine, loratadine, astemizole, terfenadine

Common side effects

One of the common side effects of antihistamines is its *sedatory effects*. They may also cause excessive *dryness of the mouth* and *nose. Rebound rhinitis* is seen when the antihistamines given for allergic rhinitis is discontinued. Systemically, these drugs can cause *irritability, insomnia* and *hypertension*.

Antihypertensives

The aim of antihypertensive treatment is to prevent the long-term sequelae such as strokes, myocardial infarction etc. Although mild forms of hypertension can be controlled by alteration of life style and dietary habits, moderate to severe forms require treatment with drugs that need to be taken over a long periods.

In general, antihypertensive drugs reduce the blood pressure by relaxing the smooth muscles of blood vessels. This is done by reducing the activity of the sympathetic nervous system - by affecting the areas in the brain regulating the system or by giving drugs that reduce the availability of the neurotransmitters secreted by the sympathetic nervous system at its nerve endings. Calcium channel blockers are other mechanisms by which the smooth muscle of blood vessels can be relaxed. Diuretics may also be given to reduce blood pressure. This acts by reducing the blood volume and the plasma level of sodium. Some drugs act by inhibiting hormones that normally tend to increase blood pressure. All of the above have the potential to produce adverse effects that are due to excessive sympathetic suppression.

Examples

Atenolol, betaxolol, metoprolol, nadolol, timolol, amlodipine, diltiazem, isradipine, nicardipine, nifedipine, verapamil, captopril, doxazosin, prazosin, clonidine, guanfacine, methyldopa, hydralazine, minoxidil, reserpine

Common side effects

Slowing of heart rate (bradycardia), drowsiness, dry mouth, postural hypotension, sexual dysfunction, dizziness, headache and *depression* are some adverse effects. *Gastrointestinal dysfunction* in the form of nausea and constipation may also be seen. Specifically, the massage therapists should remember that these clients are prone to postural hypotension and ensure that clients are well supported when they get up from the massage table. Antihypertensives can cause *bronchospasm* and precipitate an *asthma* attack. (This is the opposite effect of the sympathetic system that causes dilation of the bronchus). In the renal system, antihypertensives can cause *urinary retention.*

Antiinflammatories – Non-steroidal antiinflammatory drugs (NSAID)

Antiinflammatory drugs can be nonsteroidal or steroidal and the side effects vary accordingly. They are used in any condition where inflammation has to be reduced. They may be used for short or long periods according to the disease. The nonsteroidal antiinflammatories act by reducing the synthesis of prostaglandin. Some of the agents also have an antipyretic effect.

Examples

aspirin (acetyl salicylate), mobidin (magnesium salicylate), magan, arthropan liquid, trilisate, tylenol, dsalcid, voltaren (diclofenac sodium), dolobid (diflunisal), lodine, nalfon, ansaid, motrin, rufen (ibuprofen), indocin (indomethacin), indocin, orudis (ketoprophen), meclomen (meclofenamate sodium), relafen, naprosyn (naproxen), anaprox, daypro (oxaprozin), butazolidin (phenylbutazone), feldene (piroxicam), clinoril (sulindac), tolectin (tolmetin)

Common side effects

The major side effects are related to the gastrointestinal system in the form of *nausea, indigestion* and development of *peptic ulcers.* The gastrointestinal

irritation can be reduced by intake of these drugs after food or by using enteric coated drugs. All NSAIDs reduce the functioning of platelets resulting in *bleeding tendencies.* Some people may be allergic to aspirin and the drug may produce *hypersensitivity* reactions like bronchospasm(asthma), generalized swelling. NSAIDs can be *toxic to the kidney* and *liver* and should be used very cautiously in those with already existing renal/ kidney disease.

Antiinflammatories - steroidal drugs

These are among the most potent antiinflammatory drugs available and are used in severe inflammatory diseases like arthritis of multiple joints (eg. rheumatoid arthritis) and in those with severe, chronic symptoms (eg. SLE) or those not responding to NSAIDs. Steroids may be given orally, as injections or applied topically.

Example

glucocorticoids - hydrocortisone (cortisol), cortisone, prednisone, prednisolone, methylprednisolone, triamcinolone, paramethasone, dexame-thasone, betamethasone

Cmmon side effects

Since the steroids are similar in structure to those secreted by the adrenal cortex, externally administered steroids *suppress the normal interaction between the hypothalamus, pituitary and adrenal cortex.*This adrenal suppression may present as *weight loss, lethargy, fever* and *postural hypotension* especially at the time of severe stress. In the massage clinic, postural hypotension may manifest as dizziness on climbing off the table. The Therapist should ensure that the client gets up slowly after a massage and is well supported when climbing off the table.

Steroids also suppress immunity (*immunosuppression*) and the resistance to infections is reduced. Thus exposure to even minor local infections may manifest as a severe systemic forms. Also, infections that do not harm a normal individual may be harmful in those on steroids.The situation is made worse by the fact that steroids suppress local and systemic signs of infections such as inflammation. Infections that have been in an inactive stage - such as tuberculosis (TB) may surface as active forms when the immunity is suppressed. The Massage Therapist should therefore ensure that clients on steroids are not exposed to any form of disease in the clinic. Also, it should be ensured that these clients are not carriers of diseases such as TB, that may be harmful to the Therapist.

Endocrine abnormalities are other adverse effects. It includes *Diabetes mellitus, fluid and electrolyte imbalances - edema*, and *hypertension*. The individual tends to become obese with the accumulation of fat more in the trunk (*trunkal obesity*). The face becomes round and fat accumulating behind the neck appears like a hump.

The effect on the musculoskeletal system results in *osteoporosis*. Fractures are common in these individuals and the Therapist should take care that only light pressure is used during massage. The muscles may be weak. Other adverse effects include *changes in mental status* ranging from nervousness, euphoria, insomnia to severe depression.

Antimalarial drugs

The antimalarial drugs act by interacting with the DNA and killing the parasite. They may be taken as part of the treatment or for prophylaxis. For the later, the drug has to be started 1 week before the possible exposure and continued during the stay and for 6 weeks after leaving the place where malaria is endemic.

Examples

Chloroquine, mefloquine salt

Common side effects

Some of the side effects associated with this drug are *dizziness, headache, nausea, vomiting, diarrhea*, and *anorexia*. Some may develop a *rash*.

Antimicrobial - antibacterial agents

Antimicrobials are prescribed by a physician after careful consideration, as they are expensive and have side effects. Also, due to the increasing incidence of resistant organisms, care is taken to prescribe an antimicrobial that has an effect on as narrow a spectrum of microorganisms as possible.

Depending on the seriousness of the infection, antimicrobials are given intravenously, intramuscularly or orally. The dosage is altered according to the condition of the person - eg. if there is associated kidney or liver disease there are chances of the drug

being metabolized and excreted at a much slower rate so the dosage has to be reduced. In pregnant women, care has to be taken that the drug does not cross the placenta and affect the development of the fetus.

In general, in acute, uncomplicated infections, the duration of therapy is continued till the person has no fever for at least 72 hours. However, in complicated diseases like infections of the heart, bone and joints, treatment may have to be continued for a very long period.

Examples

Penicillins, cephalosporins, erythromycin, tetracyclines, chloramphenicol, sulphonamides, trimethoprim, metronidazole, aminoglycoside

Common side effects

Hypersensitivity is the most common side effect of the penicillin, cephalosporin groups. If a client gives a history of hypersensitivity to penicillin it is likely that they may be allergic to other substances in addition, so special precautions should be taken while treating these clients.

The cephalosporin group may produce *inflammation of the veins* and increase the *tendency of blood to clot*. In high doses *seizures* may occur in susceptible individuals.

Other side effects include *gastrointestinal upsets*, and with prolonged use, *candidiasis* in the oral/ vaginal mucosa. The later is due to the destruction of the microorganisms that are normally present in the body. The aminoglycosides tend to produce *toxic effects in the kidney and the inner ear* especially with prolonged use(>14 days). *Hearing loss, giddiness* and *gait imbalance* are some of the other adverse effects.

Antimicrobial - antifungal agents

Examples amphotericin, flucytosine, azoles (ketoconazole, fluconazole, miconazole, itraconazole)

Common side effects

Acute side effects include *fever, chills, headache, muscle pain, nausea* and *vomiting*. Amphoterecin which is given intravenously tends to cause *thrombophlebitis* and *renal toxicity*.

Antimicrobial - antitubercular agents

Due to the higher incidence of resistance, a minimum of two drugs are given to treat tuberculosis. Also, since the bacilli takes a long time to multiply, treatment is continued over a long period (6-12 months).

Examples

Isoniazid (INH), rifampicin, pyrazinamide, ethambutol, streptomycin

Common side effects

One of the adverse effects is the *hepatotoxicity* (toxicity to the liver). Hepatitis can occur especially in those who are alcoholics. *Peripheral Neuropathy* is a a dose-related complication of INH therapy. Care should be taken by the Therapist to ensure that undue pressure is not used in these individuals as the sensations are lower in the periphery. Rarely, ethambutol can produce *inflammation of the optic nerve* leading to decreased green color perception, and diminished sight. Streptomycin can result in *inner ear problems* such as loss of hearing, gait imbalance, giddiness and ringing in the ear (tinnitus).

Antimicrobial - antiviral agents

Examples

Amantidine, rimantidine, acyclovir, ganciclovir, foscarnet, zidovidine

Common side effects

In general, side effects are *uncommon*. They may be associated with *gastrointestinal complaints* such as nausea and vomiting. Some of the antivirals may cause *nephrotoxicity* (ie affect the normal functioning of the kidney).

Antipsychotics

Antipsychotics, also known as neuroleptics, are used to treat symptoms of psychosis including hallucinations, delusions, thought disorders etc. The drugs have an effect on the receptors for dopamine, blocking them and reducing the transmission of impulses.

Examples

Chlorpromazine (Thorazine), triflupromazine, chlorprothixene, haloperidol (Haldol), Molindone (Moban), Loxapine hydrochloride (Loxitane C)

Common side effects

Since these drugs affect the neurotransmitter dopamine, the side effects are related to deficiency of dopamine – a neurotransmitter also found in the basal ganglia (involved with motor function). The side effects are related to the dosage of the drug. Some of the side effects are *facial grimacing, abnormal eye movements, involuntary muscle movements, restlessness, difficulty in sitting still,* and symptoms of *Parkinsonism* (dopamine is deficient in Parkinsonism). The general depression of the nervous system brought about can produce *sedation. Dryness of mouth, hypotension, tachycardia, weight gain* and *photosensitivity* are other side effects that may be seen.

Antipyretics

Antipyretics are drugs that are used to reduce fever. The toxins produced by infective organisms, or the products of immune reaction have an effect on the hypothalamus heat-regulating center causing fever. These drugs act by resetting the temperature in the "thermostat" located in the hypothalamus. The temperature is brought down by vasodilation and sweating.

Examples

Aspirin, acetaminophen, other salicylates

Common side effects

Aspirin can have an effect on the mucosal barrier in the stomach and lead to *ulcer formation* and *bleeding.* Prolonged use can reduce platelet aggregation and lead to *bleeding tendencies. Nausea* and *vomiting* are other common symptoms.

Antithyroid drugs

Antithyroid drugs are used to treat hyperthyroidism. The drugs reduce/prevent the synthesis of thyroid hormones.

Examples

Propylthiouracil, methimazole, radioactive iodines (get concentrated in the thyroid and destroy tissue by emitting rays), potassium iodide, sodium iodide

Common side effects

Some of the common side effects are *nausea, vomiting, skin rash* and *loss of taste.*

Appendix C

Antitoxins

It is a collection of serum, which has been collected from an individual who has been immunized against a toxin-producing organism.

Examples

Diphtheria antitoxin, botulism antitoxin, tetanus antitoxin

Common side effects

Since the body fluid is used, there is a danger of *blood-borne diseases* being transmitted. *Hypersensitivity reactions* are other problems that may be encountered. Some people may experience *fever, chills, headache* and general *malaise*.

Bronchodilators

Bronchodilators are drugs that result in relaxation of the bronchial smooth muscles. There are three major categories of bronchodilators – the sympathomimetics, anticholinergics and xanthines. Since the stimulation of the sympathetic nervous system causes the bronchi to dilate, drugs that mimic this effect can be used - sympathomimetics. Stimulation of the parasympathetic nervous system causes constriction of the bronchi. Therefore, drugs that oppose this effect can be used – anticholinergics. Xanthines act by increasing the availability of the chemical cyclic AMP (adenosine mono phosphate), the lack of which produces bronchospasm.

As the mode of action is different in each of these groups, drugs from one or more groups can be used.

Examples

Sympathomimetics – epinephrine (adrenaline), ephedrine, isoproterenol

Anticholinergics – atropine, ipratropium bromide

Xanthines – theophyline, aminophylline

Common side effects

The side effects resemble the symptoms of overstimulation of the sympathetic stimulation – *tachycardia, dryness of mouth, anxiety, urinary retention, increase in blood pressure* etc. *Nausea* and *vomiting* are other side effects.

Cancer chemotherapy

Chemotherapy is given to treat many different types of cancer either alone or in combination with radiotherapy and/or surgery. The dosage is calculated based on the body surface area. They may be given orally, intravenously or injected directly into the affected site. They act by suppressing the rapid multiplication of cells. Since they target multiplying cells, in addition to the cancer cells, they tend to suppress the activity of the bone marrow, gastrointestinal tract, ovaries and testis where multiplication of normal tissue occurs.

Examples

Ara-C, cytosine arabinoside, fludarabine, 5-Fluorouracil, methotrexate, busulfan, chlorambucil, cyclophosphamide, melphalan, limustine, bleomycin, dosorubicin, etoposide, vinblastine, vincristine, carboplatin, L-Asparaginase, procarbazine

Common side effects

The most common side effects are *suppression of the bone marrow* and *toxicity to the gastrointestinal tract*. The reduction in the white blood cells make these individuals more prone to infections. The Therapist should ensure that the clients on chemotherapy are not exposed to any form of infection in the clinic. The suppression of the platelet formation affects the clotting process, increasing the *tendency to bleed*. The Therapist should therefore closely monitor the pressure used to prevent bleeding under the skin. The suppression of red blood cell formation leads to *anemia*.

The gastrointestinal effect presents as *stomatitis, diarrhea, nausea* and *vomiting*.

Most of the agents produce *alopecia* (loss of hair). In general chemotherapy agents are *toxic to almost all systems* and require careful monitoring and alteration of dosage.

In those clients where the agent is given intravenously, leak into the local tissue can produce *pain* and *redness at the injection site*. Hot /cold compresses are used to minimize the symptoms. The death of tissue at the local site may require surgery and skin grafting.

Chelating agents

These are substances that form ringlike complexes that bind to metal ions. They are used in various types of metal poisoning. After binding with the metal ion in the body, the chelating agent is excreted, usually via the kidneys. For example, the chelating agent deferoxamine is used to remove iron build up in patients who have recurrent blood transfusions. Deferoxamine enters the cells and binds with the iron, after which the complex moves extracellularly to be eliminated in the urine. Chelating agents are usually administered intravenously or subcutaneously.

Examples

Deferoxamine

Common side effects

There may be *irritation* and *rash formation at the site* of administration. *Abdominal discomfort* may be experienced. Rarely, a variety of *visual* and *auditory effects* may occur.

Cholinergic drugs

Cholinergic drugs are those that mimic the effects of acetylcholine. Acetylcholine is the neurotransmitter that is secreted at the neuromuscular junction. It is also the neurotransmitter secreted by the parasympathetic nerves – between the nerve and the effector cells. As well, it is the neurotransmitter secreted between the pre and postganglionic cells of the sympathetic and parasympathetic neurons. Since the receptors in each of these regions are different, the effects of the drugs are different depending on which of these receptors they affect. For example, for treating the condition myasthenia gravis, drugs that affect the neuromuscular junction are used. For treating conditions such as urinary retention, reduced intestinal motility or glaucoma, drugs that affect the receptors at the parasympathetic nerve ending are used. Some drugs have a more generalized effect (on more than one type of receptor).

Examples

Carbachol, pilocarpine, neostigmine

Common side effects

The side effects resemble the symptoms of overstimulation of the parasympathetic nervous system - *Hypotension, bradycardia, bronchoconstriction, increased intestinal motility, constriction of the pupil* and *excessive secretions from exocrine glands.*

Contraceptives - oral

Contraceptive pills are similar to steroid hormones given in varying combinations and concentrations throughout the menstrual cycle. The combination and dosage of hormones are adjusted to suppress ovulation in the female and yet resemble the normal cyclical secretion. The pills contain a combination of estrogen and progestogen.

Examples

Ortho-Novum (mestronol, norethindone combination), Norinyl, Ovcon, Ovral, Demulen, Norlestrin, Nordette, micronon, Nor Q.D., Ovrette

Common side effects

The incidence of *deep vein thrombosis* and pulmonary embolism is higher in those women using oral contraceptives. A Therapist should be alert regarding symptoms of deep vein thrombosis in these women and refer them to a physician if there is a suspicion of this. A small *increase in blood pressure* is also common.

Some women may have *abnormal glucose tolerance.* Incidence of *gall stones* have been found to be higher in women on oral contraceptives. Other effects include *breast discomfort, weight gain, development of pigmentation of the face,* and *psychological symptoms* like depression and alteration in sexual function.

Diuretics

Diuretics are drugs that increase the excretion of water and electrolytes in the urine. They are usually given in conditions that increase the load on the heart, renal failure and edema.

Examples

Thiazides (chlorothiazide, benzthiazide), loop diuretics (furosemide, ethacrynic acid), spironolactone, amiloride, triamterene

Common side effects

Diuretics can lead to *dehydration* and *electrolyte imbalances.*

Eye drops

Eye drops are used to treat a wide variety of eye ailments. Therefore, the contents of the eye drops vary according to the ailments. Antibacterial, antifungal, antiviral and antiinflammatory medications are often used to treat infective conditions and those that result in inflammation. To enable proper examination of the eye or to do eye surgery, anaesthetics may be used in

Appendix C

the form of eye drops. To dilate the pupils for examination, eye drops (mydriatics) containing medications that oppose acetylcholine (neurotransmitter secreted by parasympathetic nerves) – anticholinergics, or mimic the action of sympathetic nerves – sympathomimetics, may be used.

In patients who have lost the ability to blink, lubricants may be used to replace tears or to prevent damage to the cornea. Cholinergics – drugs that cause pupillary constriction (miotics) are used to treat and control glaucoma. Drops impregnated with dye such as fluorescein sodium are used for diagnostic purposes.

Examples

Antibacterial – bacitracin, erythromycin, neomycin
Antifungal – Natamycin
Antiviral – idoxuridine (IDU, Herplex)
Antiinflammatories – dexamethasone, medrysone
Anesthetics – proparacaine
Lubricants – polyvinyl alcohol (Tears plus)
Miotics – pilocarpine, carbachol
Mydriatics – atropine, cyclopentolate

Common side effects

For all drops there is a danger of contamination by microorganisms. Many products produce initial stinging and burning sensations.

The side effects depend on the type of medication. Miotics tend to produce effects similar to overstimulation of the parasympathetic nerves. Mydriatics tend to produce symptoms of sympathetic stimulation. Blurring of vision and intolerance to light are common symptoms when the pupils are dilated.

Immunosuppressants

Immunosuppressants are drugs that reduce the activity of T lymphocytes. T lymphocytes are responsible for the rejection of transplanted organs. Immunosuppressants act by reducing the production of these cells and/ or their response to chemical mediators that stimulate them to destroy foreign cells.

Examples

Cyclosporine (Sandimmune), Antithymocytic globulin equine (Atgam)

Common side effects

Immunosuppressants increase the *susceptibility* of the individual *to infections*. There is also an increased risk of *malignancies*, especially lymphomas.

Keratolytics

Keratolytics are substances that dissolve keratin. They soften scales and loosen the horny layer of skin. In addition to callosities, they are used to treat conditions like psoriasis, superficial fungal infections, and acne among others. Keratolytics are available as creams, gels, plasters etc.

Examples

Salicylic acid (Wart-Off, Freezone), resorcinol (Sebulex), podophyllum resin (Pod-Ben), cantharidin

Common side effects

Side effects vary with the medication used. Salicylic acid can get absorbed into the body through the skin and should not be used over large surfaces or for prolonged periods. If absorbed, it can produce *dizziness* and *ringing in the ear* (tinnitus). *Tingling, burning* and *itching* may be experienced at the site of application of cantharidin.

Laxatives

Laxatives or cathartics are medications that are used to treat constipation or to clear the bowel before diagnostic procedures or surgery. They may be used to hasten the expulsion of poisons or parasites. Depending on the consistency of the stools resulting from their use, they may be classified as laxatives, cathartics or purgatives. The mode of action varies from one laxative to another and they may be classified accordingly as contact laxative or stimulant, bulk-forming laxative, saline or osmotic cathartics, lubricants etc.

In general, laxatives promote fluid accumulation within the lumen of the bowel. Contact laxatives, obtained from the bark, seed pods, leaves of many plants irritate the wall of the intestines and increase peristalsis. Bulk-forming agents are natural or semisynthetic cellulose derivatives (eg. Bran, agar). They absorb water and increase the bulk of the feces, which in turn promote peristalsis. Osmotic laxatives are very powerful and draw water into the bowel lumen by osmosis. Lubricant laxatives soften the stool and retard water absorption.

Examples

Contact laxative – bisacodyl (Dulcolax), castor oil,
Senna products
Bulk-forming agents – plantago seed (psyllium seed),
psyllium hydrophilic mucilloid (Metamucil)
Saline or osmotic cathartics – magnesium salts, sodium
salts, potassium salts
Lubricants – mineral oil

Common side effects

Excessive bowel activity such as *diarrhea, nausea,
vomiting, abdominal cramps, bloating* and *flatulence*
are some side effects that may be seen.

Muscle relaxants

Increased skeletal muscle activity presents as spasm
or spasticity. Here, the muscle tone is increased and
may be seen in many types of neurological disorders
like cerebral palsy, stroke etc. The increased tone
interferes with rehabilitation in these patients and/or
produce contractures, pain and psychosocial problems.
Acute muscle injury, severe cold or lack of blood flow
may cause spasm. In such cases muscle relaxants are
used. Some muscle relaxants act on the central nervous
system at the site of the interneurons in the brain and
spinal cord, inhibiting the transmission of impulses.
Some other direct-acting skeletal muscle relaxants
interfere with the release of calcium ions by the
sarcoplasmic reticulum in the muscle fiber.

Muscle relaxants are often required during surgery and
are used by anaesthetists. In this situation, the drugs
paralyse the skeletal muscles and produce total
relaxation. They act at the level of the neuromuscular
junction preventing stimulation of the muscle by
affecting the action of acetylcholine on the muscle
receptors.

Muscle relaxants used in the operating room are of
two kinds. One prevents the muscle from depolarizing
by competing with acetylcholine for the receptors. By
itself, it does not depolarize the muscle. The other type
resembles acetylcholine and occupies the site of the
receptors producing prolonged, uncoordinated
depolarization. The muscle relaxants do not produce
anaesthesia and the patient is paralysed but conscious.
These drugs are given intravenously or intramuscularly.

Examples

Centrally acting muscle relaxants – carisoprodol (Soma,
Rela), chlorphenesin carbamate (Maolate), metaxalone
(Skelaxin)
Direct-acting muscle relaxants – dantrolene sodium
Nondepolarizers – metocurine, pancuronium
Depolarizers - Succinylcholine.

Common side effects

Drowsiness, dizziness and *lightheadedness* are some
common side effects of centrally acting muscle
relaxants.

Nose drops / Nasal decongestants

These are used to constrict the blood vessels in the
nose and thereby relieve congestion and blockage. The
decongestants are sympathomimetic drugs – ie. they
produce their effect by having the action of the
sympathetic nervous system. The duration of action
drops is short and may result in overuse.

Examples

Oxymetazoline hydrochloride, phenylephrine
hydrochloride, ephedrine

Common side effects

With repeated use, there could be vasodilation and
"rebound congestion" after the effect of the drug wears
off. If absorbed into the system in large amounts, the
drug can produce a *sympathomimetic effect in other
organs.* This includes tachycardia, irritability, anxiety,
increase in blood pressure, dryness of mouth etc.

Painkillers

The best treatment for pain is to remove the cause.
However, most often the cause cannot be identified
easily. Therefore, analgesics (pain killers) are resorted
to even before diagnosis is made (see Analgesic).

Nonsteroidal antiinflammatory agents (NSAIDs) are
most commonly used (see under antiinflammatories).
These reduce pain by reducing the inflammatory
reaction. Opiod analgesics are the most potent pain
relievers currently available.

The opioid act on the central nervous system and
activate pain-inhibitory neurons and directly inhibit
neurons that transmit pain. For chronic pain as in
postherpetic neuralgia, tension headache, migraine

Appendix C

headache, chronic low back pain and cancer, antidepressant medications, anticonvulsants and antiarrythmics may be used.

Examples

NSAIDs (see under antiinflammatories), opioid - codeine, oxycodone, morphine, levorphanol, methadone, meperidine, fentanyl, butorphanol; antidepressants - doxepin, amitriptyline, imipramine, nortriptyline, dsipramine; anticonvulsants and antiarrhythmics - phenytoin, carbamazepine, clonazepam, mexiletine

Common side effects

For the side effects of NSAIDs see under antiinflammatories. The opiods can produce *sedation, itching, constipation* and rarely *respiratory depression*. There is a risk of *addiction* to the pain killers - especially the opioids (narcotics). Massage therapists have to obtain a detailed history of the use of pain killers as injury to the tissue may be inflicted inadvertently by excessive use of pressure in these individuals with lowered sensitivity to pain.

Suppositories

These are masses impregnated with medication that can be easily melted and absorbed across the mucosa of the urethra, vagina or rectum. Rectal suppositories are cone-shaped or spindle shaped; vaginal suppositories are globular or egg shaped and the urethral ones are pencil-shaped. Suppositories are of particular use in patients who are uncooperative, who have severe vomiting or have digestive disorders that affect proper absorption of oral drugs.

Common side effects

The rate of absorption cannot be controlled precisely. Side effects may be due to rapid absorption of the drug into the system.

Sympatholytic drugs

Also known as antiadrenergic, they inhibit the sympathetic nervous system. They cause relaxation of smooth muscles and thereby increased peripheral circulation and drop in blood pressure. Specific drugs that are available have an effect on the alpha, beta or both receptors. They are used in hypertension.

Examples

Ergotamine derivatives, phenoxybenzamine, phentolamine

Common side effects

The side effects are similar to the action of cholinergic drugs and include *hypotension, drowsiness, nasal congestion, dry mouth, constipation* etc.

Sympathomimetic drugs

These are drugs that produce the same effect as stimulation of the sympathetic nervous system. They may act by promoting the release of neurotransmitters at the sympathetic nerve endings or by attaching to the receptors of noradrenaline and stimulating the neurons. These drugs may be used to reduce congestion in the nose, to dilate the bronchi (eg. Asthma, bronchiectasis, emphysema), to stimulate the heart in acute hypotension or shock, or to maintain the blood pressure.

Examples

Cyclopentamine, naphazoline, terbutaline sulphate, epinephrine

Common side effects

The side effects are due to overactivity of the sympathetic nervous system and include *dryness of mouth, hypertension, tachycardia, anxiety, headache, nausea, vomiting, anxiety, dilation of pupils* etc.

Tranquillizers

These are drugs that are given to reduce the anxiety and agitation of the individual without decreasing consciousness. They depress the central nervous system by facilitating the action of neurotransmitters that inhibit the CNS.

Examples

Diazepam, pentobarbital, hydroxyzine, chlordiazepoxide, phenothiazine, butyrophenone.

Common side effects

These drugs tend to cause *drowsiness* and *ataxia* and have *addictive* potential.

Vasoconstrictors

Also known as vasopressors, these drugs reduce the diameter of the blood vessels by stimulating the smooth muscles. Epinephrine, norepinephrine, angiotensin among others, are some vasoconstrictors produced in the body. Drugs that mimic the action of the sympathetic nervous system - sympathomimetic drugs have the same effect. They are used to treat severe hypotension.

Examples

Methoxamine hydrochloride, metaraminol bitartrate, norepinephrine.

Common side effects

Increased blood pressure, anxiety, headache, tachycardia, and *anginal pain* are some of the side effects. The side effects are similar to overstimulation of the sympathetic nervous system.

Vasodilators

Vasodilator drugs are primarily used to treat angina. They may also be used by people with Raynaud's syndrome. Vasodilators may be used to facilitate the healing of non-healing ulcers. These drugs directly relax smooth muscles and relieve spasm. By dilating the veins and causing pooling of blood, they reduce the volume of blood returning to the heart and thereby the load on the heart. Since they are absorbed easily through the skin and mucous membrane, they may be administered under the tongue, or used as patches on the skin. Coated tablets that release the drug slowly may be taken orally.

Examples

Nitrates – nitroglycerin, isosorbide, amyl nitrite, verapamil

Common side effects

Due to the dilatation of cerebral blood vessels, the person may have a *headache. Pounding pulses, flushing, hypotension, dizziness, fainting, nausea* and *vomiting* are some side effects. The Therapist has to watch for hypotension in these clients, especially when they get off the table.

Therapies

Biofeedback

It is a process where feedback in the form of visual or auditory stimuli is given in response to autonomic physiologic changes such as blood pressure, muscle tension, brain activity etc. By trial and error, the person learns to control these involuntary functions based on the stimuli. Biofeedback can be used to treat many conditions like hypertension, paralysis, bowel or bladder control, migraine headache etc.

Craniosacral therapy

It is a form of therapy where the bones of the cranium and other bones are manipulated gently to produce relief. The technique is used by trained practitioners to treat conditions such as headache, temporomandibular joint dysfunction syndrome, whiplash, facial neuralgias etc.

Defibrillators

It is a device that produces an electric shock at a specific voltage to the heart through the chest wall. It is used to bring normal rhythm and rate back to a heart that has stopped beating or that is fibrillating. One of the "paddles" of the defibrillator is applied just below the right clavicle to the side of the sternum while the other is placed in the left midaxillary line in the lower part of the rib cage. The defibrillator is usually set to deliver a shock equivalent to 200 – 400 joules, but the voltage is varied according to the type of tachycardia. Defibrillators are also available for implantation. These devices are programed to give an electrical shock if fibrillation or other forms of arrhythmias are detected.

Electrotherapy/ Electroconvulsive therapy (ECT)

Also known as electric shock therapy or electroshock therapy or electrotherapy, it is a form of treatment where electric current is passed through the brain for a brief moment. It is used for treating certain affective disorders where drugs have no effect. After sedating and restraining the patient, electrodes are placed on the forehead and 70-130 millivolts current is delivered for less than half a second.

Appendix C

Hormone therapy/replacement

Also known as endocrine therapy, it indicates the treatment of diseases by using hormones obtained from endocrine glands or substances that simulate the effects of specific hormones.

Hyperbaric oxygen therapy

This is a form of therapy where a person is exposed to oxygen at increased pressures ie. more than that of the atmosphere. This way, the dissolved oxygen in blood can be markedly increased. Hyperbaric oxygen may be used during surgery for some forms of congenital heart disease. It is also beneficial in treating those with gas gangrene since the microorganisms producing this condition are anaerobic. It is used to treat carbon monoxide poisoning. The high concentration of oxygen can displace the carbon monoxide that is bound to hemoglobin molecules. In cyanide poisoning, the higher concentration of dissolved oxygen in plasma that results from this form of therapy is beneficial to the hypoxic tissues. However, prolonged exposure to oxygen at high pressure ie. more than 5 hours can result in oxygen toxicity with muscle twitching, ringing in the ear, dizziness, convulsion and coma.

Imagery

A form of therapy where the person is encouraged to form mental concepts and figures in order to treat specific disorders.

Immunization

This is a therapeutic procedure where a person is exposed to the antigens of a pathogen in order to stimulate the body to develop antibodies against the specific antigen. Later. when the person is exposed to the actual pathogen, the body responds quickly because of the previous exposure. Many diseases which produce severe symptoms or that are potentially fatal can be prevented in this way. Some of the disorders for which immunization exists are measles, poliomyelitis, diphtheria, whooping cough, tetanus, mumps etc. Sometimes, already developed antibodies against a pathogen are used to prevent infection on a temporary basis. Usually, the reaction to immunization is minimal. Rarely, some people may develop severe symptoms. (See also Vaccination and skin tests - appendix B)

Immunotherapy

This is a form of therapy where the serum of an immunized individual containing antibodies against a specific disease is used to treat certain acute infections in another unimmunized individual. It is used in conditions where the infecting microorganism produces toxins that are very harmful to the body. Since antimicrobial agents destroy the organism and not the already produced toxin, immunotherapy is used to neutralize the toxins and prevent irreparable damage to tissues. Concurrent administration of antimicrobials destroys the organism that produces the toxins.

Laser therapy

Laser is an acronym for "Light amplification by stimulated emission of radiation". Here, intense radiation of a part of the light spectrum (visible, ultraviolet or infrared) is used to divide tissue, destroy tissue and produce adhesions or to fix tissue.

Mechanical ventilation

It is a form of intervention where mechanical devices are used to support ventilation (the movement of air in and out of the lungs). It is used in different forms of respiratory failure. Mechanical ventilation is administered in various ways – where the rate, volume and pressure of air are controlled and maintained by the machine or patient triggered. The air that is administered is warmed and humidified.

Prolonged use of mechanical ventilation can result in complications such as pneumonia, oxygen toxicity, hypotension etc.

Oxygen treatment

It includes any procedure where oxygen is used to relieve hypoxia. There are many methods for administering oxygen and the method used depends on the condition of the patient and what causes hypoxia. Low amounts of oxygen may be administered to a patient by using a nasal catheter. In those with chronic obstructive airway disease, a mask may be used. For patients with cardiac disease, oxygen in higher concentrations may be used. It may be necessary to frequently measure the levels of blood gases in some patients. Oxygen toxicity is complication that has to be prevented.

Phototherapy

It is a form of therapy where light – especially ultraviolet light is used to treat some conditions. It may be used to treat acne, certain ulcers, psoriasis, vitiligo and jaundice. In jaundice of the newborn, the baby is exposed to intense fluorescent light after covering the eye and the genitalia. The light speeds up the excretion of bilirubin that has accumulated under the skin by oxidizing it. Dehydration is a complication that has to be addressed.

In psoriasis, phototherapy is combined with application of certain compounds. The light produces changes in the compounds, which in turn affect the function of the cells. Certain compounds along with exposure to light stimulate the synthesis of melanin, the rationale for its use in vitiligo.

Plaster cast

It is a form of intervention where a part of the body is immobilised by encasing it in a cast. Plaster of paris – a white powder (calcium sulfate hemihydrate) is impregnated in guaze. The gauze is dipped in warm water and used to encase the body. Recently, casts made of glass fibers or plastic are used to immobilize the injured part.

Radiation therapy

Radiation therapy is given to treat many types of cancer. Often it is given alone, or in combination with chemotherapy and /or surgery. Like chemotherapy, radiation suppresses rapidly multiplying cells. To reduce its effects on the bone marrow, gastrointestinal tract and the gonads (ovary and testis), radiation is targeted to local sites by shielding the normal surrounding tissue from radiation.

Radiation can be toxic to the local area. The severity depends on the dose, location of therapy and the rate of delivery. Acute toxicity develops within the first 3 months and presents as an inflammatory reaction. This may be treated with antiinflammatories and cold compresses to the local site.

The therapist should ensure that oil is not used at the radiation site as it may affect the rate of radiation delivery. By suppressing the immune cells, radiation may also make the individual more prone to infection.

The therapist should ensure that these clients are not exposed to even mild infections in the clinic. Associated bleeding tendencies and anemia may also be seen. While massaging, only light pressure should be used to prevent small bleeds under the skin.

Gastrointestinal toxicity can present as loss of appetite, nausea, vomiting and diarrhea. Radiation may result in subacute/chronic toxicities where fibrosis and scarring can occur at the injection site. Techniques such as transverse friction can be used to reduce adhesions.

Sclerosing agents

It is a liquid that causes inflammation and fibrosis by irritating the tissue. These agents may be used to treat conditions such as hemangiomas, certain types of ulcers, arrest bleeding and to collapse varicose veins.

Sunscreen

Sun screen or suntan preparations are creams that have the ability to occlude ultraviolet rays. They are rated generally on a scale of 1-35 with 1 being least occlusive. Ratings of 35 are total sun-blocking agents. The index used is termed "sunscreen protective factor index (SPF)". For example, a factor of 15 indicates that the preparation provides protection 15 times more than that of unprotected skin.

While the ultraviolet rays are less harmful early in the morning and in late afternoons, they too have been implicated in skin cancer. It has been estimated that there would be a decrease of about 78% of skin cancers if children under 18 used sunscreen with a blocking agent of at least 15.

TENS

It is an abbreviation for Transcutaneous Electric Nerve Stimulation. It is a method used to control pain. Here, electrodes are placed on the skin over the site of pain. The electrodes are connected by means of wire to a stimulator that generates impulses similar to that produced in the body. The impulses stimulate nerve endings of afferent nerves that alter the perception of pain by the brain. This method of pain control has no side effects and unlike many other painkillers is not addictive. However, it is contraindicated in patients who have implanted pacemakers.

Appendix C

Investigations

Doppler technique

It is a technique used to detect the flow of blood in blood vessels or the heart. The principle used is that when light or sound waves from a source are reflected by a moving object, the frequency of the reflected waves changes. The shift in frequency between the waves from the source and the reflected waves is used to find out the speed of flow. It is a useful non-invasive technique used in people with circulatory problems.

Genetic testing/counselling

It is a process of testing and/or counselling people with regard to the risk or occurrence of a specific inherited disorder. Special biochemical tests or cytological tests may have to be done to arrive at a diagnosis. Based on this, information and advice as to the options available are given to the patient. Usually, a team approach is taken with involvement of the physician, nurse, psychologist, social worker, and geneticist, among others.

Lumbar puncture/spinal tap

Lumbar puncture or spinal tap is done to obtain a sample of cerebrospinal fluid (CSF) for examination. After using a local anaesthetic, with the spine flexed to increase the space between the vertebrae, a sufficiently large bore needle is inserted between the 3rd and 4th lumbar vertebrae until the subarachnoid space is reached and CSF flows out in drops. Since the spinal cord ends at the L2 level, it is not injured by the introduction of the needle. The spinal nerves in this location float away from the needle (like hair in water) and are unlikely to be pierced. The patient may have a headache after the spinal tap due to the reduction in volume of CSF and traction on the meninges. Vomiting, infection and leakage of CSF are some of the complications that may be encountered.

Lumbar puncture may be done to inject a radiopaque substance for radiological visualisation of structures in the nervous system, to inject an anesthetic or drug etc.

The sample of CSF can give useful information. If pink or red it indicates fresh bleeding (normal CSF is clear and colorless). If yellow, it could indicate an old bleed and presence of bilirubin. The type of meningitis ie bacterial, viral or tuberculous can be diagnosed by examining CSF. Increase in intracranial pressure is reflected by the flow of CSF during the spinal tap.

Pap smear

This is an investigative procedure where cells or tissue from the cervix is removed for microscopic examination and examined for cancerous changes. It is a routine screening method used to detect cervical carcinoma. Pap smear can also identify the presence of certain sexually transmitted pathogens and to assess hormonal changes. This test should be done periodically for all sexually active women and especially those who have multiple partners, who have had intercourse at an early age and those with a history of sexually transmitted disease.

A speculum is inserted into the vagina to visualise the cervix and a wooden spatula or a cotton-tipped applicator is used to obtain the cervical cells. A smear is then made on a slide, fixative added and the slide sent to a cytologist for examination.

Procedures

Amputation

This is a surgical procedure where a part of the body, the whole limb or part of the limb is removed. This procedure may be resorted to in those with limbs that are crushed beyond repair, extensive cancer, vascular dysfunction with gangrene formation, severe infection of bone etc. Today, the level of amputation is mainly determined by the viability of the skin. During surgery, a skin flap is made to cover the exposed surface and the dimension of the stump altered to fit the prosthesis. Different types of prosthesis are available eg. Above-knee prosthesis, below-knee prosthesis, upper extremity prosthesis fitted with a hook or a hand terminal device etc.

Some of the problems with amputation and prosthesis include loss of socket fit, formation of neuroma (a ball shaped mass of axons at the point where the nerve is cut). Phantom limb pain and skin lesions such as blisters and abrasions at the site of attachment of prosthesis. Since, the absence of the body part is visible, this procedure has tremendous psychological implications.

Angioplasty

It is a surgical procedure where damaged or injured blood vessels are reconstructed. Percutaneous Transluminal Angioplasty (PTA) is the full name given to the procedure where a catheter is introduced into the lumen of the blood vessel and the defective region of the blood vessel is dilated using catheters of varying sizes or inflating a balloon present at the tip of the catheter. With the advances made in refining the procedure, angioplasty is very common. It is used to dilate the coronary blood vessels, renal vessels or other vessels such as the femoral artery that are stenosed due to accumulation of atheromatous plaques. The procedure does not require prolonged hospitalization and the cost is low as compared to a surgical procedure.

Some of the complications include rupture of the blood vessel at the site of dilatation, dislodgement of emboli, aneurysm formation etc. The effects of PTA may not be long lasting and patients sometimes have to return for another PTA.

Arthroscopy

This is a procedure where an endoscope is inserted into a joint through a small skin incision. It is possible to visualize the inside of the joint, obtain biopsies of the cartilage or synovial membrane, do specific surgery and even remove loose bodies from the joint space. Use of this procedure is advantageous as it can be easily performed in the outpatient setting.

Balloon tamponade

It is one of the procedures used to control bleeding from esophageal blood vessels (esophageal varices) - a complication of cirrhosis of the liver. Here, a three or four lumen catheter is introduced into the stomach. A balloon is inflated in the stomach through one of the lumens. After inflation, this balloon is pulled tight against the cardia of the stomach to apply counterpressure and stop the bleeding. If this is not successful, another balloon is inflated in the esophagus. The contents can be aspirated through one of the other

lumens. The patient is intubated to prevent aspiration.

One of the complications of this procedure is rupture of the esophagus and pneumonia due to accidental aspiration of the stomach contents.

Blood/plasma expanders

These are substances that are infused into a patient intravenously to quickly bring the blood volume to normal. Expanders are usually high molecular weight dextrans that increase the oncotic (osmotic) pressure in the circulation, thus retaining water in the blood vessels and maintaining blood volume.

Blood transfusion

This is a term used to denote infusion of blood or products of blood into a recipient. Blood, when used for transfusion should be considered as a drug, a biological product or as a transplant. Whole blood is used in patients who are bleeding acutely. A red cell concentrate where most of the plasma has been removed is used in severely anemic patients. In some cases, washed red cells, where the plasma is completely removed is used. Frozen red cells may also be used. The latter increases the duration or preservation of red cells. Platelet concentrates are used in patients with certain bleeding disorders. Here concentration of platelets obtained from a single or multiple donors, suspended in plasma is used for transfusion. Leukocyte (white blood cell) concentrates, plasma, albumin, plasma protein fractions are other blood products that may be used for transfusion.

Some of the complications of blood transfusion are hyperkalemia (potassium levels tend to increase in stored blood), hypothermia (due to improper warming of the transfusion blood), hypocalcemia etc. It is important to screen the donor for hepatitis, AIDS, syphilis, malaria and other disorders that can be transmitted through blood. The blood of the donor has to be matched with that of the recipient to avoid antigen antibody reactions.

Autotransfusion, where the blood donated by a patient two weeks prior to his/her own operation is stored and reused if necessary, eliminates many of the complications of blood transfusion.

Appendix C

Bypass grafting / Arterial bypass

In this procedure extraneous material is used to help bypass the flow of blood from defective segments of arteries. Arteries, veins or synthetic materials may be used for the bypass. Arteries and veins may be from another individual (allograft) or from self (autograft). Rarely, Xenografts – vessels from another species may be used. The internal mammary artery, the great saphenous vein, cephalic vein, basilic vein and umbilical vein are blood vessels that are commonly used as autografts. Prosthetic or synthetic grafts made of Teflon or Dacron, among others may be used in some occasions. Some of the complications that may occur are infections, rupture, aneurysm, thrombus formation and deterioration with time.

Catheterization

A procedure where a tube (catheter) is introduced into the body through a lumen eg, cardiac catheterization, urinary catheterization or parenteral catheterization. Cardiac catheterization may be done for diagnosing heart disease or determining the severity of disease that will help with the selection of optimal treatment. Cardiac catheterization may be done prior to surgery to help the surgeon plan the procedure and also to identify any other disease that may coexist. Sometimes it is done to measure volumes and pressures in order to determine the efficacy of the treatment. Usually, the catheter is passed through the femoral artery or vein. Sometimes the brachial artery, brachial vein, subclavian vein or jugular vein is used. A vein is used to approach the right side of the heart while an artery is used to approach the left side. The incidence of complications due to catheterization is low. Some of the complications of left heart catheterization include myocardial infarction, stroke, and arrhythmias, among others. Some of the complications of right heart catheterization are hematoma, inadvertent arterial puncture, pneumothorax, arrhythmia, cardiac perforation, introduction of infection etc.

Urinary catheters are used to help empty the urinary bladder usually when there is an obstruction or when a patient is unable to void due to nervous or muscular insufficiencies. The catheter may be used on a temporary basis or for longer durations. One of the common problems is urinary tract infection.

Parenteral catheterization is used to introduce nutritional fluids into the body. This may be resorted to if the patient is unable to take adequate nutrition by mouth and are in danger of severe malnutrition. Here the internal or external jugular vein is used to reach the superior vena cava. Infection, thrombosis and thrombophlebitis are some of the complications that may be occur.

Cesarean section

This is a surgical procedure where the baby is delivered after incising the abdominal wall and the uterus. It is used in situations where the condition of the mother or the fetus is not conducive to vaginal delivery. The abdominal incision may be transverse or vertical.

Some of the complications include infections, and excessive loss of blood.

Cholecystectomy

A surgical procedure where the gall bladder is removed. It is one the treatments used for patients who have gallstones that produce symptoms. Here, the gall bladder is approached through a midline, paramedian or subcostal incision. The artery supplying the gallbladder is ligated along with the cystic duct and the gallbladder dissected out. Infection is a complication that may be encountered. Cholecystectomy may be done endoscopically, through a small incision near the umbilicus. An endoscope is introduced to determine if the surgery is feasible. If feasible, using three other openings – one to irrigate, another to hold the gall bladder, and yet another to introduce instruments to dissect and apply clips, the gall bladder is removed. Bleeding, injury to surrounding organs and bile duct injury are some of the complications. However, hospital stay and postoperative recovery is much faster.

Since the gall bladder only stores the bile and bile is actually manufactured by the liver, fat digestion is not unduly affected.

Colostomy

This is a procedure where the bowel is opened on to the surface of the abdomen. Colostomies may be temporary or permanent. It is done when a site for elimination of the feces is necessary in situations where the colon or rectum has been removed. Other indications for colostomies are: when the feces has to be diverted while a distal anastomosis heals; as a diversion or "vent" when there is obstruction distally; or to temporarily divert the feces from a pathological process that will be addressed at a later date.

Usually, the distal part of the colon is brought to the surface after closing the other end (depending on the type of surgery). The opening is usually situated in the left iliac fossa and the colon brought through the rectus muscle. The opening is raised above the surface of the skin to facilitate the application of appliances to collect the feces. The frequency of elimination varies from individual to individual and can be regulated to some extent by the diet.

Some of the complications include stenosis (narrowing) of the opening, hernias around the opening, bleeding, perforation, prolapse etc. Many hospitals that regularly perform such surgery have trained specialists who can help the individual maintain and manage these abdominal openings.

Cryotherapy

It is a form of treatment where intense cold is used to destroy tissue. Liquid nitrogen or solid carbon dioxide is used and applied over the tissue that is to be destroyed using an applicator. The intense cold freezes the cells and the cells get dehydrated, with rupture of the cell membrane. A blister forms in the area, followed by scab formation. This form of therapy is often used to treat lesions such as warts.

Curettage

It is a procedure where the inner lining or wall of a cavity is scraped off using a blunt or sharp instrument and sometimes by suction. It is usually done in the uterus after an abortion or to obtain tissue for microscopic examination. The term is also used to indicate such procedures used to clear dead tissue from fistulas or sites of chronic infection.

Dialysis

This is a procedure used to remove poisons, excessive amounts of drugs, correct electrolyte imbalances and to remove waste products like urea, uric acid, and creatinine (in patients with kidney failure). The

principle used is diffusion – where solutes move from an area of higher to lower concentration across a semipermeable membrane and water moves from an area of lower concentration of solutes to an area with higher concentration. By altering the concentration of solutes in the fluid (dialysate) separated from blood by a semipermeable membrane, the content of the blood can be altered.

Hemodialysis

In hemodialysis, an artery and a vein are accessed. The blood from the artery passes through the dialyzer (the machine that exposes the dialysate to the blood across the semipermeable membrane), while the temperature, pressure etc are monitored. Then the blood is infused back into the body through the vein. The duration of the procedure varies from 3-8 hours and depending on the condition of the patient may be required daily or 2-3 times per week. Infection at the infusion site, clotting, inflammation of the skin around the infusion site are some of the complications.

Peritoneal dialysis

In peritoneal dialysis, the peritoneum is used as the semipermeable membrane and the dialysate is infused into the peritoneal cavity and left there for exchange to occur between the blood in the abdominal blood vessels and the dialysate (across the peritoneum). The dialysate is then removed from the peritoneal cavity. Some of the complications that may be encountered are peritonitis, hypervolemia (increase in blood volume) leading to cardiac failure, adhesions between abdominal organs due to local reaction, pneumonia and atelectasis due to the volume of dialysate reducing the respiratory excursions, etc.

Exchange transfusion

Exchange transfusion is done in infants who have severe hemolysis (rupture of red blood cells) due to blood incompatibility to Rh or ABO antigens. This may happen to infants who have the Rh antigen in their red blood cell membrane (Rh positive) and are born to Rh negative mothers who have developed antibodies to the Rh antigen. The antibodies from the mother cross to the fetus across the placenta resulting in antigen-antibody reaction in the fetus with resultant hemolysis and severe jaundice that is life threatening.

Appendix C

In this procedure, 75-85% of blood from an infant is exchanged for fresh, compatible blood. A small amount of the infant blood is removed repeatedly, with replacement of an equal amount of donor blood while carefully monitoring the infant. In this way, the antibodies, bilirubin and sensitized red blood cells are replaced with blood that has a higher oxygen-carrying capacity.

Gastrectomy

This is a surgical procedure where part of or the whole stomach is resected. It may be done for gastric tumors. The type of resection depends on the location and extent of the gastric tumor. The spleen and other surrounding organs may be removed along with the stomach in some cases. Continuity is established by anastomosing the duodenum or the jejunum to the remnant of the stomach or esophagus.

Ileostomy

It is a surgical procedure where an opening of the small intestine – the ileum is brought to the surface of the abdomen to facilitate drainage of the fecal matter. This kind of operation is done in those who have extensive ulcerative colitis, Crohn's disease or cancer of the large intestines. Before the surgery, the diet is altered to reduce the amount of fecal matter formed. Antibiotics are also given to reduce the bacterial count in the intestines. The ileum is usually brought through the rectus abdominus muscle at a point below the umbilicus and the opening raised above the skin surface to facilitate attachment of appliances to collect the fecal mater. Collecting bags have to be worn day and night. Trained specialists (enterostomal therapists) are available in hospitals that do such surgery on a regular basis, to help the patient cope with this new device. The presence of an ileostomy has tremendous psychological and social implications.

Since the fecal mater contains intestinal enzymes, the skin around the opening has to be cared for to prevent ulceration. More recently, the ileum is made into a pouch inside the abdomen, with a valve between the pouch and the abdominal opening. This eliminates the use of an external bag. The patient can use a tube to empty the pouch on a regular basis. Some of the complications that may follow include inflammation of the pouch, infection, ulceration around the stoma etc.

Intubation

This is a procedure where a tube is inserted into a body aperture. Intubation usually denotes the passage of a tube through the mouth or the nose into the trachea to facilitate breathing or administration of anaesthetics or oxygen or to prevent entry of secretions from the digestive tract into the trachea in a patient who is unconscious or paralyzed. The tube is passed into the trachea through the larynx with the help of the laryngoscope to help visualize the passage. If the patient cannot breathe by himself/herself, the tube is attached to a ventilator and the vital signs monitored on a regular basis. Introduction of infection, aspiration – entry of secretions into the lung with resultant inflammation and necrosis of the trachea are some of the complications that may be encountered (rarely).

Joint replacement

This is also known as Arthroplasty. It is an operation where a new movable joint is constructed. Usually such a surgical procedure is done in the hip, knee, shoulder, elbow, and some metacarpophalangeal and metatarsophalangeal joints. It may be used in those with severe osteoarthritis, rheumatoid arthritis, some types of bony deformities, unhealing fractures of the neck of femur etc.

Arthroplasty may be done in three ways. In one of the methods, the whole joint is removed. The gap eventually fills with fibrous tissue. Sometimes soft tissue like muscles from the surrounding area is interspersed between the bones. In another method, only one of the articular surfaces is replaced by prosthesis (usually metal). In the more common method, both articular surfaces are replaced by prosthesis. One of the complications that may be encountered is the tendency for the prosthesis to work loose with time.

Laparoscopy

This is a procedure where a type of endoscope (laparoscope), an illuminated tube, is inserted into the abdominal cavity through a small incision in the abdominal wall to visualize the contents. It is often used to examine the ovaries and the fallopian tube. Using this technique, ligation of the fallopian tube can be done (laparoscopic sterilization).

Lithotripsy

Known as Extracorporeal Shock Wave Lithotripsy, this procedure is used on highly selected patients who have gallstones. Special criteria exist for selecting patients in whom this procedure can be done. Here, large amplitude acoustic waves are focussed on the stones. The stones fragment and are expelled into the duodenum via the cystic duct and common bile duct. It may be necessary to repeat the procedure if the fragmented stones are more than 5mm in size. Lithotripsy can be done in an outpatient setting. Some of the complications include bruising at the site of passage of waves, pain on passage of the stones and sometimes blood in urine due to injury to the right kidney that lies proximal to the gallbladder.

Lithotripsy is used for fragmenting kidney stones too. Here the waves may be administered as above or using a scope to directly access the stones and then fragment them by ultrasound waves – ultrasonic lithotripsy.

Nasogastric suction

It is a procedure where a tube is passed through the nose into the stomach to suction out solids, liquids or gases from the stomach. Standard plastic nasogastric tubes are used. The length of the tube that has to be inserted is approximated by measuring the distance from the xiphoid sternum to the tip of the nose and then to the ear and around the ear once. This level is marked off on the tube. After application of lubricant to the tube, it is inserted through the nose to about 7.5 cms, at which point it reaches the pharynx. Then the tube is moved through the esophagus as the patient swallows until it reaches the measured distance. Suction is used intermittently or directly connected to a suction pump.

Some of the complications that may occur due to the use of the nasogastric tube and suction are: discomfort, interference with coughing and build up of secretions in the lungs, drying of the mouth and pharynx due to mouth breathing, inflammation of the esophagus – esophagitis due to reflux of gastric secretion into the esophagus, necrosis of the nares, electrolyte imbalance (due to loss of hydrogen, potassium, chloride and other ions through the suctioned out secretions) etc.

Mammography

It is a radiological procedure where the soft tissue of the breasts is screened for abnormal growths. It may be used to diagnose tumors or to screen women for tumors. Here, a low energy radiation beam is passed through the breast tissue before it falls on a film, screen or plate. Tissue that is dense shows up as opaque areas. Abnormal tissue is visualized as calcification spots, distortion in architecture, asymmetry or as a dense mass.

Guidelines from the American Cancer Society recommend annual mammograms for women over 50 years. Mammogram, as a screening procedure for women below 40 is controversial. It may be advisable for younger women at risk eg. With family history of breast cancer, to undergo regular screening.

Mastectomy

It is a surgical procedure where one or both breasts are removed. It is usually done as a therapeutic intervention for breast cancer. The extent of tissue removed is related to the size, location and type of cancer. In simple mastectomy, only the breast tissue is removed. In radical mastectomy, some of the muscles underlying the breast along with the lymph nodes that drain the breast are removed. The patient may be fitted with prosthesis soon after surgery or after healing has occurred.

Many social, psychological and other factors affect the adaptation of the individual to the disfigurement (actual and perceived) caused by this surgery. All these factors have to be taken into account before, during and after the procedure to help the individual adapt to the physical changes.

Organ transplantation

This is a procedure where an organ from one individual is transplanted into another. It is undertaken in patients where all other interventions have failed. With the advent of drugs to suppress immunity, matching of tissue antigenic properties of the donor and recipient is not as critical as it used to be. Organs such as the kidney, liver, heart, lung, pancreas, intestines among

Appendix C

others are being used for transplantation. The organ is kept viable by perfusing with standardized solutions and by reducing the temperature (hypothermia) to reduce the metabolic rate.

One of the complications of transplantation is rejection of the organ. Here, the recipients' white blood cells recognize the transplanted tissue as foreign and antigen-antibody reactions occur. Other complications include infection, functional problems because of mismatch of size of the recipient and donor organs etc.

Today, there are numerous networks that have developed organ-sharing plans and coordinate better matching of donors and recipients using their large pool of individuals across the globe.

Plasmapheresis

This is the process of removing the plasma from blood that has been withdrawn from the body. The remaining cellular components can be reused by suspending them in isotonic solutions.

Shunts

A procedure where the flow of body fluid (eg. blood, cerebrospinal fluid) is redirected from one vessel or cavity to another. *Portocaval shunts* are those where the blood in the portal vein is redirected to the inferior vena cava. *Portal systemic shunt* diverts the blood from the portal vein to the systemic blood vessels. These types of shunts are used when the pressure in the portal system (portal hypertension) is high resulting in esophageal varices, which may happen in cirrhosis of the liver. In some cases, where fluid accumulation in the peritoneal cavity is abnormally increased (ascites), peritoneovenous shunt where a plastic tube with a one-way valve directs the peritoneal fluid into the superior vena cava may be done.

In the case of some individuals with hydrocephalus, the cerebrospinal fluid may be diverted to the peritoneal cavity or right atrium using a catheter, with the flow regulated by a valve. This is known as the ventriculoperitoneal/ventriculoatrial shunt.

Some of the complications of shunt operations are infection and obstruction of the shunt or injury to abdominal organs by the peritoneal catheter (in ventriculoperitoneal shunts).

Skin graft

This is a procedure where skin from another region is used to cover wounds where insufficient skin is available to allow skin closure. It may be used after extensive burn injury or after surgery where a large area of skin has to be removed, or to cover very large non-healing ulcers. Usually autografts (skin from the same person) is used.

Skin grafts are of many types. A *pedicle graft* is one where the blood supply to the skin from the donor site is not cut until revascularization has occurred in the recipient site. Here, the skin is cut on three sides with one side continuous with the rest of the skin. The flap is then sutured immediately to the site requiring the graft. A *free graft* is one where the skin is separated from its blood, nerve and lymphatic supply completely. The whole skin including the dermis and epidermis (*full-thickness graft*) or the whole epidermis and part of the dermis (*partial* or *slit-thickness graft*) may be used in areas where quick vascularization is possible. The donor site is chosen taking the texture, color match and visibility of scar into consideration. Infection is one of the important complications that has to be addressed.

Surgical sympathectomy

It is a surgical procedure where the sympathetic nerves are cut. This may be used to relieve certain types of chronic pain, or to produce vasodilation as may be required in conditions such as Raynaud's phenomenon, Buerger's disease etc. Before the surgery, an anesthetic may be injected into the sympathetic ganglion to temporarily stop the passage of impulses in order to determine the effect on the blood vessel. The sympathetic nerves, which lie along the spinal column, are accessed via the back or the neck.

By doing this procedure other functions of the sympathetic nerves such as sweating will be affected in the region supplied by the nerve.

Tracheostomy

This is a surgical procedure where a tube is inserted through the neck into the trachea to facilitate passage of air into the lungs. It is used to relieve obstruction in the upper respiratory tract, control secretions (in very sick patients), and support ventilation in those with respiratory failure. It may be done as an emergency (rarely) or as an elective procedure eg. in patients with laryngeal cancer. After making a horizontal (or vertical) incision in the neck, the second and third tracheal ring is cut to introduce the tube. Suction has to be done intermittently to remove the tracheobronchial secretions

and the patency of the tube constantly checked. The air breathed in has to be sufficiently humidified to prevent dehydration and warmed to body temperature.

Some of the complications include pneumothorax, lung infection, tracheoesophageal fistula, mediastinal emphysema (air in the mediastinum), and bleeding.

Appendix C

Resources
Organisations & Support groups

ACHALASIA

United States of America

National Institute of Diabetes and Digestive and Kidney Diseases of the National Institutes of Health,
Bethesda, Maryland.
URL: http://www.niddk.nih.gov/

ACQUIRED IMMUNODEFICIENCY SYNDROME

Australia

Australian Federation of AIDS
PO Box 876 Darlinghurst 1300
Level 4-74 Winworth Ave
Surrey Hills NSW 2010
Tel: 61-02-9281 1999 Fax: 61-02-9281-1044

E-mail: afa@rainbow.net.au

Aids Information Line/Advice
Tel: 61-3-224-5526

Canada

AIDS Calgary Awareness Association
Social Service Agency
200 1509 Centre St. SW
Calgary AB T2R 0B7
Tel: (403) 508-2500

AIDS Committee of Toronto
399 Church St 4th Floor
Toronto Ont M5B 2J6
Tel: (416) 340-2437 Fax: (416) 340-8224

AIDS & HIV Services
Community AIDS Treatment Information Exchange
517 College St
Toronto ON M6G 4A2
Tel: (416) 944-1916 Fax:(416) 928-2185

AIDS Information and Support Services
885 Dunsmuir St Suite 1000,
Vancouver BC V6C 1N5
Tel: (604)-688-7294 Fax: (604) 689-4888

AIDS Information Line
STD Centre
Edmonton General Hospital
11111 Jasper Avenue 3B20
Edmonton AB T5K 0L4
Tel: 1-800-772-2437

Canadian Infectious Disease Society
Hospital Saint-Luc 1058 rue Saint Denis St.
Montreal PQ H2X 3J4
Tel: (514) 281-2121 Fax: (514) 281-2443

Immunology Research Center
531 Boulevard des Prairies
Laval PQ H7N 423
Tel: (514) 686-5332 Fax: (514) 686-5501

United Kingdom

British Infection Society
c/o Dept of Microbiology
Friarage Hospital
Northallerton DL6 1JG
Tel: 44-1609-779911 or 44-1609-763035
Fax: 44-1609-778656

Institute of Public Health
University of Cambridge

Appendix D

Forvie Site, Robinson Way
Cambridge CB2 2SR
Tel: 44-223-330300

United States of America

Centre for disease control – national
prevention and information network
CDC NPIN P.O. Box 6003
Rockville, MD 20849-6003
Tel: 1-800-458-5231
URL: http://www.cdcnpin.org/start.htm

American Foundation for AIDS Research
120 Wall St. 13th Floor
New York NY 10005
Tel: (212)806-1600 Fax: (212) 806-1601

AIDS Service Center
Lower Manhattan 80 5th Ave
New York NY
Tel: (212) 645-0875

Body Positive
19 Fulton St. Suite 308B
New York NY 10038
Tel: (212)566-7333 Fax: (212) 566-4539

American Association of Immunologists
9650 Rockville Pike
Betheda MD 20814-3994

Centers for Infectious Disease Control
1600 Clifton Rd NE
Atlanta GA 30333
Tel: (404) 639-3311 or (404) 639-3535

National Foundation for Infectious Diseases
4733 Bethesda Ave, Suite 750
Bethesda MD 20814
Tel: (301) 656-0003 Fax: (301) 907-0878

National Vaccine Information Center
512 Maple Ave W Suite 206
Vienna VA 22180
Tel: (703) 938 3783 or (800) 909 SHOT
Fax: (703) 938-5768

ADHESIVE CAPSULITIS

United States of America

The Centre for Orthopedics and Sports
Medicine. Frozen shoulder (adhesive
capsulitis).

URL: http:/www.arthroscopy.com

ADULT RESPIRATORY DISTRESS SYNDROME

United States of America

American Lung Association
Tel: 1-800-LUNG-USA.
URL:http://www.lungusa.org/

ALCOHOLISM

Canada

Alcoholics Anonymous
Support Group for Alcoholics
200 L 200 Haddon Rd SW
Calgary AB T2V-2Y6
Tel: (403) 252-6817

Alcoholics Anonymous
234 Eglington Ave E
Toronto ON M4P 1K5
Tel: (416) 487-5591 Fax: 487-5855

United States of America

Alcoholics Anonymous
475 Riverside Dr.
New York NY 10115
Tel: (212) 254-7230

Alcoholics Anonymous (AA) World Services
PO Box 459 Grand Central Station
New York NY 10163
Tel: (212) 870-3400

ALZHEIMER'S DISEASE

Canada

Alzheimer's Society of Alberta
Association 218-2323 32nd Ave NE
Calgary AB T2E 6Z3
Tel: (403) 250-1303 Fax:(403) 250-8241

Alzheimer Society of Calgary
Education /Support
1920-11 St SE
Calgary AB T2G 3G2
Tel: (403) 290-0110 Fax: (403) 269-8836

Alzheimer Society of Canada
1320 Yonge St Suite 201
Toronto ON M4T 1X2
Tel: (416) 925-3552 Fax: (416) 925-1649

United States of America

Alzheimer's Association
919 N Michigan Ave Suite 1000
Chicago IL 60611
Tel: (312) 335-8700 or (1-800) 272-3900
Fax: (312) 335-1110

Alzheimer's/Aging Resource Center
2351 Brigham
Brooklyn NY
Tel: (718) 646-7001

AMYOTROPHIC LATERAL SCLEROSIS

Canada

Amyotrophic Sclerosis Society of Canada
220-6 Adelaide St E
Toronto ON M5C1H6
Tel: (416) 362-0269 Fax: (416) 362-0414

United States of America

Amyotrophic Lateral Sclerosis Association
21021 Ventura Bld. Suite 321
Woodland Hills CA 91364
Tel: (818) 340-7500 or (800) 782-4747

The ALS Association National Office
27001 Agoura Rd, Suite 150
Calabasas Hills CA 91301-5104
Tel: 1-800:782-4747
E-Mail: alsinfo@alsa-national.org

ANAPHYLAXIS

Canada

Allergy Asthma & Information Association
30 Eglinton West Suite 750
Mississauga ON L5R 3E7
Tel: (416) 783-8944 Fax: (905) 712-2245

United States of America

American Allergy Association
PO Box 7273, Menlo park
CA 94026
Tel: (415) 855-8036

Allergic Diseases Research Lab
Mayo Clinic & Foundation
200 SW 1st
Rochester Minnesota
Tel: (507) 284-2511 Fax: (507) 284-5771

National Institute of Allergy and Infectious
Diseases
9000 Rockville Pike Bldg. 31
Bethesda MD 20892-2520
Tel: (301) 496-2263 Fax: (301) 496-4409

ANEMIA

Canada

Aplastic Anemia Association of Canada
22 Aikenhead
Etobicoke ON M9R 2Z3
Tel: (416) 235-0468

Appendix D

ANEURYSM

United States of America

Brain Aneurysm foundation Inc
66 Caual St.
Boston Massachusetts 02144
Tel: (617) 723-3870 Fax: (617) 723-8672

American Heart Association
National Center
7272 Greenville Ave
Dallas Texas 75231
Tel: 1-800-AHA-USA1
URL: http://www.americanheart.org/

ANGINA PECTORIS

United States of America

American Heart Association
National Center
7272 Greenville Ave
Dallas Texas 75231Tel: 1-800-AHA-USA1
URL: http://www.americanheart.org/

ANGIOEDEMA

See Anaphylaxis

ANTHRAX

Canada

Canadian Infectious Disease Society
Hospital Saint-Luc 1058 rue Saint Denis St.
Montreal PQ H2X 3J4
Tel: (514) 281-2121 Fax: (514) 281-2443

Immunology Research Center
531 Boulevard des Prairies
Laval PQ H7N 423
Tel: (514) 686-5332 Fax: (514) 686-5501

United Kingdom

British Infection Society
c/o Dept of Microbiology
Friarage Hospital
Northallerton DL6 1JG
Tel: 44-1609-779911 or 44-1609-763035
Fax: 44-1609-778656

Institute of Public Health
University of Cambridge
Forvie Site, Robinson Way
Cambridge CB2 2SR
Tel: 44-223-330300

United States of America

American Association of Immunologists
9650 Rockville Pike
Betheda MD 20814-3994
Centers for Infectious Disease Control
1600 Clifton Rd NE
Atlanta GA 30333
Tel: (404) 639-3311 or (404) 639-3535

National Foundation for Infectious Diseases
4733 Bethesda Ave, Suite 750
Bethesda MD 20814
Tel: (301) 656-0003 Fax: (301) 907-0878

National Vaccine Information Center
512 Maple Ave W Suite 206
Vienna VA 22180
Tel: (703) 938 3783 or (800) 909 SHOT
Fax: (703) 938-5768

APHASIA

United States of America

Paraquad 311 North Lindbergh Boulevard
St. Louis, Missouri 63141
Tel: 314 567 1558; Fax: 314 567 1559
Website: http://www.paraquad.org
email: paraquad@paraquad.org

ARRHYTHMIAS

See Angina Pectoris

ARTHRITIS

Canada

Arthritis Society
Education & Support Association
200 1301 8 St SW
Calgary AB T2R 1B7
Tel: (403) 228-2571 Fax: (403) 229-4232

Arthritis Society
393 University Avenue Suite 1700
Toronto ON M5G 1E6
Tel: (416) 979-7228 Fax: (416) 979-1149

Arthritis Society
895 W 10th Avenue
Vancouver BC V5Z 1L7
Tel: (604) 879-7511#3 Fax: (604) 871-4500

United Kingdom

British Arthritis Care
18 Stephenson Way
London NW1 2HD
Tel: 44-171-3231531 Fax: 44-171-6373644

Arthritis and Rheumatism Council
Stopford Bdlg Oxford Rd
Manchester M13 9PT
Tel: 44-161-2755037 Fax: 44-161-2755043

Rheumatology and Rehabilitation Research
Unit
University of Leeds
36 Clarendon Rd
Leeds West Yorkshire LS2 9NZ
Tel: 44-113-2334940 Fax: 44-113-2446066

University of Manchester
Rheumatic Diseases Centre
Hope Hospital Stott LN, Salford
Greater Manchester M68 HD
Tel: 44-161-7874369 Fax: 44-161-7874687

United States of America

Arthritis Foundation
1314 Spring St. NW
Atlanta GA 30329
Tel: (800) 283-7800

Arthritis Foundation
1330 West Peachtree St.
Atlanta GA 30329
Tel: (404) 872-7100 Fax: (404) 872-0457
Tel: (1-800)-283-7800

ARTHRITIS - OTHERS

See Arthritis - gouty

ASTHMA - BRONCHIAL

See also Anaphylaxis

Canada

Asthma Society of Canada
130 Bridgeland Ave Suite 425
Toronto ON M6A 1Z4
Tel: (416) 787-4050 Fax: (416) 787-5807

United States of America

Asthma and Allergy Foundation of America
1125 15th St. NW Suite 502
Washington DC 20005
Tel: (202) 466-7643 or (800) 7 ASTHMA
Fax: (202) 466-8940

ATHEROSCLEROSIS

See Angina Pectoris

AUTISM

Paraquad 311 North Lindbergh Boulevard
St. Louis, Missouri 63141
Tel: 314 567 1558; Fax: 314 567 1559
URL: http://www.paraquad.org
email: paraquad@paraquad.org

Appendix D

BACK PAIN

United Kingdom

Pain Relief Foundation
Rice Lane
Liverpool L91AE
Tel: 44-151-5231486 Fax: 44-0151-5216155

BELL'S PALSY

United States of America

American Academy of Neurology
1080 Montreal Avenue, St. Paul,
Minnesota 55116
Tel: 651.695.1940

URL: http://www.aan.com/

BOTULISM

See Anthrax

BRONCHIECTASIS

Also see Anthrax

United States of America

American Lung Association
Tel: 1-800-LUNG-USA.
URL:http://www.lungusa.org/

BRONCHITIS

See Bronchiectasis

BRUCELLOSIS

See Anthrax

BURNS

MedicineNet: Burns. Information Network
Inc.
URL: http://www.medicinenet.com/

BURSITIS

Bursitis: Common inflammation responds to
simple care.
Mayo Foundation for Medical Education
and Research.
URL: http://www.mayohealth.org/mayo/
9506/htm/bursitis.htm

CANCER

Australia

Centenary Institute of Cancer
Lockedbag
Newtown NSW 2042
Tel: 61-2-9565-6156 Fax: 61-2-9565-6101

Bldg. 93- Royal Alfred Hospital
Missenden Rd Camperdown NSW 2050

Cancer Centre
Ludwig Institute for Cancer Research
PO Box 2008 Royal Melbourne Hospital
Parkville Victoria 3050
Tel: 61-3-9341-3155 Fax: 61-3-9341-3104

Canada

Alberta Cancer Foundation
1331 29 St. NW
Calgary AB T2N 4N2
Tel: (403) 670-2433

Canadian Cancer Society
Cancer Information Service
20 Holly St Suite 302
Toronto ON M4S 3B1
Tel: (416) 440-3330 TF: 1-888-939-3333

Cancer Information Service
National Office
10 Alcorn Avenue Suite 200
Toronto ON M4V 3B1
Tel: (416) 961-7223

Appendix D

United Kingdom

British Association for Cancer Research
Institution of Cancer Research
15 Cotswold Rd, Sutton
Surrey, London SW7 2DZ
Tel: 44-181-6438901 Ext 4247
Fax: 44-181-7701395

Imperial Cancer Research Fund
PO Box 123 Lincolns Inn Fields
London WC2A-3PX
Tel: 44-0171-2693333

Paterson Institute for Cancer Research
Christie Hospital NHS Trust
Wilmslow Road
Manchester M20 4BX
Tel: 44-161-4463101 Fax: 44-171-4463109

United States of America

American Association for Cancer Education
MD Anderson Cancer Centre
Department of Epidemiology
1515 Holocombe Blvd.
Houston TX 77030
Tel: (713) 792-3020 Fax: (713) 792-0807

American Association for Cancer Research
150 Independence Mall W Suite 826
Philadelphia PA 19106
Tel: (215) 440-9300 Fax: (215) 440-9313
URL: http://www.aacr.org/

American Cancer Society
1599 Clifton Rd NE
Atlanta GA 30329
Tel: (404) 320-3333 or (800) 227-2345
Fax: (404) 329-7985

Cancer Research Center
Albert Einstein College of Medicine
1300 Morris Park Ave
Bronx NY 10461
Tel: (718) 430-2302 Fax: (718) 430-8550

Cancer Research Center
University of Chicago
Maryland Ave
Chicago IL MC1 140
Tel:(773) 702-6180 Fax: (773) 702-9311

National Coalition for Cancer Research
426 C St. NE
Washington DC 20002
Tel: (202) 544-1880 Fax: (202) 543-2565
Mayo Foundation for Medical Education
and Research.
URL: http://www.mayohealth.org/mayo/
common/htm/canhpage.htmCancer

Prevention: Tips to lead a healthy life.
Cancer Research foundation of America.
URL: http://www.preventcancer.org/

CANCER - BONE

See Cancer

CANCER - BREAST

See Cancer

United States of America

National Alliance of Breast Cancer
Organizations
9E 37th St. 10th Floor
New York NY 10016
Tel: (212) 719-0154 or (800) 719-9154
Fax: (212) 689-1213

CARBOHYDRATE INTOLERANCE

See Achalasia

CARDIOMYOPATHIES

See Angina Pectoris

CARPAL TUNNEL SYNDROME

A patient's guide to carpal tunnel syndrome.
Medical multimedia group.
URL: http://www.sechrest.com/mmg/cts/
ctsintro.html

Appendix D

CELLULITIS

See Anthrax

CEREBRAL PALSY

Canada

Cerebral Palsy Association of Alberta
10-8180 Macleod Tr SE
Calgary AB T2H 2B8
Tel: (403) 543-1161 Fax:(403) 543-1168

Cerebral Palsy Parent Council
9 Butternut Lane
Markham ON L3P 3M1
Tel: (905) 294-0944 Fax: (905) 294-4378

United States of America

United Cerebral Palsy Association
1660 L St. NW Suite 700
Washington DC 20036
Tel: (202) 776-0406 Fax: (202) 776-0414
1-800-872-5827

URL: http://www.ucpa.org/

CHAGAS' DISEASE

See Anthrax

CHICKEN POX

See Anthrax

CHOLECYSTITIS

See Achalasia

CHOLERA

See Anthrax

CHRONIC FATIGUE SYNDROME

United States of America

National Chronic Fatigue Syndrome &
Fibromyalgia Association
PO Box 18426
Kansas City MO 64133
Tel: (816) 313-2000 Fax: (816) 313-2001

The CFIDS Association of America Inc.
URL: http://www.cfids.org/

CIRRHOSIS

See Achalasia

The American Liver Foundation
URL: http://sadieo.ucsf.edu/alf/alffinal/
infocirrh.html

COMMON COLD

See Anaphylaxis

CONGENITAL HEART DISEASE

See Angina Pectoris

CONJUNCTIVITIS

See Anthrax

CONSTIPATION

See Achalasia

CONTACT DERMATITIS

See Anaphylaxis

CREUTZFELDT-JAKOB DISEASE

See Anthrax

CYSTIC FIBROSIS

Canada

Cystic Fibrosis Foundation
512 206 7ave SW
Calgary AB T2P 0W7
Tel: (403) 266-5295 Fax: (403) 262-7556

Cystic Fibrosis Foundation
2221 Yonge St Suite 601
Toronto ON
Tel: (416) 485-9149 or (800) 378-2233
Fax: (416) 485-0960

United States of America

Cystic Fibrosis Foundation
6931 Arlington Rd Suite 200
Bethseda MD 20814
Tel: (301) 951-4422 or (800) 344-4823
Fax: (301) 951-6378
URL: http://www.cff.org

American Lung Association.
URL: http://www.lungusa.org

DECUBITUS ULCERS

United States of America

The Agency for Health Care policy and
Research. URL: http://text.nlm.nih.gov/
DermaSafe systems
URL: http://www.dermasafe.com/

DIABETES MELLITUS

Australia

International Diabetes Institute
WHO Center for Epidemiology of Diabetes
Mellitus and Health
260 Kooyony Rd, Caulfield,
South Victoria 3162
Tel: 61-3-9258-5050 Fax: 61-3-9258-5090

Canada

Canadian Diabetes Association
15 Toronto St Suite 800
Toronto ON, M5C 2E3
Tel: (416) 363-3373 Fax: (416) 214-1899

United Kingdom

British Diabetic Association
10 Queen Anne St
London W1M 0BD
Tel: 44-171-3231531 Fax: 44-171-6373644

United States of America

American Association of Diabetes Educators
444 N Michigan Ave Suite 1240
Chicago IL 60611 3901
Tel: (312) 644-2233 or (800) 338 DMED
Fax: (312) 644-4411

American Diabetes Association
1660 Duke St.
Alexandria VA 22314
Tel: (703) 549-1500 or (1-800) 542-2383
Fax: (703) 549-6995
URL: http://www.diabetes.org

Juvenile Diabetes Foundation International
120 Wall St. 19th Floor
New York NY 10005
Tel: (212) 785-9500 or (800) 533-2873
Fax: (212)785-9595

Diabetes Research Center of Pennsylvania
36th Hamilton Walk Stemmler Hall
Rm. 501 Philadelphia, PA 19104
Tel: (215) 898-4365 Fax: (215) 898-2178

DIARRHEA

See Anthrax

DIPHTHERIA

See Anthrax

DIVERTICULAR DISEASE

National Digestive Diseases Clearinghouse.
URL: http://www.mediconsult.com/

Appendix D

DOWN'S SYNDROME

United States of America

National Association for Down Syndrome
P.O. Box 4542
Oak Brook, IL 60522
URL: http://www.nads.org/

DYSENTERY

See Anthrax

EATING DISORDER - ANOREXIA NERVOSA

United States of America

Anorexia Nervosa and Related Eating
Disorders
PO Box 5102
Eugene OR 97405
Tel: (541) 344-1144

Anxiety Disorders Association of America
11900 Parklawn Dr. Suite 100
Rockville MD 20852
Tel: (301) 231-9350 Fax: (301) 231-7392

EATING DISORDER - BULIMIA

See Eating disorder – anorexia nervosa

EBOLA VIRUS INFECTION

See Anthrax

EMPHYSEMA

See Bronchiectasis

ENCEPHALITIS

See Anthrax

ENDOMETRIOSIS

MedicineNet Information Network Inc.
URL: http://www.medicinenet.com

ENDOMETRITIS

See Endometriosis

EPILEPSY

Canada

Epilepsy Association of Calgary
4112 4 St NW
Calgary AB T2K 1A2
Tel: (403) 230-2764

Epilepsy Canada
1470 Peel St Suite 745
Montreal PQ H3A 1T1
Tel: (514) 845-7855 Fax: (514) 845-7866

United Kingdom

British Epilepsy Association
Anstey House 40 Hanover Square
Leeds L53 1BE
Tel: 44-113-2439393 or 1-44-0800-309030
Fax: 44-113-2428804

National Society for Epilepsy
Chalfont St Peter
Chasmem, Buckinghamshire
Gerrards Cross SL9 ORJ
Tel: 44-1494-601300 Fax: 44-1494-871927

United States of America

American Epilepsy Society
638 Prospect Ave
Hartford CT 06105
Tel: (860) 585-7505 Fax: (860) 586-7550

Epilepsy Foundation of America
4351 Garden City Dr.
Landover MD 20785
Tel: (301) 459-3700 or (800) EFA-1000
Fax: (301) 577-4941
URL: http://www.efa.org

ESOPHAGEAL VARICES

See Cirrhosis

FIBROMYALGIA

United States of America

Fibromyalgia Alliance of America
PO Box 21990
Columbus OH 43221-0990
Tel: (614) 457-4222 Fax: (614) 457-2729

National Chronic Fatigue Syndrome &
Fibromyalgia Association
PO Box 18426
Kansas City MO 64133
Tel: (816) 313-2000 Fax: (816) 313-2001

The fibromyalgia network.
http://www.fmnews.com

Oregon fibromyalgia foundation.
http://www.myalgia.com

National fibromyalgia research association.
http://www.teport.com/~nfra

FUNGAL INFECTIONS

See Anthrax

GALL STONES

See Cirrhosis

GASTROESOPHAGEAL REFLUX

See Achalasia

GASTRITIS

See Achalasia

GERMAN MEASLES

See Anthrax

GIARDIASIS

See Anthrax

GLAUCOMA

United States of America

Glaucoma Research Fund
200 Pine St., Suite 200
San Francisco, CA 94104
Tel: (415) 986-3162

GLOMERULONEPHRITIS

National Institute of Diabetes and Digestive
and Kidney Diseases of the National
Institutes of Health, Bethesda, Maryland.
URL: http://www.niddk.nih.gov/

GONORRHEA

See Acquired Immunodeficiency Syndrome

GUILLAIN-BARRÉ SYNDROME

United States of America

Guillain-Barre Syndrome Foundation
International
PO Box 262
Wynnewood PA 19096
Tel: (610) 667-0131 Fax: (610) 667-7036

HAY FEVER

See Anaphylaxis

HEADACHE – CLUSTER

United States of America

National Headache Foundation
5232 N Western Ave
Chicago IL 60625
Tel: (312) 388-6399 or (800) 843-2256
Fax: (312) 907-6278

Appendix D

National Headache Foundation
428 W St. James PL 2nd Floor
Chicago IL 60614-2750
Tel: (773) 388-6399 or 1(888) NHF-5552
Fax: (773) 525-7357

HEADACHE - MIGRAINE

See Headache - cluster

United Kingdom

British Migraine Association
178 A High Rd Byfleet
West Byfleet KT14 7ED
Tel: 44-1932-352468 Fax: 44-1932-351257

HEART ATTACK

See Angina Pectoris

HEART FAILURE

See Angina Pectoris

HELMINTHIC INFECTION

See Anthrax

HEMOPHILIA

Canada

Canadian Hemophilia Society
625 President Kennedy Ave Suite 1210
Montreal PQ H3A 1K2
Tel: (514) 848-0503 Fax: (514) 848-9661

United States of America

National Hemophila Foundation, Greene
Street, Suite 303, New York, NY 10012.
URL: http://www.hemophilia.org

World Federation of Hemophilia.
URL: http://www.wfh.org

HEPATITIS

See Anthrax and Cirrhosis

HERPES SIMPLEX

See Anthrax

HERPES ZOSTER

See Anthrax

HODGKIN'S DISEASE

See Cancer - bladder

HUNTINGTON'S DISEASE

Canada

Huntington Society of Canada
13 Water St N Suite 3 PO Box 1269
Cambridge ON N1R 7G6
Tel: (519) 622-1002 Fax: (519) 622-7370

HYDROCEPHALUS

Canada

Spina Bifida & Hydrocephalus Association
of Ontario
69 Yonge St
Toronto ON M4R 3C1
Tel: (416) 214-1056

United States of America

Spina Bifida Association of America
4590 MacArthur Blvd. NW Suite 250
Washington DC 20007
Tel: (202) 944-3285 or (800) 621-3141
Fax: (202) 944-3295

HYPERTENSION

See Angina Pectoris

Canada

Canadian coalition for high blood pressure
prevention and control
Stroke Research Centre U of Saskatchewan
Saskatoon SK S7N 0W0
Tel: (306) 966-7695 Fax: 966-7685

IMPETIGO

See Anthrax

INFECTIOUS MONONUCLEOSIS

See Anthrax

INFLAMMATORY BOWEL DISEASE (IBD) - CROHN'S DISEASE

Canada

Crohn's and Colitis Foundation of Canada
21 St. Clair Avenue East Suite 301
Toronto ON M4T 1L9
Tel:(416) 920-5035 or (800) 387-1479

United States of America

National Institute of Diabetes and
Digestive and Kidney Diseases
of the National Institutes of Health,
Bethesda, Maryland.
URL: http://www.niddk.nih.gov/
Tel:(416) 920-5035 or (800) 387-1479

INFLAMMATORY BOWEL DISEASE (IBD) - ULCERATIVE COLITIS

See Inflammatory Bowel Disease (IBD) - Crohn's
disease

INFLUENZA

See Anthrax

IRRITABLE BOWEL SYNDROME

See Achalasia

LEPROSY
See Anthrax

LEUKEMIA

United States of America

International Association for Comprehensive
Research on Leukemia & Related Disases
665 Huntington Ave Boston MA 02115
Tel: (617) 432-1023 Fax: (617) 739-8

Leukemia Society of America
600 3rd AveNew York NY 10016
Tel: (212) 573-8484 or (800) 955 4LSA
Fax: (212) 856-9686

LIVER FAILURE

See Cirrhosis

LUNG ABSCESS

See Bronchiectasis and Anthrax

MALABSORPTION SYNDROME

Canada

Celiac Canada
190 Britannia Rd E
Malton ON
Toronto Helpline
Tel: (905) 507-6208 Fax: (905) 507-4673

United States of America

See Achalasia

MALARIA

See Anthrax

MALIGNANT LYMPHOMAS

See Cancer - bladder

MEASLES

See Anthrax

Appendix D

MENINGITIS

See Anthrax

MOLLUSCUM CONTAGIOSUM

See Anthrax

MULTIPLE MYELOMA

United States of America

International Myeloma Foundation
2129 Stanley Hills Dr
Los Angeles CA 90046
Tel: (800) 452 CURE Fax: (213) 656-1182

MULTIPLE SCLEROSIS

Canada

Multiple Sclerosis Society of Canada
238-2116 27 ave NE
Calgary AB T2E 7A6
Tel: (403) 250-7090 Fax: (403) 264-6408

Multiple Sclerosis Society of Canada
250 Bloor St E Suite 1000
Toronto ON M4W 3P9
Tel: (416) 922-6065 Fax: (416) 922-7538

United States of America

National Multiple Sclerosis Society 733
Third Ave 6th Floor
New York NY 10017
Tel: (212) 986-3240 or (800) 344-4867
Fax: (212) 986-7981

MUMPS

See Anthrax

MUSCULAR DYSTROPHY

Australia

University of Sydney-Muscle Research Unit
Rm. 150, Bldg. Code F13,
Sydney University 2006 NSW
Tel: 61-02-9351-3209 Fax: 61-02-9351-2813

Canada

Muscular Dystrophy Association of Canada
2345 Yonge St Suite 900
Toronto ON M4P 2E5
Tel: (416) 488-0030 or (800)567-2873
Fax: (416) 488-7523

United States of America

Muscular Dystrophy Association
3300 E Sunrise Dr
Tucson AZ 85718
Tel: (520)529-2000 or (800) 572-1717
Fax: (520) 529-5300

MYASTHENIA GRAVIS

Canada

Myasthenia Gravis Association
2805 Kingsway
Vancouver BC V5R 5H9
Tel: (604) 451-5511 Fax: (604) 451-5651

United States of America

Myasthenia Gravis Association
1820 S 75th St. Suite 120
West Allis WI 53214
Tel: (414) 938-9800 or (800) 541-5454

NECROTIZING FASCIITIS

See Anthrax

NEPHROTIC SYNDROME

See Achalasia

NEUROFIBROMATOSIS

Canada

Neurofibromatosis Society of Ontario
923 Annes St
Whitby ON L1N 5K7
Tel: (905) 430-6141 Fax: (905) 430-46141

United States of America

Neurofibromatosis Inc
8855 Annapolis Rd Suite 110
Lahnam MD 20706 2924
Tel: (301) 577-8984 Fax: (301) 577-0016

National Neurofibromatosis Foundation
95 Pine St. New York NY 10005
Tel: (212) 344-6633 or (800) 323-7938
Fax: (212) 529-6094

OBESITY

See Achalasia

OSTEOMYELITIS

See Anthrax

OSTEOPOROSIS

Canada

Osteoporosis Society of Canada,
33 Laird Drive, Toronto, ON,
Canada M4G 3S9.

United States of America

North American Menopause Society
94527 Cleveland OH 44101
Tel: (440)-442-7550 Fax: (440)-442-2660

National Osteoporosis Foundation
1232 22nd St., NW
Washington DC 20037-1293
Tel: (202)-223-2226
URL: http://www.nof.org/BoneHealth.html

PAGET'S DISEASE

United States of America

The Paget Foundation
120 Wall Street, Suite 1602, New York,
NY 10005
Tel:212-509-5335 Fax: 212-509-8492
URL: http://www.osteo.org/paget.html

PANIC DISORDER

United States of America

Anxiety Disorders Association of America
11900 Parklawn Dr. Suite 100
Rockville MD 20852
Tel: (301) 231-9350 Fax: (301) 231-7392

PARKINSON'S DISEASE

Canada

Parkinson's Society of Southern Alberta
480 D 36th Avenue SE
Calgary AB T02G 1W4
Tel: (403) 243-9901 Fax: (403) 243-8283

Parkinson Foundation of Canada
390 Bay St Suite 710
Toronto ON M5H 2Y2
Tel: (416) 366-0099 or (800) 565-3000
Fax: (416) 366-9190

United States of America

American Parkinson's Disease Association
1250 Hylan Blvd. Suite B4
Staten Island NY 10305
Tel: (718) 981-8001 or (800) 223-2732
Fax: (718) 981-4399

Parkinson's Disease Foundation
710 West 168th St. New York
NY 10032
Tel: (212) 923-4700 Fax: (212) 923-4778

American Academy of Neurology
1080 Montreal Avenue,
St. Paul, Minnesota 55116
Tel: 651.695.1940
URL: http://www.aan.comCanada

PEDICULOSIS

See Anthrax

PELVIC INFLAMMATORY DISEASE

See Anthrax

Appendix D

PEPTIC ULCER

See Achalasia

PERICARDITIS

See Angina Pectoris

PERIPHERAL NEURITIS

United States of America

American Academy of Neurology.
1080 Montreal Avenue,
St. Paul, Minnesota 55116
Tel: 651.695.1940
URL: http://www.aan.com

PLAGUE

See Anthrax

PLEURAL EFFUSION

See Bronchiectasis

PLEURISY

See Bronchiectasis

PNEUMOCONIOSIS - ASBESTOSIS

See Bronchiectasis

PNEUMOCONIOSIS - BERYLLIOSIS

See Bronchiectasis

PNEUMOCONIOSIS - COAL WORKER'S

See Bronchiectasis

PNEUMOCONIOSIS - SILICOSIS

See Bronchiectasis

PNEUMONIA

See Anthrax

POLIOMYELITIS

See Anthrax

United States of America

International Polio Network
4207 Lindell Blvd.
No. 110St Louis MO 63108
Tel: (314) 534-0475 Fax: (314) 534-5070

PORTAL HYPERTENSION

See Cirrhosis

POLYPS

See Achalasia

PSORIASIS

Canada

Canadian Psoriasis Foundation
1306 Wellington St Suite 500 A
Ottawa ON K1Y 3B2
Tel: (613) 728-4000 or (800) 265-0926
Fax: (613) 7288-8913

United States of America

National Psoriasis Foundation
6600 SW 92nd Ave Suite 300
Portland OR 97223 7195
Tel: (503) 244-7404 or (800) 723-9166
Fax: (503) 245-0626
URL:http://www.psoriasis.org/

National Institute of Arthritis and
Musculoskeleral and Skin Diseases
National Institutes of Health
Bethesda, Maryland 20892-2350
URL: http://www.nih.gov/niams/

PULMONARY EDEMA

See Bronchiectasis

PULMONARY EMBOLISM

See Bronchiectasis

PULMONARY HYPERTENSION

See Bronchiectasis

Q FEVER

See Anthrax

RABIES

See Anthrax

RAYNAUD'S SYNDROME

United States of America

National Institute of Arthritis and Musculoskeleral and Skin Diseases National Institutes of Health
Bethesda, Maryland 20892-2350
URL: http://www.nih.gov/niams/

RELAPSING FEVER

See Anthrax

RENAL FAILURE

See Achalasia

RENAL STONES

See Achalasia

RHEUMATIC HEART DISEASE

See Anthrax

RINGWORM

See Anthrax

Scabies

See Anthrax

SCLERODERMA

United States of America

Scleroderma Federation
Peabody Office Bldg.
1 Newbury St.Peabody MA 01960
Tel: (508) 535-6600 or (800) 422 1113
Fax: (508) 535-6696

Scleroderma Research Foundation
Box 200 Columbus
New Jersey NJ 08022
Tel: (609) 723-2600 Fax: (609) 723-6700

SCOLIOSIS

United Kingdom

Scoliosis Association
2 Ivebury Ct
323-327 Latimer Road
London W10 6RA
Tel: 44-181-9645343 Fax: 44-181-9645343

United States of America

Scoliosis Association
PO Box 811705 Boca Paton
FL 33481-1705
Tel: (407) 994-4435 or (800) 800-0669
Fax: (407) 368-8518

Scoliosis Research Society
6300 N River Rd Suite 727
Rosemont IL 60018-4226
Tel: (847) 698-1627 Fax: (847) 823-0536

SLEEPING SICKNESS

See Anthrax

SPINA BIFIDA

Canada

Spina Bifida Association of Canada
388 Donald St Suite 220
Winnipeg MB R3B 2J4
Tel: (204) 957-1784 or (800) 565-9488
Fax: (204) 957-1794

Appendix D

Spina Bifida & Hydrocephalus Association
of Ontario
69 Yonge St
Toronto ON M4R 3C1
Tel: (416) 214-1056

SPINAL CORD INJURY

Paraquad 311 North Lindbergh Boulevard,
St. Louis, Missouri 63141
Tel: (314) 567 5222 Fax: 567 1559.
Website: http://www.paraquad.org
email: paraquad@paraquad.org

STILL'S DISEASE

See Arthritis - gouty

STROKE

United States of America

American Paralysis Association
500 Morris Ave
Springfield NJ 07081
Tel: (201) 379-2690 Fax: (201) 912-9433

National Stroke Association
96 Inverness Dr. E Suite 1
Englewood CO 80112
Tel: (303) 649 9299 or (800)787-6537
Fax: (303) 649-1328

Stroke Clubs International
805 12 St.Galveston TX 77550
Tel: (409) 762-1022

SYPHILIS

See Anthrax

SYSTEMIC LUPUS ERYTHEMATOSUS

Canada

Lupus Canada
Box 64034 5512 4th St NW
Calgary AB T2K 6J1

Tel: (403) 274-5599 or (800) 661-1468
Fax: (403) 274-5599

United States of America

Lupus Foundation of America1
300 Piccard Dr. Suite 200
Rockville MD 20850 3226
Tel: (301) 670-9292 or (800) 558-0121
Fax: (301) 670-9486

Lupus Network
230 Ranch Dr
Bridgeport CT 06606
Tel: (203) 372-5795

TETANUS

See Anthrax

TINEA VERSICOLOR

See Anthrax

TORTICOLLIS

National Spasmodic Torticollis Association.
9920 Talbert Avenue Suite 233
Fountain Valley, CA 92708
Tel: (714) 378-7838 (800) 487-8385
(800) HURTFUL
Fax: (714) 378-7830
URL: http://www.bluheronweb.com/NSTA/
NSTA.htm

TRACHOMA

See Anthrax

TRANSIENT ISCHEMIC ATTACK

United States of America

American Academy of Neurology.
1080 Montreal Avenue,
 St. Paul, Minnesota 55116
Tel: 651.695.1940
URL: http://www.aan.com#

TRIGEMINAL NEURALGIA

United States of America

Trigeminal Neuralgia Association
PO Box 785 Barnegat Light
NJ 08006
Tel: (609) 361-1014 Fax: (609) 361-0982

TUBERCULOSIS – LUNG

See Anthrax

TUBERCULOSIS – BONE

See Anthrax

TULAREMIA

See Anthrax

TYPHOID FEVER

See Anthrax

TYPHUS FEVER

See Anthrax

WARTS

See Anthrax

YAWS

See Anthrax

Appendix D

Glossary

A

abdomen   the region of the trunk lying between the diaphragm and pelvis

abduction   to move a body part away from the midline of the body; to move digits away from the axis of limb

abscess   a cavity containing pus, surrounded by inflamed tissue

absorption   the active or passive uptake of material

acid   a compound that dissociates into hydrogen ion and an anion; an acid solution has a pH below 7.0

acquired   a change in an organ or tissue that occurs during the lifetime of the individual, which is not inherited but due to environmental effects, use, disuse etc.

action potential   nerve impulse; a conducted change in the potential across the cell membrane of excitable cells like neurons and muscle

acute disease   disease beginning suddenly/ abruptly, and subsiding after a short period

addiction   a state where a person is physically or mentally dependant on a particular substance and experiences adverse effects if s/he stops taking it

adduction   to move a body part towards the midline of the body; to move digits towards the axis of the limb

adhesion   fusion of two layers that may occur after irritation or damage; results in restriction of movement of involved parts

afferent   going towards; eg. Afferent nerve – impulses go towards the spinal cord or brain

agonist   a muscle that produces the same movement as another muscle

aldosterone   a hormone secreted by the adrenal cortex involved in regulation of minerals like sodium and potassium and water; has an effect on the kidney

alkali   a compound that releases hydroxide ions when dissolved in water; the pH of an alkali is more than 7.0

allergen   a substance that produces a hypersensitivity response

allergy   state of hypersensitivity caused by exposure to an antigen. It causes histamine and other molecules to be liberated in the site by the action of the immune system

alveolus/alveoli   sacs found at the end of the respiratory tree where gas exchange occurs; also denotes tooth socket

amenorrhea   failure to commence menstruation or cessation of menstruation

androgen   a sex hormone primarily produced by the testis; also manufactured in small quantities by the adrenal cortex (both sexes)

antacid   a substance that reduces the acidity in the stomach

antagonist   a muscle that opposes the movement of another muscle

antibiotic   a chemical agent that acts against microorganisms that are harmful

antibodies   proteins secreted by B lymphocytes that target specific antigens

anticoagulants   substances that inhibit the clotting (coagulation) of blood

antidepressants   drugs that are given to treat depression

antigen   a molecule - usually a protein that triggers the production of antibodies

antihistamines   drugs that inhibit the action of histamine

antipyretics   drugs used to prevent or reduce fever

aponeurosis   a broad sheet of connective tissue/tendon which serves as a point of insertion or origin of a muscle

appendicectomy   removal of the vermiform appendix

arteriosclerosis   any one of a group of diseases that cause the wall of arteries to thicken and harden

artery   a blood vessel that carries blood away from the heart

arthroscopy   visualising the inside of a joint using a fibre-optic device

articulation   a joint

ascites   abnormal volume of fluid in the peritoneal cavity

atrium   the right/left chamber of the heart that receive blood from the veins

atrophy   a decrease in the size of a cell/tissue/organ

autoimmune   immunity acting against self

autoinoculation   to introduce under the skin or mucous membrane by self; usually used in relation to spread of disease from one area of the body to another by self

autonomic nervous system   the part of the nervous system that controls the internal organs and skin; consists of the sympathetic and parasympathetic systems

B

B lymphocytes   a type of white blood cells that produce antibodies

baroreceptor   nerve receptors that monitor the pressure in the blood vessels

basal ganglia   gray mater located near the center of the brain; responsible for stability and coordinated movement

basophil   a type of white blood cell, similar to mast cell that releases histamine, serotonin etc.; participates in inflammatory responses

benign   not malignant; used in reference to tumors that increase very slowly in size and do not spread

bile   secretion from the liver that is stored in the gall bladder and released into the gut through the common bile duct; helps with the digestion of fat

bilirubin   a pigment that is a breakdown product of hemoglobin

Appendix E

biofeedback a process where artificial signals are used to give a person feedback on physiological activities that are involuntary / the person is not conscious of

blister damage to the skin between the superficial and deep layers of the epidermis without an open wound, resulting in accumulation of interstitial fluid in small pockets

bony spurs a bony, pointed projection

brain stem part of the central nervous system that lies between the spinal cord and the brain; includes the medulla oblongata, pons and mid brain

breech delivery a form of vaginal delivery of the baby where the legs or lower part of the body exit first

bronchospasm constriction / narrowing of the bronchus

bronchus a branch of the trachea that conducts air into the lungs

bulla a large fluid-filled lesion

bursa a sac filled with synovial fluid which serves to reduce friction between muscle and joints/ muscle and muscle/ skin and muscle/ bone and muscle

C

calcification deposition of calcium salts in tissue

calcitonin a hormone secreted by certain cells in the thyroid gland; it helps to reduce calcium levels in the blood

calculus / calculi formation of stones by insoluble material inside the body fluids; may be found in the kidney, gall bladder, urinary bladder

cancer a tumor characterized by abnormal and rapidly multiplying cells; refers to malignant tumors

capillary the smallest blood vessel that allows exchange of substances; it connects an arteriole with a venule

carcinogen a substance that is capable of causing cancer

cardiac output The volume of blood pumped out of the left ventricle in one minute; approximately 5 liters

cardiomegaly abnormal enlargement of the heart

carnivorous an animal that feeds on other animals

carrier a person or animal that transmits infection to others without showing signs of infection

cartilage a type of connective tissue that has more elastic matrix and less calcium than bone

cataract a condition where the lens in the eye becomes cloudy resulting in blurred or loss of vision

catecholamine includes a group of chemicals having a similar molecular structure; epinephrine (adrenaline), norepinephrine (noradrenaline), dopamine etc. are examples

catheter a tube inserted into a body cavity or into a blood vessel or passageway

catheterization a procedure where a flexible tube is inserted into a body cavity through its external opening eg. inserting into the bladder through the urethra

cecum a pouch-like area that lies at the junction of the small intestine and ascending colon

cell the smallest structure of the body that is capable of performing all the functions necessary for life

central nervous system part of the nervous system which includes the brain and the spinal cord

cerebellum part of the brain involved with the coordination of the skeletal muscles

cerebrospinal fluid circulating fluid that fills the ventricles of the brain, surrounds and bathes the brain and spinal cord

cerebrum the largest portion of the brain made up of the two cerebral hemispheres

cervix the narrow necklace portion of an organ; in the uterus it is the part that projects into the vagina

chelating agent a chemical agent that combines with unwanted metal ions. It is often used to treat heavy metal poisoning

chemotherapy treating illnesses using specific chemicals

chorea a neurological disorder that results in jerky, involuntary movements

chromosomes structures in the nucleus of a cell that contain the genes

chronic disease developing slowly and lasting for a long time

cilia thin threadlike projections that are present in certain epithelial cells

cilia a part of the cell that projects above the epithelial surface and undergoes rhythmic movement, aids movement of secretions eg. mucus in the respiratory tract

clitoris a small organ in the external genitalia of the female, which is erectile; it is the embryological equivalent of the penis in males

clotting factors substances in the blood that participate in the process of clotting; many of the factors are in an inactive form and are converted to an active form by specific chemical reactions

coagulation clotting of blood

cognitive pertains to the intellect and the mental process involved in problem-solving ie. obtaining and processing information

colic/colicky severe, fluctuating, spasmodic pain in the abdomen

collagen a type of insoluble protein found in connective tissue

collateral running parallel or side by side

colostomy a surgical procedure where a part of the colon (large intestine) is connected to the body wall to enable discharge of fecal material

congenital present at the time of birth

congestion abnormal accumulation of fluid in an area

connective tissue binding and supportive tissue

consolidation a process of becoming solid

contagious a disease that is communicable - spread from one person to another

contracture an abnormal, permanent contraction of a muscle which can occur in paralyzed muscle

cornification the formation of keratin (a type of fibrous protein) by stratified squamous epithelium; also known as keratinization

coronary circulation the arterial and venous circulation that supply the walls of the heart

corticosteroids hormones secreted by the adrenal cortex that affects the metabolism of fat, carbohydrates and proteins

craniosacral therapy a form of therapy where the skull (cranium), spine and sacrum are manipulated

crust accumulation of dried secretions eg. scabs

cryotherapy a form of treatment in medicine where extreme cold is used

curettage a procedure where the wall of a cavity (eg. uterus) is scraped using a spoon-shaped instrument

cyanosis blue discoloration of the mucous membranes due to excess of deoxygenated hemoglobin

D

deep towards the core of the body

defecation the process of evacuating the bowels

definitive host the organism that houses another (eg. parasite) at its own expense; the parasite requires the presence of this organism for its life cycle

degeneration the slow death/deterioration of cells

dementia a chronic mental disease

demyelination the loss of the myelin sheath that surrounds some axons of neurons

dendrite a process of the neuron that conducts impulses towards the cell body of the neuron

dermis the inner layer of the skin where the glands, nerve endings and blood vessels are located

diastole the period of the cardiac cycle when the chambers are relaxed

distal away from the trunk

diuretic an agent that promotes excretion of urine

dominant describes a gene that imparts its characteristics to the individual even if it is derived only from one parent

dorsal refers to the posterior portion of a body part

dorsal root ganglion a region close to the posterior aspect of the spinal cord where the cell bodies of the sensory neurons that enter the spinal cord are located

dorsiflexion movement of the ankle where the dorsum is elevated

dyspnea subjective difficulty in breathing

E

effleurage a massage technique where broad, light or firm strokes are used

ejaculate the expulsion of semen from the penis as a result of contraction of muscles in the pelvic floor

EKG / ECG electrocardiogram; a record of the electrical changes of the heart that is monitored from specific locations on the surface of the body

electrolytes ions and molecules that can carry positive or negative electric charges

encephalin morphine-like substances found in many parts of the brain and spinal cord; have pain-killing function

endemic refers to the presence of a disease in the local population or geographical area

endocrine gland a gland without ducts that secretes hormones directly into the blood

endorphin morphine-like substances found in many parts of the brain and spinal cord; have pain-killing function

endoscope an instrument introduced into a body cavity that helps to visualize the inside

enzyme a protein that facilitates a specific biochemical reaction

eosinophil one of the white blood cells whose granules stain pink in standard staining fluids; it participates in the immune reactions increasing in number specially in allergic conditions

epidemic refers to the spread of disease rapidly through a population affecting a large number of people at the same time

epidermis the superficial layer of the skin

epithelium type of tissue that lines or covers body surfaces

erythropoietin the hormone that regulates the formation of red cells, which is secreted by the kidney

estrogens any of the many hormones secreted by the follicles of the ovary

eversion a movement of the foot where the sole of the foot faces outwards

exacerbation an increase in the severity of the disease

exocrine gland a gland that secretes onto the body surface or into a passage that is connected to the exterior of the body eg. sweat gland; salivary gland

extension a movement that results in an increase in the angle between the parts of a joint

external located on or towards the body surface

extravasation escape of fluid (usually blood) into the tissues

F

fascia a tough sheet of fibrous connective tissue that surrounds/supports muscles or binds skin to underlying muscle

fetus a prenatal human after 8 weeks of pregnancy

fibroblasts connective tissue cells that produce fibrous protein

fibrosis thickening and scarring of tissue with accumulation of collagen fibres; usually following injury

fissure cut through epidermis and dermis eg. athlete's foot

flaccid soft; limp; flabby; lack of muscle tone

flexion a movement that decreases the angle between the parts of a joint

forceps delivery a procedure where the delivery of the baby is assisted by the use of a pair of forceps - a pincer-like instrument

G

gall bladder a sac lying beneath the liver that stores bile

ganglion a collection of the cell bodies of nerve cells outside the central nervous system

gastrectomy a surgical procedure where the whole or part of the stomach is removed

Appendix E

gene   a unit of heredity that is part of the chromosome, which holds the code that determines a specific characteristic of an individual

gene therapy   a form of treatment where genes (units of heredity found in chromosomes) are used to treat specific diseases

genetics   the study of the mechanism of heredity

gestational   the period between conception and birth (during pregnancy)

glans penis   the enlarged distal, sensitive portion of the penis

glomerulus   a tuft of capillaries that are surrounded by a cup-shaped capsule found in the kidney that filters urine from the blood

growth factor   chemical substance secreted by the body, which results in an increase in growth of the tissue

H

habituation   the condition where the response to a frequent, repeated stimulus is diminished

hallucination   an experience where the person perceives something that is not present or happening

hematoma   a swelling filled with blood

hemiplegia / hemiparesis   paralysis affecting one side of the body

hemodialysis   a process where there is diffusion between blood and another solution of different concentration, separated by a semipermeable membrane; used to regulate the composition of blood

hemoglobin   the (iron containing protein) pigment in the red blood cell responsible for carrying oxygen and carbon dioxide

hemolysis   the breakdown of red blood cells (erythrocytes)

hereditary   determined by genetic factors; can be passed on to children from parents

hormone   a chemical secreted by an endocrine gland into the blood; it causes an effect in a specific organ away from the site of origin of the hormone

host   an organism which supports another organism at its own expense

hyperextension   the movement where the angle between two bones is increased excessively, beyond its normal range

hyperplasia   an increase in the size of the organ due to an increase in the number of cells

hypertrophy   increase in the size of organ due to increase in size of individual cells

hypothalamus   the region in the brain located inferior to the thalamus, responsible for numerous vegetative functions like hunger, thirst etc; it secretes many hormones that regulate the function of the pituitary gland

hypothenar muscles   muscles that produce the bulge observed on the medial side of the palm of hand (proximal to the little finger)

hypoxia   a low concentration of oxygen in the blood

I

ileum   the last portion of the small intestine that connects the jejunum with the cecum

immunization   the process of increasing the resistance of the body to pathogens

immunocompromised   an individual whose immunity is low

immunodeficient   unable to produce normal numbers and types of antibodies and lymphocytes to fight infection; inadequate immunity

immunosuppressants   substances that inhibit the immunity of an individual

immunosuppressive   a drug, exposure to toxic chemicals, radiation or infection that results in suppression of immune responses

immunotherapy   treating an illness using antibodies that block the specific antigen

incidence   the number of new cases that appear in a particular period of time

incubation period   the period between the exposure to the disease and the onset of disease

inflammation   a local reaction of the body to cell injury characterized by redness, swelling, pain, increase in temperature and loss of function

inguinal canal   a canal located in the groin area through which structures that enter/leave the abdomen pass; in male fetuses, the testis, along with its blood vessels and nerves pass through the canal to reach the scrotum

inoculation   to introduce a substance into the body through the skin

inorganic   pertaining to chemical elements and their compounds other than those containing carbon atoms (ie. organic)

insertion   the place where the muscle is attached; indicates the part that is most mobile (opposite of origin)

insidious   slow onset; proceeding gradually

insomnia   a persistent inability to fall asleep

intervertebral disc   the cartilage that lies between two vertebrae

intercostal   between the ribs

intermediate or intermediary host   in the life cycle of a parasite, a secondary host which carry the young forms or resting stage of the parasite between the adult stages in the primary host

interstitial compartment   the fluid space between the cells but outside the blood and lymph vessels

inversion   a movement where the sole of the foot is turned inwards

iris   the pigmented, circular part of eye lying in front of the lens with an opening (the pupil) in the center

ischemia   an inadequate supply of oxygen to the tissue

isometric   muscle contraction in which there is no lengthening of muscle fibers but an increase in tension occurs

isotonic   muscle contraction in which there is lengthening of muscle fibers and same amount of tension is maintained

J

jejunum   part of the small intestine that lies between the duodenum and ileum

K

keratinocytes   cells from which the fibrous protein keratin is formed

keratolytic   breakdown of the fibrous protein - keratin, found in the superficial layer of skin

L

labia a part of the external genitalia of the female consisting of two longitudinal folds that extend inferiorly and posteriorly; two pairs of labia major and labia minor are present

large intestine part of the gastrointestinal tract that includes the cecum, colon, rectum and anal canal

lasers device that generates and emits an intense stream of electromagnetic radiation; used in surgery and in many other applications

latent a period when the infection is lying dormant

lateral towards the side of the body

laxatives substances that are used to treat constipation; facilitates/ stimulates evacuation of the bowel

lesion a wounded or damaged area

leukocyte white blood cell; includes eosinophils, basophils, neutrophils, lymphocytes and monocytes

ligament a tough cord or band that binds bone to bone

lipids organic compounds that contain carbon, hydrogen and oxygen in a ratio other than 1:2:1; eg. wax, oil, fat

lobectomy a surgical procedure where the nerve fibers connecting the thalamus and the frontal lobe are cut

lordosis an exaggeration of the curvature in the lumbar region

lumen the space within a tubular structure through which substances pass

lymph the fluid that flows through the lymph vessels

lymph node an oval mass with a collection of lymphocytes through which the lymph pass

lymphocyte a type of white blood cell involved in immunity; constitutes 20-25% of all white blood cells

M

macrophage a large white blood cell capable of phagocytosis

macule an irregular lesion, not raised, on the surface of the skin with localized color change eg. freckle

malaise a general feeling of illness or discomfort

malignant virulent; refers to a tumor that grows and spreads at a rapid rate

mammography a technique where X-ray is used to locate tumors in the breast

mast cell a cell found in the connective tissue that secretes histamine and participates in local inflammation

mastectomy a surgical procedure where the breast is removed

medial closer or towards the midline of the body

mediastinum the central mass of tissue in the thorax that divide the thoracic cavity into two pleural cavities; it includes the heart and great vessels, esophagus, thymus, nerves and lymphatics in this location

mediators chemicals involved as intermediate agents in physiological process/es

menarche the beginning of the first menstrual cycle; occurs at puberty

meninges the fibrous membrane that covers the brain; consists of three membranes - the dura, arachnoid and pia mater

meniscus wedge-shaped cartilage that is found in certain types of synovial joints eg. knee

menopause the period when a female ceases to have menstrual cycle

menstruation the discharge of blood and tissue from the uterus in the first few days of the menstrual cycle; the first day of bleeding is considered day 1

metabolism the chemical changes that occur in a cell

metastasis spread from one organ or body part to another; usually refers to spread of a malignant tumor

micturition the process of passing urine; urination

monocyte a white blood cell that is capable of phagocytosis; forms 3-8% of all white cells

motor neuron a neuron carrying impulses away from the spinal cord/ brain

mucous membrane membrane that lines cavities and tubes that are exposed to the external environment

mucus a lubricating fluid containing water and proteoglycans (mucins); secreted in the respiratory, urinary, digestive and reproductive tracts

mutation the changing of the structure of a gene resulting in a variant form that may be passed on to the offspring

myelin a lipoprotein substance that covers nerve fibers

myocardium the muscle layer of the heart

myoneural junction the contact area between the motor nerve and the muscle; also known as neuromuscular junction

N

necrosis cell or tissue death

neoplasm a new abnormal growth

neuroendocrine cells special cells that are from the same embryonic origin as sympathetic ganglion and adrenal medulla that are capable of producing hormones

neurotransmitter a chemical stored in nerve endings that is released in the synapses; it enables communication across neurons

neutrophil a type of white blood cell that is capable of phagocytosis; it constitutes about 60-70% of all white blood cells

nodule a small, rounded swelling

nucleic acid regulates the synthesis of proteins; the genetic material in cells

nystagmus an involuntary, continuous movement of the eyeball

O

omentum part of the peritoneum (the lining of the abdominal cavity) that hangs like an apron from the stomach, over the intestines; it contains a lot of adipose (fat) tissue

omnivorous an animal that eats food of plant and animal origin

oncotic pressure the osmotic pressure produced by proteins; in the plasma it helps counteract the tendency of the capillary hydrostatic pressure to push fluids into the interstitial space

Appendix E

opportunistic infection an infection that does not affect normal individuals; affects patients in unusual circumstances eg. when the immunity is low

organic denotes compounds containing many carbon atoms

origin the place where the muscle is attached; indicates the part that is stationary (opposite of insertion)

ovarian follicle the developing ovum along with the surrounding epithelial cells in the ovary

P

pacemaker a device that sets the pace of cardiac contraction; cardiac cells that have the same function are also known as pacemakers

pallor a palè appearance

palmar relates to the palm of the hand

palpitation an uncomfortable sensation where the rapid/strong/irregular beating of the heart is perceived

pancreas a gland that secretes enzymes into the intestines; it also has an endocrine component that secretes insulin and glucagon into the blood

papule solid elevation of epidermis and dermis eg. insect bites

paralysis loss of muscle function and/or sensation

paranasal sinus a chamber filled with air and lined with mucous membrane that communicates with the nasal cavity

paraplegia paralysis of the legs and lower body

parasite an organism that lives on or in another organism and benefits at that organism's expense

parasympathetic part of the autonomic nervous system that opposes the effect of the sympathetic system in general

parathyroid endocrine glands located posterior to the thyroid glands that secrete parathormone; regulates calcium metabolism

perforation formation of a hole

pericardium the membrane covering the heart; it consists of two membranes - the visceral pericardium close to the myocardium and the parietal pericardium that is the outermost membrane; the space between the two membranes contains fluid known as the pericardial fluid; the pericardium prevents the heart from dilating excessively

peristalsis waves of contractions seen in the gut that proceed towards the anus

peritoneal cavity the cavity lined by peritoneum - the membrane that lines the abdominal cavity and covers the abdominal organs

peritoneum the membrane that lines the abdominal cavity and covers the abdominal organs

petrissage a massage stroke where the skin is lifted and squeezed as in kneading

pH a measure of the acidity/alkalinity of a solution; ranges from 0-14, with 7 denoting neutral, 7-14 denoting alkalinity and < 7 denoting acidity

phagocytosis the ability of certain white blood cells to engulf and digest large particles

photophobia extreme sensitivity to light

placenta the organ that helps transport nutrients/ oxygen from mother to fetus

plantar sole of foot

plantar fascia a thick sheet of connective tissue found in the sole of the foot, stretching from the heel towards the toes

plaque a layer of amorphous (without a clearly defined shape or form) material adhering to the surface

plasma the fluid in the blood which remains after the removal of cells

platelets small fragments of certain cells in the bone marrow which primarily take part in the clotting of blood

pleural cavity a potential cavity found between the two layers of the pleura of the lungs

polydipsia excessive thirst

polyp a smooth, soft, rounded growth with a neck, that grows from mucous membrane

polyphagia excessive hunger

polyuria passage of excessive urine

popliteal the region behind the knee

posterior towards the back

precursor a substance from which another is formed by a metabolic reaction

predisposition are more prone to; have the potential to

prognosis prediction of the probable outcome of the disease

prolapse abnormal projection/protrusion or slipping forward/down of an organ of the body eg. uterine prolapse, umbilical cord prolapse

pronation the movement that turns the palm of the hand towards the back

prophylaxis measures taken to prevent an illness

prostaglandins a group of complex fatty acids secreted by most tissues of the body that act as local hormones regulating blood supply, acid secretion (in the stomach), temperature regulation etc.

prostate a gland located below the urinary bladder, surrounding the male urethra

proteinuria presence of protein in the urine

proximal closer to the core of the body

pruritis itching

psychosis a major mental disorder

puberty a growth period when there is sexual maturation and secondary sexual characteristics appear; normally between the ages of 10 and 15

purines nitrogen compounds that have a double-ring structure eg. adenine, guanine

pustule pus-filled papule (solid elevation of epidermis and dermis) eg. infected acne

Q

quadriplegic paralysis of all four limbs

Appendix E

R

radiating having a radial pattern; proceeding outward from a central area

radiation emission of energy as electromagnetic waves eg. X-ray; commonly used to treat cancer

radioactive relates to the emission of ionizing radiation or particles

rectum the part of the gastrointestinal tract that lies between the colon and the anus

regeneration growth of new tissue to replace lost or old tissue

regurgitation to bring up again to the mouth; also denotes back flow eg. aortic regurgitation

remission a decrease in the seriousness of the illness

renin an enzyme released by special cells in the kidney when the blood pressure drops; it converts angiotensinogen to angiotensin I(a vasoconstrictor)

reticular activating system (RAS) the region of the central nervous system that is responsible for maintenance of consciousness and arousal

rotated to move around an axis

S

scales abnormal keratinization (transformation from live to dead cells in the superficial layer of skin) eg. psoriasis

Schwann cells special supporting cells located around axons of myelinated neurons; they manufacture myelin

sclera the fibrous outer layer that forms the white of the eye

sclerosing agent an irritant substance injected into a blood vessel to cause inflammation, clotting of blood, hardening and narrowing of the vessel

sebaceous gland a gland located near a hair follicle that secretes sebum (responsible for the oil on the skin)

sedentary inactive; tending to spend more time seated

serum plasma of the blood without the substances that cause clotting

sign an objective finding made by the examiner

sinusoids an extensive network of blood vessels found in areas such as the liver, spleen and pancreas

sloughed the dropping off of dead tissue

spastic uncontrolled contraction of a muscle

sphincter a ring of muscle around the entrance or exit of internal passages that contracts/relaxes to close/open the passageway

spleen large blood-filled organ located in the upper left quadrant of the abdomen

sputum secretion from the lungs

stasis stagnation of fluid movement

stenosis narrowing; constriction of a passageway

sterility not able to produce children

strabismus squint eye; cross eye; abnormal alignment of the eye

subcutaneous the layer of connective tissue below the dermis; also known as hypodermis or superficial fascia

subluxation a partial separation of the articulating surface of one bone of a joint from the other

superficial towards the outer surface; on or near the skin

superinfection infection that occurs over an already existing condition

superior above; towards the upper part

supination the movement that turns the palm upward/ anterior

suppository a solid, cylindrical or conical material that is inserted into the rectum or vagina

surgical sympathectomy a surgical procedure that destroys the action of the sympathetic nervous system to a specific region of the body; eg. cervical sympathectomy - where the cervical sympathetic ganglion is destroyed

sutures joints between the flat bones of the skull

sympathetic part of the autonomic system that is responsible for the 'fight or flight' reaction

symptom a subjective perception of a disease by the person with the disease

syndrome a condition characterized by a set of specific symptoms that occur together

synovial cavity space between the bones of a synovial joint; filled with synovial fluid

synovial joint a freely movable joint that is lined by synovial membrane, having a synovial cavity

systole the period of the cardiac cycle when the chamber of the heart contracts

systolic pressure the blood pressure that is recorded inside an artery when the ventricle contracts

T

T cell type of lymphocyte that is responsible for the type of immunity mediated by cells

tender points painful spots usually located in the muscle, that are painful on applying pressure

tendon tough cord-like connective tissue that connects muscle to bone

thalamus an oval gray area in the brain that serves as the sensory relay station

thenar eminence the bulge produced by muscles and other tissues on the lateral aspect of the palm of the hand (proximal to the thumb)

thrombus a blood clot formed inside a blood vessel

thymus an organ located posterior to the sternum which is part of the lymphatic system

topical to apply on the surface of the skin

toxin poisonous substance

tracheostomy a surgical opening made in the anterior aspect of the trachea to facilitate airflow into the lungs

tranquillizer a drug that reduces tension and anxiety

trigger points points on the surface of the body that are very sensitive to touch and cause referred pain (pain that travels or spreads when palpated)

Appendix E

trunk the thorax and abdomen together

U

ulcer erosion; loss of epidermis of skin

umbilicus the site where the umbilical cord was attached in the fetus (navel; belly button)

ureter the tube connecting the kidney to the urinary bladder

urethra the tube that transports the urine to the exterior from the urinary bladder

urticaria an itchy, red rash associated with swelling

V

vaccine a substance used to stimulate the production of antibodies to immunise a person against one or more diseases

valgus angulation of bone away from the body

varus angulation of bone towards the body

vasoconstriction narrowing of the lumen of a blood vessel by contraction of the smooth muscles

vasodilation widening of the lumen of a blood vessel by relaxation of the smooth muscles

vasomotor center a collection of cell bodies of neurons located in the brainstem responsible for regulating blood pressure

vein a blood vessel that carries blood to the heart

ventral towards the front; anterior

vesicle a fluid-filled lesion eg. blister

vestibular apparatus the structures in the inner ear responsible for balance of the body; responds to acceleration, deceleration and gravitational forces

viscera organs inside the abdominal/thoracic cavity

visual acuity sharpness of vision

vulva refers to the external genitalia of the female

System-wise Index

CARDIOVASCULAR

Acquired Immunodeficiency Syndrome - 7
AIDS - 7
Alcoholism - 13
Alcohol dependence - 13
American Trypanosomiasis - 85
Amyloidosis - 17
Anaphylaxis - 19
Anemia - 20
Aneurysm - 21
Angina pectoris - 22
Angioedema - 24
Anthrax - 27
Arrhythmias - 30
Atherosclerosis - 42
Beryllium disease - 264
Beryllium poisoning - 264
Brucellosis - 53
Buerger's Disease - 54
Cardiac failure - 160
Cardiomyopathies - 79
Chagas' disease - 85
Congenital Heart Disease - 94
Cyanosis - 104
DIC - 115
Disseminated Intravascular Coagulation - 115
Down's syndrome - 116
Dyspnea - 120
Ebola virus infection - 122
Edema - 124
First rib syndrome - 326
Gangrene - 144
German Measles - 148
Headache - others - 157
Heart attack - 160
Heart Failure - 160
Hemangiomas - 173
Hemophilia - 173
Hemorrhoids - 174
High blood pressure - 190
Human Immunodeficiency Virus infection - 7
Hypertension - 190
Hypotension - 196
Hypoxia - 199
Icterus - 209
Ischemic Heart Disease - 22
Jaundice - 209
Leukemia - 216
Lyme arthritis - 219

Lyme disease - 219
Malaria - 221
Marfan's Syndrome - 224
Myocardial Infarction - 160
Nicotine addiction - 238
Nutritional deficiencies - Vitamin B - 240
Nutritional deficiencies - Vitamin C - 241
Nutritional deficiencies - Vitamin K - 243
Oedema - 124
Pericarditis - 256
Piles - 174
Pneumoconiosis - Berylliosis - 264
Polycythemia - 271
Raynaud's disease - 282
Raynaud's phenomenon - 282
Raynaud's syndrome - 282
Relapsing fever - 283
Rheumatic fever - 287
Rheumatic heart disease - 287
Rubella - 148
Scalenus syndrome - 326
Scurvy - 241
Shock - 296
SLE - 313
Stasis ulcers - 338
Systemic Lupus Erythematosus - 313
Thoracic Outlet Syndrome - 326
Thromboangiitis obliterans - 54
Trisomy 21 - 116
Varicose ulcers - 338
Varicose veins - 339
Venous thrombosis - 341
Volkmann's ischaemic contracture - 343

ENDOCRINE

Acromegaly - 189
Addison's disease - 193
Adrenal hypofunction - 193
Adrenal insufficiency - 193
Adrenogenital syndrome - 10
Basedow's disease - 191
Conn's syndrome - 188
Cretinism - 198
Cushing's syndrome - 103
Diabetes Insipidus - 110
Diabetes Mellitus - 111
Dwarfism - 195
Gigantism - 189
Goiter - 152

Grave's disease - 191
High blood pressure - 190
Hyperaldosteronism - 188
Hyperparathyroidism - 188
Hyperpituitarism - 189
Hypertension - 190
Hyperthyroidism - 191
Hypoadrenalism - 193
Hypoparathyroidism - 194
Hypopituitarism - 195
Hypothyroidism - 198
Impotence - 201
Multiple neuroma - 237
Myxedema - 198
Neurofibroma - 237
Neurofibromata - 237
Neurofibromatosis - 237
Neuromatosis - 237
NF - 237
Nontoxic goiter - 152
Obesity - 244
Panhypopituitarism - 195
Parry's disease - 191
Pheochromocytoma - 259
Simple goiter - 152
Thyrotoxicosis - 191
Von Recklinghausen's disease - 237

GASTROINTESTINAL

Achalasia - 4
Acidosis - 5
African eye worm - 167
Alcoholism - 13
Alcohol dependence - 13
American Trypanosomiasis - 85
Amyloidosis - 17
Anthrax - 27
Appendicitis - 29
Beryllium disease - 264
Beryllium poisoning - 264
Cancer - colon - 68
Cancer - gallbladder - 69
Cancer - liver - 70
Cancer - oral - 71
Cancer - pancreas - 73
Cancer-stomach - 75
Carbohydrate Intolerance - 77
Carcinoid tumors - 78
Chagas' disease - 85

Appendix F

INTEGUMENTARY

LYMPHATIC

MUSCULOSKELETAL

Appendix F

Nervous

RENAL

REPRODUCTIVE

Appendix F

Fibroadenoma - breast - 135
Fibrocystic disease - breast - 135
Fibroid - 136
Fibromyoma - 136
Gonorrhea - 153
Hydrocele - 186
Impotence - 201
Leiomyoma - 136
Lung abscess - 218
Mammary dysplasia - 135
Miscarriage - 1
Myoma - 136
Ovarian cysts - 248
Pelvic Inflammatory Disease - 254
PID - 254
Placental abruption - 2
PMS - 276
Preeclampsia - 330
Pregnancy - induced hypertension - 330
Premenstrual dysphoria disorder - 276
Premenstrual syndrome - 276
Prostatic hyperplasia - 277
Prostatitis - 277
Salpingitis - 289
Syphilis - 312
Toxemia of pregnancy - 330
Undescended testis - 101
Vulvitis - 344

RESPIRATORY

Acidosis - 5
Acquired Immunodeficiency syndrome - 7
AIDS - 7
Adult Respiratory Distress Syndrome - 11
Allergic rhinitis - 155

Amyloidosis - 17
Anaphylaxis - 19
Anthracosilicosis - 265
Anthracosis - 265
Anthrax - 27
ARDS - 11
Aspergillosis - 141
Asthma - bronchial - 38
Atelectasis - 41
Bends - 49
Beryllium disease - 264
Beryllium poisoning - 264
Black lung disease - 265
Bronchiectasis - 51
Bronchitis - 52
Bronchogenic carcinoma - 71
Brucellosis - 53
Caisson disease - 49
Cancer - lung - 71
Coal miner's disease - 265
Collapsed lung - 41
Common cold - 93
Consumption - 335
Cystic fibrosis - 105
Decompression sickness - 49
Deer fly fever - 336
Diptheria - 114
Dyspnea - 120
Emphysema - 126
Flu - 207
Fungal infections - 141
Grippe - 207
Hay fever - 155
Human Immunodeficency Virus Infection - 7
Hyaline membrane disease - 287
Hypoxia - 199
Infectious mononucleosis - 204
Influenza - 207
Kissing disease - 204
Laryngitis - 212

Lung abscess - 218
Measles - 225
Miner's asthma - 265
Mucormycosis - 141
Mucoviscidosis - 105
Mycosis - Systemic Pneumocystosis - 141
Nasal polyps - 233
Nicotine addiction - 238
Phthisis 335
Plague - 260
Pleural effusion - 262
Pleurisy - 263
Pleuritis - 263
Pneumoconiosis - Asbestosis - 263
Pneumoconiosis - Berylliosis - 264
Pneumoconiosis - Coal Worker's - 265
Pneumoconiosis - Silicosis - 266
Pneumonia - 267
Pneumothorax - 268
Pulmonary edema - 279
Pulmonary embolism - 279
Pulmonary hypertension - 280
Q fever - 281
Rabbit fever - 336
RDS - 287
Respiratory Distress Syndrome - 287
Rhinitis - 93
Rubeola - 225
Shock lung - 11
Sinusitis - 296
SLE - 313
Sleep apnea - 298
Systemic candidosis - 141
Systemic Lupus Erythematosus - 313
TB - 335
Tonsillitis - 328
Tropical pulmonary eosinophilia - 333
Tuberculosis - lung 335
Tularemia - 336

Word Index

Appendix G

Appendix G

Cerebrum
5, 41, 83, 91, 92, 108, 130, 134, 140, 185, 187, 222, 244, 293, 309
Cervical
25, 34, 66, 67, 114, 120, 157, 159, 181, 205, 207, 212, 301, 326, 329, 345, 346, 347
Cervicitis 84
Cervix 1, 67, 84, 289
Cesarean section 287
description of 388
CFIDS 89
Chagas' disease 85, 367
Chagoma 85
Chancre 299, 314
Charcot's arthropathy 38
Chelating agents 213
description of 378
Chemotherapy
description of 378
Chest pain
Achalasia 4
Cancer - lung 71
Chagas disease 85
Esophageal stenosis 133
Heart attack 160
Lung abscess 218
Panic disorder 251
Pericarditis 256
Pleural effusion 262
Pleurisy 264
Pneumoconiosis 266
Pneumonia 267
Pulmonary edema 279
Pulmonary embolism 280
Pulmonary hypertension 281
Chicken pox 86, 362, 367
Chilblains 86
Chlamydiae
description of 361
Chlamydial infection 95, 289, 331
Cholecystectomy 87
description of 388
Cholecystitis 87
Cholelithiasis 142
Cholera 88, 362, 367
Cholinergic drugs
description of 379
Chondrodystrophia fetalis 4
Chondromalacia 88
Chorea 185
Chromosome
1, 100, 116, 117, 174, 231, 237
Chronic Epstein-Barr virus infection 89
Chronic Fatigue & Immune Dysfunction Syndrome 89
Chronic Fatigue Syndrome 89
Chronic Obstructive Pulmonary Disease (COPD)
Bronchitis 53

Emphysema 127
Chylothorax 262
Cilia 51, 238
Cirrhosis 90, 392
Clavus 65
Cleft palate 5
Clinic
care of 365
Clitoris 11, 103, 344
Clotting factors
21, 91, 115, 173, 217, 342
Clubfoot 91
Coagulation
Disseminated intravascular coagulation 115
Heart attack 160
Hemangioma 174
Hemophilia 173
Nephrotic syndrome 235
Nutritional deficiencies - Vitamin K 243
Pulmonary embolism 279
Relapsing fever 284
Toxemia of pregnancy 330
Venous thrombosis 341
Coal 71, 265, 266, 278
Coal miner's disease 265
Coarctation of the aorta 95
Cochlea 346
Cold sore 182
Colitis 205, 206
Collagen
Carpal tunnel syndrome 81
Cushing's syndrome 103
Ehlers-Danlos syndrome 126
Homocystinurias 185
Malnutrition 224
Marfan's syndrome 224
Nutritional deficiencies - Vitamin C 241
Collapsed lung 41
Collateral ligament 146, 305
Colon 362
Back pain 44
Cancer 68
Chagas' disease 85
Constipation 96
Diverticular disease 115
Dysentery 118
Helminthic infection 170, 172
Indigestion 203
Intestinal obstruction 209
Polyp 272
Ulcerative colitis 206
Colostomy 68, 115
description of 388
Coma
5, **91**, 92, 99, 108, 128, 193, 198, 213, 218, 222, 227, 249, 267, 282, 309, 338, 373, 384

Common cold 93, 367
Compartment syndrome
26, 139, 274, 295
Compression chambers 49
Concussion 93
Conduction defects 31, 224
Condyloma acuminata 345
Congenital 329
Adrenogenital syndrome 10
Albinism 12
Aneurysm 22
Arrhythmias 31
Bronchiectasis 51
Club foot 91
Diverticular disease 115
Dysphagia 120
Emphysema 127
German measles 148
Heart disease 94, 104
Hydrocele 186
Hydrocephalus 187
Incontinence 202
Muscular dystrophy 231
Pulmonary hypertension 280
Sciatic nerve lesions 290
Spina bifida 44
Tendinitis 317, 321
Torticollis 329
Congenital heart disease 95, 384
Congestion
brain 309
general 125, 276
leg 27
liver 90
lungs 39
nasal 155, 207, 225, 296
nose 93, 155
portal circulation 217, 275
varicose veins 339
Congestive cardiomyopathy 81
Conjunctiva
53, 85, 95, 150, 155, 239, 283, 331, 336
Conjunctivitis 95, 366
Connective tissue
Arthritis 35
Compartment syndrome 27, 274
Dupuytren's contracture 118
Ehlers-Danlos syndrome 126
Fibromyalgia 137
Hyperpituitarism 190
Hyperthyroidism 192
Marfan's syndrome 225
Nutritional deficiencies - vitamin C 241
Osteogenesis imperfecta 245
Scleroderma 292
Torticollis 330
Volkmann's ischaemic contracture 343
Conn's syndrome 188

Appendix G

Appendix G

Hepatitis
 8, 13, 24, 70, 90, 91, 154, 174, **175**, 176, 210, 211, 218, 226, 281, 367, 377, 387
Hepatocarcinoma 71
Hepatotoxicity 377
Hereditary
 4, 15, 18, 19, 82, 117, 137, 173, 1 85, 210, 271, 272, 285. *See also* Genetic
Hereditary chorea 185
Hernia 389
 femoral 177
 hiatal 177
 incisional 178
 inguinal 179
 umbilical 180
Herniated disc 181
Herniated nucleus pulposus 181
Herpes simplex
 16, 67, 72, 132, 182, 183, 307, 308, 367
Herpes zoster 86, 183
Hiatus hernia 177
Hide bound disease 292
High blood pressure 371.
 See also Hypertension
High risk pregnancy 124
Hip
 Ankylosing spondylitis 25
 Arthritis 34, 308
 ataxia 40
 bursitis 58, 59, 63
 cancer 65
 Coxa plana 99
 disc prolapse 182
 innervation 302, 303
 sciatic nerve lesions 291
Hirschsprung's disease 96
Histoplasmosis 141
HIV 7, 8, 46
Hodgkin's disease 184
Hoffman's disease 322
Homan's sign 341, 342
Homocystinurias 185
Hookworm infection 166
Hormone therapy 110, 119, 195, 198
 description of 384
Housemaid's knee 62
Human Immunodeficiency Virus infection. *See* AIDS
Humerus
 9, 65, 101, 237, 246, 321, 322, 343
Huntington's chorea 185
Huntington's disease 185
Hyaline membrane disease 287
Hydatid cysts 171
Hydrocele 186
Hydrocephalus
 41, 108, 109, 187, 227, 300, 392

Hyperaldosteronism 188
Hyperglycemia 373. *See also* Diabetes mellitus
Hyperkalemia 387
Hypernephroma 69
Hyperparathyroidism 188
Hyperpituitarism 189
Hyperplasia 10, 106, 277, 285
Hypersensitivity 376, 378
Hypertension
 3, 21, 22, 23, 30, 32, 42, 43, 47, 90, 124, 133, 134, 160, 161, 169, 188, **190**, 191, 218, 231, 238, 244, 270, 271, 273, 274, 280, 285, 309, 330, 339, 370, 371, 372, 374, 376, 378, 379, 381, 382, 383
Hyperthyroidism 191, 377
Hypertrophic cardiomyopathy 81
Hypertrophy 23, 79, 95, 152, 161, 290
Hyperuricemia 32
Hypervitaminoses - Vitamin A and D 192
Hypoadrenalism 193
Hypocalcemia 387
Hypoglycemia
 92, 108, 109, 111, 112, 151, 152, **194**, 196, 197, 222, 276, 373
Hypoparathyroidism 194
Hypopigmentation 215, 342
Hypopituitarism 195
Hypotension
 28, 79, 88, 93, 108, 111, 112, 154, 191, 193, **196**, 197, 259, 282, 284, 285, 301, 302, 309, 338, 370, 371, 372, 373, 374, 375, 377, 379, 382, 383, 384
Hypothalamus 134, 195, 244, 375, 377
Hypothermia 30, 197, 198, 387
Hypothyroidism 198
Hypoxia
 92, 108, 109, 127, 199, 271, 309, 384

I

IBD 205, 206
IBS 209
Ichthyosis 199
Icterus 209
Idiopathic compartment syndrome 295
Idiopathic polyneuritis 153
Ileostomy 206, 207
 description of 390
Ileum 20, 205, 206, 207, 240
Imagery
 description of 384
Immunization
 114, 148, 282, 325, 326, 362, 378
 description of 384
 schedule 363
Immunocompromised

 3, 86, 141, 170, 184, 207, 228, 260, 290
Immunosuppressants
 description of 380
Immunosuppressive 33, 36, 267
Immunotherapy 20, 65, 70, 155, 216
 description of 384
Impetigo 200, 367
Impingement syndrome 321
Impotence
 13, 112, 196, 201, 217, 285, 298
Incontinence
 15, 201, 202, 203, 310, 383
Indigestion 203, 371, 375
Infantile paralysis 269
Infection
 transmission of 361
Infectious diseases
 15, 54, 86, 88, 100, 113, 130, 132, 139, 153, 154, 175, 182, 183, 184, 200, 204, 205, 215, 219, 230, 234, 269, 299, 312, 313, 314, 334, 335, 337, 348
Infectious hepatitis 175
Infectious mononucleosis 204, 367
Infectious polyneuritis 153
Inflammatory Bowel Disease (IBD)
 Crohn's disease 205
 Ulcerative coli 206
Influenza 207, 362, 367
Inguinal 45, 59, 101, 126, 179
Inherit
 12, 14, 24, 117, 126, 130, 174, 185, 224, 231, 237, 242, 245, 270, 272.
See also Hereditary
Inoculation 208, 227, 337, 344, 348.
See also Immunization
Insecta
 description of 361
Insomnia 295, 298, 346, 376
Insulin
 20, 111, 112, 188, 194, 244, 373
Intercostal
 40, 41, 105, 127, 212, 263, 301, 302
Intercourse
 7, 67, 84, 129, 153, 254, 289
Intermittent fever 135
Intervertebral disk 25, 181, 345
Intestinal flora 373
Intestinal obstruction
 79, 96, 97, 105, 116, 163, 208
Intubation 20, 212
 description of 390
Intussusception 208
Inversion 226, 304
Iris 12, 149
Irritable bowel syndrome (IBS) 209
Ischemia 274, 283, 296
Ischemic heart disease 22

Appendix G

Malnutrition
1, 20, 82, 83, 121, 122, 123, 125, 141, 163, 194, 206, 207, **223**, 224, 262, 267, 388
Mammary dysplasia 136
Mammogram 391
Mammography 66
description of 391
Mandibular pain dysfunction syndrome 315
Mantoux test 335, 363
Marasmus 224
Marfan's syndrome 224
Marie-Strumpell disease 25
Mask-like face 252, 293
Mast cell 20, 24, 38, 372
Mastectomy 135
description of 391
Maturity onset diabetes 111
Measles 225, 362, 367, 384
Mechanical ventilation
description of 384
Medial epicondylitis 320
Medial tibial stress syndrome 226
Median nerve 80, 81, 236
Mediastinum 28, 262, 263, 268
Mediators 24, 38
Melanin 12, 214, 385
Melanoma 74, 76
Melena 255
Memory
13, 16, 29, 93, 94, 99, 100, 109, 110, 137, 186, 213, 309
Meninges
47, 157, 227, 230, 260, 299, 300
Meningitis **227**, 366, 367, 386
Meningocele 299
Menopause 66, 152, 248
Menstrual cycle
21, 66, 84, 103, 119, 121, 128, 129, 130,
135, 156, 158, 182, 192, 193, 196, 224, 248, 276, 285
Mental retardation
43, 83, 84, 148, 185, 187, 198, 213, 300
Metastasis 44, 65, 67, 70, 108
Metazoa
description of 361
Micturition 74, 201, 202
Milwaukee brace 294
Miner's asthma 265
Miotics 380
Miscarriage 1
Mites 38, 290, 337
Mole 76
Molluscum contagiosum 227, 367
Moniliasis 78
"moon" face 103
Morton's metatarsalgia 236

Mosquito 85, 128, 165, 221, 222, 364
Motor neuron
18, 19, 154, 269, 272, 275, 325
Mouse 219
MS 229, 230, 345
Mucormycosis 141
Mucous membrane
23, 77, 85, 104, 105, 110, 114, 115, 127, 131,
132, 182, 210, 217, 225, 239, 281, 283, 284, 287, 312, 345
Mucoviscidosis 105
Mucus
39, 40, 41, 51, 52, 53, 88, 105, 106, 113, 118, 127, 154, 172, 206, 238, 255, 302
Multiple myeloma 228
Multiple neuritis 257
Multiple neuroma 237
Multiple sclerosis 96, 109, 229, 333
Mumps 230, 362, 367, 384
Muscle relaxants
description of 381
Muscular dystrophy 41, 79, 231
Mutation 4, 224, 237
Myalgic encephalomyelitis 89
Myasthenia gravis 231, 379
Mycosis - Systemic pneumocystosis 141
Mydriatics 380
Myelin 154, 213, 229
Myeloma 228
Myelomatosis 228
Myelomeningocele 299
Myocardial infarction 160, 388
Myocarditis 81
Myocardium 31, 160
Myofascial pain syndrome 315
Myoma 136
Myositis ossificans 233
Myxedema 198

N

Nasal decongestants
description of 381
Nasal polyps 234
Nasogastric suction
description of 391
Nausea
20, 28, 30, 50, 94, 113, 116, 118, 119, 130, 145, 150, 156, 157, 160, 162, 170, 171, 172, 176, 177, 178, 179, 180, 192, 193, 199, 204, 205, 260, 273, 282, 284, 285, 286, 336, 337, 346, 372, 374, 375, 376, 377, 378, 381, 382, 383, 385
Necrosis 99, 112, 114, 144
Necrotizing fasciitis 234
Nephroblastoma 69
Nephrocalcin 286
Nephrolithiasis 286

Nephrotic syndrome 235
Nephrotoxicity 371, 375, 376, 377
Nerve entrapment syndromes 235
Neuroendocrine cells 78, 79
Neurofibroma 237
Neurofibromata 237
Neurofibromatosis 237
Neuroma 237
Neuromatosis 237
Neurotransmitters
15, 137, 213, 251, 259, 294, 325
Neutrophils 134
Nevus 76
NF 237
Nickel 71
Nicotine addiction 238
Night blindness 239
Nit 253
Nodules
6, 36, 117, 168, 215, 265, 266, 287
Non-Hodgkin's Lymphoma 223
Noradrenaline 31, 251, 259, 370.
See also Norepinephrine
Norepinephrine 15, 373, 383.
See also Noradrenaline
North American blastomycosis 141
Nose drops
description of 381
NSAID 375
Nutritional deficiencies
Vitamin A 239
Vitamin B 240, 241
Vitamin C 241
Vitamin D 242
Vitamin E 242
Vitamin K 243
Nystagmus 12, 346, 377

O

Obesity
23, 32, 41, 103, 122, 178, 179, 191, **244**, 280, 340, 376
Oedema. *See* Edema
Ohio Valley disease 141
Omentum 177, 179, 180
Onchocerciasis 168
Opiates
examples of 371
Opportunistic pathogens
definition of 361
Optic nerve 190, 377
Organ transplantation
description of 391
Orgasm 73, 301
Orthopnea 121
Orthostatic hypotension 196
Osgood-Schlatter disease 245
Osteitis deformans 249
Osteoarthrosis 34

Appendix G

Polycystic kidneys 270
Polycystic renal disease 270
Polycythemia 271, 280
Polydipsia 110, 112
Polyneuritis 153, 257
Polyphagia 112
Polyposis 272
Polyps
  gastrointestinal 68, 214, 272
  nasal 233, 297
Polyuria 110, 112
Popliteal 46, 47, 236, 291, 320
Popliteal cyst 47
Popliteal entrapment syndrome 236
Porphyria 272
Portal hypertension
  90, 133, 134, 169, 218, **273**, 274, 392
Postmenopausal
  32, 42, 43, 66, 202, 247
Postpolio syndrome 269, 275
Postpoliomyelitis neuromuscular atrophy 275
Postural hypotension 196
Pott's disease 334
Preeclampsia 330
Pregnancy 376
  abortion 1
  abruptio placenta 2
  anemia 20
  anticoagulants 372
  birth injury 83
  breast cancer 66
  calcium requirements 247
  carpal tunnel syndrome 80
  constipation 96
  diabetes mellitus 111
  Disseminated Intravascular Coagulation 115
  ectopic 123, 255
  embolism 280
  epilepsy 130
  estrogen therapy 76
  facial palsy 47
  fetal abnormalities
    91, 94, 101, 148, 299, 300, 331
  fibroid 136
  goitre 152
  Gonorrhea 153
  Hemorrhoids 175
  hernia 178, 179
  high risk 2, 124
  hypothyroidism 198
  nutritional deficiencies 223, 240
  poliomyelitis 270
  smoking 238
  thrombosis 342
  toxemia 330
  tubal 124
  urinary tract infection 338

varicose veins 340
Pregnancy - induced hypertension 330
Premenstrual dysphoria disorder 276
Premenstrual syndrome 276
Pressure sores 107
Pressure ulcers 107
Prion 100
Progesterone
  96, 128, 136, 248, 276, 340
Progestogen 379
Progressive chorea 185
Prolactin 195, 276
Prolapse
  44, 83, 126, 181, 290, 292, 345
Pronation 81, 303
Prostaglandin 1, 119, 255, 330, 371
Prostate
  cancer 65, 73
  hyperplasia 277
  inflammation 153, 277
  pain 44
Prostatic hyperplasia 277
Prostatitis 277
Prosthesis 386, 390
Protein-calorie malnutrition 223
Protozoa
  description of 361
Psoriasis 277, 380, 385
Psychosis 377
Ptosis 232
Puberty 11, 12, 189, 190, 224, 248
Pulmonary
  artery 95, 279
  edema 278
  embolism 279
  hypertension 280
  infarction 279
  stenosis 95
Purgatives 380
Purine 32, 286
Pustule
  6, 28, 78, 86, 107, 138, 142, 182, 200, 278, 288
Pyelonephritis 338
Pyloric stenosis 255
Pyridoxine (B6) deficiency 240
Pyrogen 134, 135

Q

Q fever 367
Quadriplegia 301
Quartan fever 135

R

Rabbit fever 336
Rabies 282, 367
Radiating pain
  45, 46, 81, 160, 250, 314, 317

Radiation
  4, 12, 20, 64, 65, 66, 67, 68, 69, 70, 71, 72, 73, 74, 75, 76, 77, 82, 95, 100, 117, 184, 194, 195, 198, 216, 217, 223, 228, 256, 278, 279, 299, 300
Radiation therapy
  description of 385
Radioactive 71, 191
Rash
  77, 86, 123, 132, 148, 167, 172, 205, 219, 225, 226, 264, 287, 313, 337, 338, 376, 377, 379
Rat 1, 260
Raynaud's disease 283
Raynaud's phenomenon 283, 392
Raynaud's syndrome 283
RDS 287
Rectum
  68, 74, 78, 174, 206, 208, 272, 273, 340, 345
Red blood cell
  20, 21, 143, 144, 209, 210, 213, 221, 241, 271, 285, 389
Referred pain 44, 45, 46, 143, 334
Reflux esophagitis 371.
See also Gastroesophageal reflux
Regeneration 56, 90, 99
Regional enteritis 205
Regurgitation 4, 85
Rejection 392
Relapsing fever 135, 283, 367
Remission
  8, 25, 206, 229, 232, 278, 313
Remittent fever 135
Renal
  calculi 286
  failure
    188, 238, 270, 271, **284**, 285, 286
  stones 286
  toxicity. *See* Nephrotoxicity
Renal failure 379
Renal stones 371
Renin 285
Respiratory Distress Syndrome 287
Respiratory failure
  49, 52, 199, 260, 384, 393
Restrictive cardiomyopathy 81
Retina 5, 81, 112, 191
Rh factor 210, 389
Rheumatic fever 287
Rheumatic heart disease 287
Rheumatoid arthritis
  9, 17, 21, 24, 33, **36**, 47, 61, 79, 80, 137, 247, 256, 257, 262, 298, 306, 307, 315, 375
Rhinitis 93, 155, 374
Rhinophyma 6
Rhomboids 159, 211, 212, 345
Riboflavin deficiency 240
'rice water' stools 88

Appendix G